Advanced Study of Child Development

Volume I

Advanced Study of Child Development Volume I

Edited by **Romana Woods**

hayle medical

New York

Published by Hayle Medical,
30 West, 37th Street, Suite 612,
New York, NY 10018, USA
www.haylemedical.com

Advanced Study of Child Development: Volume I
Edited by Romana Woods

International Standard Book Number: 978-1-63241-016-0 (Hardback)

Printed in China.

Contents

Preface

Development has many meanings for the human race. It can refer to a civilization itself, a society or an individual. Development is usually referred to in terms of changes towards a more positive outcome. Child Development therefore logically refers to the psychological, emotional and biological changes that a human being experiences from the moment they are born till the end of adolescence. This suggests that it is the time during which the individual advances from a dependent stage towards increased and eventual autonomy. This makes this stage of growth an essential one in terms of ensuring that a child has all the best the society can offer. Child Development Research is thus an extremely integral part of education in today's world. New research on teaching and development methodologies is published every year, though a few stand out because along with offering new information, they open up new ways of thinking on child development. Many of them bring freshness and a unique insight into many already well researched areas of study. Many other suddenly break out with a completely new perspective on emerging topics that are crucially important for those families looking to understand the development of their child.

This book aims at compiling such research method and papers that provide insight on child development without presuming to actually tell a parent how to raise a child. This data is an essential part of education and I am thankful to those put their hard work behind it, as well as my family who helped me through putting this book together.

Editor

The Father-Child Activation Relationship, Sex Differences, and Attachment Disorganization in Toddlerhood

Daniel Paquette[1] **and Caroline Dumont**[2]

[1] *École de Psychoéducation, Université de Montréal, Case postale 6128, Succursale Centre-Ville, Montréal, QC, Canada H3C 3J7*
[2] *Département de Psychologie, Université de Montréal, Case postale 6128, Succursale Centre-Ville, Montréal, QC, Canada H3C 3J7*

Correspondence should be addressed to Daniel Paquette; daniel.paquette@umontreal.ca

Academic Editor: Helena R. Slobodskaya

The activation relationship theory serves as a complement to Bowlby's attachment theory to better understand the impact of fathering on child development, focusing primarily on parental stimulation of risk taking and control during children's exploration. The first aim of this study was to confirm that the activation relationship as assessed with the observational procedure, the Risky Situation, is primarily determined by paternal stimulation of risk taking as assessed by questionnaire. The second aim was to verify the link between the activation relationship and attachment disorganization. The third aim was to verify the existence of a sex difference in father-toddler dyad activation relationships. The Strange Situation procedure and the Risky Situation procedure were conducted with 58 father-toddler dyads. Fathers completed questionnaires on child temperament and parental behavior. Paternal stimulation of risk taking explains activation once child sex and temperament, the attachment relationship, and emotional support are taken into account. Moreover, there is no relation between the father-child activation relationship and attachment disorganization. Finally, data confirm the existence of a sex difference in the activation relationship in toddlers: fathers activate their sons more than their daughters.

1. Introduction

Little data on father-child attachment has been collected, at least insofar as young children are concerned. What data we do possess has been obtained through the use of the Strange Situation, a method validated with mothers and used primarily with fathers who are secondary attachment figures for their children. The low stability, low transmissibility, and low predictability of father-child attachment have caused increasing numbers of researchers to question the pertinence of using the Strange Situation with fathers who have little involvement in daily caregiving [1–3]. Grossmann and Grossmann [4] and Grossmann et al. [5], for example, have suggested finding a more appropriate method to assess father-child attachment. Others agree that this relationship develops through mechanisms that may be different from those involved in mother-child attachment [6–10]. In fact, fathers' activities with their children are often unlike from those of mothers: fathers tend to excite children and to engage in more physical play with them than mothers do, especially with boys [11, 12]. According to Labrell [13], children must learn to respond to unforeseen events and it is fathers who facilitate such learning by teasing them and destabilizing them with creative, unconventional games. Fathers act as catalysts for risk taking [14], inciting children to take the initiative in unfamiliar situations, explore, take chances, overcome obstacles, be braver in the presence of strangers, and stand up for themselves. Grossmann et al. [15] have shown that paternal sensitivity in play situations with two-year-old children is a better predictor of attachment 14 years later than the father-child Strange Situation.

Drawing on this literature, Paquette [16, 17] theorized father-child attachment by developing the concept of the "activation relationship," that is, the affective bond that enables children to open up to the outside world, focusing primarily on parental stimulation of risk taking and control.

According to the attachment theory, children's feelings of confidence result from parental sensitivity to children's comfort seeking in times of distress (secure base), with parents protecting their children by maintaining a close distance between parent and child. According to the activation theory, however, children's feelings of confidence result from parental encouragement of risk-taking during children's exploration of their environment, with parents protecting their children through discipline (limit setting, control).

Paquette and Bigras [18] have developed the Risky Situation (RS), a standardized procedure designed to assess the quality of the parent-child activation relationship in children ages 12 to 18 months, and validated with both fathers and mothers. As proposed by Grossmann et al. [5], we make a distinction between attachment in the broad sense of the term and attachment in the strict sense. Broadly speaking, the attachment relationship refers to the emotional bond between adult and child that is the result of daily interaction and ensures a form of protection for the child (psychological security). The attachment relationship in the strict sense of the term concerns the child's secure base as evaluated by the *Strange Situation* [19], while the activation relationship concerns the security of exploration [5] as evaluated by the *Risky Situation* [18]. Like the Strange Situation (SS; [19]), the RS is a twenty-minute-long observational procedure that takes place in an unfamiliar room with toys and in the presence of a stranger. While the SS is divided into eight episodes including two separations from the parent, the RS is divided into six structured episodes during which the child is presented first with a social risk (an increasingly intrusive male stranger), then with a physical risk (a set of stairs), and then forbidden by the parent to climb the stairs. In the SS as conceived by Mary Ainsworth, the child's stress is gradually increased in order to trigger the attachment system; the ultimate objective is for the child to find a balance between exploring the environment and seeking comfort from the significant parent [20]. In the RS, the child is invited to take progressive risks in order to trigger the activation system, ideally a balance between exploration of the environment and acceptance by the child of limits imposed by the significant parent. In the SS, the way the child reacts when the parent returns determines the quality of the attachment relationship. Secure children (type B) welcome their parents, are comforted by them, and return to their exploration of the toys in the room. Avoidant children (type A) experience distress but do not show it and do not try to obtain the comfort they need. They continue their exploration but are less engaged than before. Resistant children (type C) are harder to comfort and stop or significantly reduce their exploration. Disorganized children (type D) act in a strange and contradictory way, both desiring comfort and rejecting it at the same time, while also exploring in a disoriented manner [21]. The scoring grid used to code the RS identifies children with underactivated relationships, activated relationships, and overactivated relationships. Underactivated children engage in little exploration, are passive and withdraw from novelty, or remain close to their parents. Activated children are confident and prudent in their exploration and conform when their parents set limits. Overactivated children are reckless and do not comply when their parents set limits. The underactivated relationship is theoretically linked to parental overprotection, while the overactivated relationship is linked to parental difficulty in applying discipline (for the child's protection). Paquette and Bigras [18] have shown that the threefold attachment typology (ABC) using the SS and the activation typology using the RS are orthogonal and evaluate different constructs. On the other hand, they have also highlighted the link between the activation typology and the attachment disorganization score. The literature demonstrates that it is primarily children with disorganized attachment who develop psychopathology [22, 23].

Depending on whether conditions in the environment are favorable, based on resource availability and the presence of potential dangers, parents would be expected to activate their children to varying degrees, preparing them for intrasex competition and to cope with adversity [16]. The activation relationship theory predicts that fathers will activate children more than mothers, and boys will be activated more than girls [18]. According to Charlesworth's evolutionist model [24], competition for limited resources may be manifested in five categories of behavior: aggression, intimidation, manipulation, deceit, and cooperation.

The activation relationship being theoretically linked to risk taking in competition for environmental resources at all ages, one might expect to find a sex difference in the prevalence of activation types early on, beginning in toddlerhood, before the appearance of sex differences in competition strategies such as aggression. Physical aggression appears in young children at an early age, around 8 or 9 months, and for the vast majority peaks at between 15 and 24 months [25]. The age of two years also corresponds to a period during which children assert their autonomy, which manifests itself through increased opposition towards adults. It is also the age at which children establish a dominance hierarchy amongst themselves. But it is only at about age three that boys engage in significantly more physical aggression and become more focused on dominance than girls [26], in Western industrial societies at least. One might conclude that the form of risk taking that constitutes aggression is modulated by the activation relationship to increase or decrease sex differences in aggression depending on whether it occurs in a society that is individualistic or collectivist. In individualistic societies, aggression would be encouraged by parents, while in collectivist societies aggression between children would be discouraged.

Using a combined sample of 21 father-child dyads and 21 mother-child dyads, Paquette and Bigras [18] have found that (1) the parent-child activation relationship is linked to parental stimulation of risk taking after controlling for child characteristics (sex, temperament) and that (2) avoidant children (as assessed with the SS) and overactivated children (as assessed with the RS) have higher disorganized attachment scores than secure children and under-activated children, respectively. This final result suggests that disorganization is tied to children experiencing an extreme lack of protection in their environment given that avoidant children tolerate being at a greater distance from the parent, and overactivated children explore their environment impulsively and recklessly. In addition, using a sample of 21 father-child dyads, Paquette and Bigras [18] demonstrated that boys are more activated than girls in toddlerhood, even though no sex differences were found in the father-child attachment relationship. However, they did not obtain a significant sex difference for the activation relationship with a second sample of 21 father-child dyads. The purpose of the current study was therefore to confirm, with a larger sample solely comprised of fathers, that the activation relationship is primarily determined by parental stimulation of risk taking after controlling for child characteristics. The second objective was to verify the link between the activation relationship and attachment disorganization. Given the instability of results for sex differences in small samples, the third objective here was to replicate the study with a larger sample to verify the existence of sex differences in the father-child activation relationship. The concept of the activation relationship would only be relevant to our understanding of the parent-child relationship, and the father-child relationship in particular, if a certain degree of stability could successfully be demonstrated in the expected results.

2. Method

2.1. Participants. The sample was comprised of 58 father-child dyads with 22 boys and 36 girls. It should be noted that the first 21 dyads recruited for this sample were used for the validation of the Risky Situation [18]. Four children (3 girls and 1 boy) were eliminated from the sample, one due to low motor skills development and the other three because their fathers were unable to comfort them when they cried during the RS.

The average age for fathers was 34.8 years (ranging between 25 and 49 years; SD = 5.16). The average number of children per family was 1.7 (ranging between 1 and 5; SD = .89) and 5.2% of the sample were single parents. Seventy-nine percent (79%) of fathers were born in North America. The average number of years of schooling was 15.4 years (ranging between 9 and 23; SD = 2.59) and 41% of the sample had an annual family income greater than CAN$80.000. Finally, fathers spent an average of 40.5 hours a week working (ranging between 20 and 80; SD = 10.55) and 13.2 hours a week alone with their child (ranging between 0 and 69; SD = 14.22).

2.2. Procedure. Fathers were recruited through monthly ads in several neighborhood newspapers and early childhood centers in the city of Montreal. Fathers were then contacted by phone to set up a first appointment at the University of Montreal. The two procedures (SS and RS) were conducted at one-month intervals in a counterbalanced manner (i.e., the RS was done first in half the cases). After having the father sign a consent form, a team of student assistants (2-3) made a video recording of one of the two observational procedures. The father then completed questionnaires while an assistant played with the child in the same room. The same sequence was followed at the second appointment. The procedures (SS and RS) were conducted in two different rooms, each equipped with three hidden cameras. The average age of children at the time of the RS was 15.8 months (ranging between 12.0 and 19.2; SD = 2.14). The average age of children at the time of the SS was 15.8 months (ranging between 12.4 and 19.4; SD = 1.92). No attrition occurred between the two time points. Fathers received $20CAN per session.

2.3. Instruments

2.3.1. The Strange Situation Procedure (SS [19]). The SS is a standardized procedure designed to assess the quality of the parent-child attachment relationship in children ages 12 to 18 months. The SS is divided into eight episodes and takes place in an unfamiliar room with toys. During the procedure, infants are exposed to mildly stressful events, including the entrance of an unfamiliar female adult and two separations from their parent followed by reunions. Infant attachment patterns are coded by trained observers and classified as secure (B), insecure avoidant (A), or insecure resistant (C), based on the Ainsworth et al. [19] scoring system. In this procedure, children must cope with the considerable distress of having their parent leave them alone for two minutes in an unfamiliar room with a complete stranger. The way the child reacts when the parent returns determines the quality of their attachment relationship. Then the Main and Solomon's [21] scoring system is used to code disorganized attachment (D). Disorganized children act in a strange and contradictory way, both desiring comfort and rejecting it at the same time, while also exploring in a disoriented manner. This system produces a disorganization score from 1 to 9, with the score of 5 being the cut-off point for the D category. Twenty-six percent (15/58) of the children in our sample were placed in the D category. Seventeen percent of the sample was coded by a second rater. Interrater agreement (Kappa) for the three- and the four-category scheme was 76%. Finally, an intraclass correlation of .73 was obtained for the disorganization scale.

2.3.2. The Risky Situation Procedure (RS [18]). The RS is a standardized procedure designed to assess the quality of the parent-child activation relationship in children ages 12 to 18 months [18]. The activation relationship theory serves as a complement to Bowlby's attachment theory to better understand the impact of fathering on child development. According to the activation relationship theory, children's feelings of confidence result from parental encouragement of risk taking during children's exploration of their environment, with parents protecting their children through discipline (limit setting, control).

The procedure lasts about 20 minutes and takes place in an unfamiliar room. It is divided into six structured episodes lasting three minutes each. After instructions have been given to the parent, the child is seated on the floor in front of available toys, while the parent reads a magazine on a chair behind the child (Episode 1). Then, a male stranger enters the room, sits on the floor, and starts playing with the toys without interacting with the child or the parent (Episode 2). After three minutes, or earlier, if the child initiates interaction with him, the male stranger starts playing with the child and becomes increasingly stimulating and intrusive (Episode 3). Toys are put away and a big colorful set of stairs that was hidden behind drapes is revealed (Episode 4); the parent is instructed to get up from the chair to make sure the child is safe during exploration only if the latter starts to climb the stairs. The parent is then asked to encourage the child to go up and down the stairs (Episode 5). Finally, the parent is asked to forbid the child to climb the stairs (Episode 6). Throughout the procedure, the parent is allowed to interact with the child when discipline is required, when giving instructions to stimulate the child, or when comfort is needed by the child; otherwise the child is to be left alone, for the same reason as in the SS. The coding grid permits children to be classified as activated, underactivated, or overactivated and also provides an activation score between 0 and 5 indicating the extent to which the child is optimally activated (with the score of 5 corresponding to the most positive activation relationship). In the RS, underactivated children tend to engage in little exploration, be passive, and withdraw from novelty or remain close to the parent. Activated children are confident and prudent in their exploration and obey when the parent sets a limit. Overactivated children are reckless and noncompliant when the parent sets limits. The coding system with its five criteria was designed for ease of use by clinicians as well as researchers, requiring an average of 30 minutes per case.

Interrater agreement (Kappa) was 70% for classification of the three types and 82% for decisions based on the five criteria. Intraclass correlation was .93 ($P < .001$) for the activation score. All cases (100% of the sample) were then discussed until a consensus could be reached by the two authors.

2.3.3. Child Temperament. Child temperament was assessed using the French version of the *Early Childhood Behavior Questionnaire* [27]. The following six scales were selected as they are theoretically closer to the concept of activation: Frustration (8 items; $\alpha = .75$); Shyness (12 items; $\alpha = .77$); Fear (7 items; $\alpha = .74$); Impulsivity (5 items; $\alpha = .77$); Inhibitory control (12 items; $\alpha = .81$); and Sociability (8 items; $\alpha = .89$). Four (4) items, 4 items, and 5 items were removed from the frustration, fear, and impulsivity scales, respectively, to obtain alphas greater than .70.

2.3.4. Parental Behavior. Parental behavior was assessed with self-report questionnaires. The Openness to the World Questionnaire (OWQ: [28]), based on the activation relationship theory, was used to assess three dimensions in the toddler period and the preschool period. Although validated with a sample of preschool children (ages 26 to 69 months), it was also used with toddlers in the current study. Stimulation of perseverance consists of encouraging the child to accomplish difficult things, overcome personal limits, and persevere in the face of adversity, introducing the child to sports and inviting the child to explore or initiate contact with an unfamiliar child: this scale has an internal consistency of .61 (7 items) for the toddler period and is significantly correlated to the same scale for the preschool period ($r = .37$, $P < .01$, $n = 48$). Punishment consists of punishing or scolding the child if the child disobeys, does not try, or breaks something: this scale has an internal consistency of .61 (6 items) for the toddler period and is significantly correlated to the same scale for the preschool period ($r = .37$, $P < .01$, $n = 48$). Finally, stimulation of risk taking consists of encouraging the child to undertake risky activities and allowing the child substantial autonomy in the child's exploration of the environment: this scale has an internal consistency of .65 (7 items) and is significantly correlated to the same scale for the preschool period ($r = .67$, $P < .001$, $n = 48$).

In order to replicate Paquette and Bigras' (2010) study, we used the same two scales from the *Montreal Father's Involvement Questionnaire* (MFIQ: [29]). Internal consistency estimates for the current study are good. Basic care (8 items; $\alpha = .76$) comprises items such as bathing, dressing, feeding, and nursing the child. Emotional support (12 items; $\alpha = .82$) comprises parental behaviors that clearly communicate to the child that he or she is appreciated, loved, supported, and protected.

3. Results

In the results section, we will first verify whether there are sex differences in the scores for the child temperament and fathers' parental behavior scales. Next, we will verify the presence of sex differences in the prevalence of types of attachment and activation. We will then verify links between temperament, parental behavior, and attachment disorganization, first using the threefold typology of attachment and then the activation relationship typology. Finally, to verify whether parental stimulation of risk taking explains the father-child activation relationship after extracting the effects of other variables, we will conduct a hierarchical regression of the activation score by first entering child's sex; followed by child temperament, father-child attachment, and emotional support; and finally stimulation of risk taking.

3.1. Sex Differences in Child Temperament and Fathers' Parental Behavior. No dimension of temperament was shown to differ by child's sex. In addition, the average scores for parental stimulation of risk taking, stimulation of perseverance, and punishment were not significantly different for girls and boys. However, girls received significantly more emotional support from their fathers than boys ($t = 2.88$, $df = 1$, $P < .01$). Girls also received more basic care than boys, but the difference was not significant ($t = 1.73$, $df = 1$, $P = .09$).

3.2. Sex Differences in the Prevalence of Activation Types and Attachment Types. Table 1 shows that 24.1% of children were both secure and activated with their fathers, indicating that children who were confident would be comforted in times of distress and protected by limit setting during their exploration of environments in which danger was present. Two groups came second in terms of size. Children who were both secure and underactivated were children who were adequately comforted in times of distress but received little encouragement to explore their environment by themselves without the parent (18.5%). Children who were both secure and overactivated were children who were comforted and soothed in times of distress but received little discipline (20.4%). Last came the children who were both avoidant and

TABLE 1: Percentage (n) of dyads as a function of three strange situation categories (A, B, C) and risky situation categories.

Risky situation	A	B	C	Total (boys; girls)
Underactivated	1.9% (1)	18.5% (10)	5.6% (3)	25.9% (1; 13)
Activated	14.8% (8)	24.1% (13)	3.7% (2)	42.6% (13; 10)
Overactivated	9.3% (5)	20.4% (11)	1.9% (1)	31.5% (7, 10)
Total (boys; girls)	25.9% (6; 8)	63.0% (15; 19)	11.1% (0; 6)	100.0% (54)

TABLE 2: Percentage (n) of dyads as a function of four strange situation categories (A, B, C, D) and risky situation categories.

Risky situation	A	B	C	D	Total (boys; girls)
Under-activated	0% (0)	18.5% (10)	3.7% (2)	3.7% (2)	25.9% (1; 13)
Activated	5.6% (3)	22.2% (12)	1.9% (1)	13.0% (7)	42.6% (13; 10)
Over-activated	3.7% (2)	18.5% (10)	1.9% (1)	7.4% (4)	31.5% (7; 10)
Total (boys; girls)	9.3% (3; 2)	59.2% (13; 19)	7.5% (0; 4)	24.1% (5; 8)	100.0% (54)

activated (14.8%), meaning children who seemed independent of the parent in times of distress but who would accept limits imposed by the latter during exploration.

Of the children in the sample, 63.0% were secure children, 25.9% avoidant children, and 11.1% resistant children (Table 1). As in the literature, chi-square analyses showed that attachment type prevalence did not differ based on the child's sex ($\chi^2 = 4.30$, $df = 2$, $P > .05$).

Forty-three percent (42.6%) of children in the sample were activated, 25.9% were underactivated, and 31.5% were overactivated (Table 1). Chi-square analysis showed that activation prevalence differed based on the child's sex ($\chi^2 = 8.98$, $df = 2$, $P < .05$): 93% of underactivated children were girls. Moreover, the average activation score for boys as a group (3.29) was significantly higher than that (2.48) of girls ($t(1, 52) = -2.54$, $P < .05$).

With respect to the fourfold typology of attachment, the results revealed that 24.1% of children displayed disorganized attachment with their father (Table 2).

3.3. *Relation of Child Temperament, Parental Behavior, and Attachment Disorganization to Father-Child Relationships*

3.3.1. Attachment Relationship. Only one dimension of temperament varied significantly among the three attachment categories (ABC): sociability ($F(2, 45) = 3.73$, $P < .05$). Scheffe tests showed that the sociability score for avoidant children was higher than the score for resistant children ($P < .05$), while the score for secure children did not differ from that for avoidant children but showed a trend toward being higher than the score for resistant children ($P = .07$). There were no significant differences in basic care and emotional support for the three categories of attachment. However, stimulation of risk taking differed significantly among the three categories ($F(2, 45) = 4.22$, $P < .05$): Scheffe tests showed that fathers of resistant children stimulated risk taking less than fathers of secure children ($P < .01$) and fathers of avoidant children ($P < .01$). It should be noted that fathers did as much risk taking stimulation with secure children as with avoidant children. On the other hand, stimulation of risk taking was not significantly different for the four categories of attachment ($F(3, 50) = 1.76$, $P > .05$).

One-way ANOVA analysis revealed significant differences among the three attachment types (ABC) for the attachment disorganization score ($F(2, 51) = 13.28$, $P < .001$); Scheffe tests showed the average score of avoidant children (5.3) to be higher than that of secure children (2.2) ($P < .001$), with the average score of resistant children (3.8) being between the scores of avoidant children and secure children.

3.3.2. Activation Relationship. One-way analysis showed no significant difference among the three types of activation relationships for any temperament scales other than frustration ($F(2, 51) = 4.08$, $P < .01$): activated children had higher frustration scores than both under- and overactivated children, but the difference was only significant with regard to overactivated children (Scheffe, $P < .05$). There was no significant correlation between the activation score and temperament scales for the sample as a whole. However, there was a significant positive correlation between frustration and activation in girls only ($r = .37$, $P < .05$; $r = -.13$ in boys).

The average stimulation of risk taking scores for activated children and overactivated children was similar, and both were higher than the average score for underactivated children although the difference was not significant. The activation score showed a trend toward being significantly correlated with stimulation of risk taking ($r = .23$, $P = .09$) and was significantly correlated with emotional support ($r = -.29$, $P = .05$). It should be noted that the correlation between activation score and emotional support remained significant for boys only ($r = -.49$, $P < .05$; $r = .02$ for girls).

One-way ANOVA analysis revealed no significant differences among the three activation types for the attachment disorganization score ($F(2, 51) = .93$, $P > .05$).

3.4. Effect of Parental Stimulation of Risk Taking after Controlling for Child's Sex and Temperament, Father-Child Attachment, and Emotional Support. Multiple regressions were conducted to verify whether paternal stimulation of risk taking explained activation once child sex and temperament, attachment relationship, and emotional support were taken into account. Multiple regression analysis was performed by first forcing child sex, then entering frustration, attachment (C versus AB), and emotional support, and finally entering stimulation of risk taking stepwise. This model explains 26% of total variance (Table 3) and confirms the importance of paternal stimulation of risk taking in the father-child activation relationship.

TABLE 3: Multiple regression on the activation score ($n = 54$).

Variables	R^2	F change	β	t	P
Step 1	.110	6.43*			
Child's sex			−.33	−2.54	.014
Step 2	.188	1.56			
Child's sex			−.23	−1.56	.126
Frustration			.22	1.64	.107
Attachment			.06	.41	.686
Emotional support			−.24	−1.68	.100
Step 3	.260	4.65*			
Child's sex			−.26	−1.87	.068
Frustration			.25	1.90	.063
Attachment			.22	1.41	.165
Emotional support			−.23	−1.68	.099
Risk stimulation			.31	2.16	.036

*$P < .05$.

4. Discussion

This study confirms that the attachment and activation relationships are two different mechanisms. It demonstrates the independence of the attachment relationship (as measured with the Strange Situation) and the activation relationship (as measured with the Risky Situation) as only 24% of children were both secure and activated with the father. Analyses with this larger sample also confirm the presence of sex differences in the activation relationship as early as toddlerhood: boys are activated more by their fathers than girls are, and this result is just as evident with respect to classification as to the activation score. Furthermore, as has been found for mother-child attachment [30], there is no sex difference in father-child attachment. The study also confirms that paternal stimulation of risk taking explains the activation score not only after controlling for child characteristics but also after controlling for father-child attachment and emotional support. Finally, we found no association between the activation relationship and attachment disorganization in this sample of father-child dyads ($n = 54$) even though Paquette and Bigras [18] found such an association in an equal mix sample of father-child and mother-child dyads ($n = 42$). Frightening behaviors from the primary caregiver have been associated with the development of disorganized attachment in children [31]. Hazen et al. [32] have shown frightening behaviors by mothers to be more problematic for child outcomes than frightening behaviors by fathers; when combined with sensitivity, such behaviors in fathers serve to surprise and destabilize children, thereby encouraging them to explore their environment.

Contrary to the first two samples in Paquette and Bigras's [18] study, the current larger sample shows no connection between the activation relationship and dimensions of temperament such as impulsivity, shyness, and sociability. Moreover, we obtained no sex difference for the six dimensions of temperament as assessed by the father. Although sex differences have been reported primarily in older children and adults in the literature, self-report questionnaires have also revealed sex differences in infancy and toddlerhood for different dimensions of temperament. Some studies have shown more shyness, fear, and withdrawal in girls and greater interest in approaching novel objects, more high-intensity pleasure, and a higher level of activity in boys [27, 33, 34]. Other studies have found more effortful control (inhibitory control and perceptual sensitivity) and sociability in girls and more impulsivity in boys [33]. Indeed, sex differences in temperament may emerge at different ages and decrease or increase over the course of development depending on maturation and socialization processes [33].

On the other hand, the current study reveals a connection between frustration and the activation relationship: activated children had higher father-rated frustration scores than overactivated children. It could be that fathers provoke more frustration in activated children by setting limits while fathers of overactivated children are more permissive. But given the significant positive correlation between frustration scores and activation only in girls, who made up the better part of the sample, it is believed that this result mainly reflects the fact that girls have a greater tendency than boys to express their frustration with limits and risk taking.

The fact that there is an early sex difference in the father-child relationship, at an age at which sex differences in temperament are difficult to detect, would seem to support the hypothesis that the father plays a unique role in amplifying or reducing children's innate tendencies, depending on the environment. It is possible that differential gender socialization, generally more pronounced in fathers [35], occurs through the activation relationship mechanism. Through the activation relationship, the father would adjust stimulation of risk taking and limit setting based on the child's temperament to encourage the child to explore the physical and social environment autonomously and carefully. Risk taking is a basic need, permitting children to explore their environment, develop skills, and therefore adapt. Children's temperaments would seem to predispose them to take more or less risks, but they need their parents to learn how to regulate their behavior. For example, parents must encourage inhibited children to explore more, but must exercise more control over impulsive children. Men, who generally take more risks than women [36], are perhaps more predisposed on average to encouraging this type of learning, provided of course that they themselves have learned to regulate their own risk taking. Jaffee et al. [37] have shown antisociality in fathers (but not mothers) to be a predictor of behavior problems in offspring, even after controlling for genetic factors. The sensation seeking and risk taking in extreme sports observed in a number of adolescents may be the result of such learning not having taken place at an early age, due to either overprotective or overly permissive parents.

To explore why fathers engage more frequently in rough-and-tumble play (RTP) with boys than with girls, Paquette and Dumont [38] tested the association of RTP with father-child attachment (as assessed with the *Strange Situation*) and with father-child activation (as assessed with the *Risky Situation*) and showed that the more optimally activated boys are by their fathers in toddlerhood, the more RTP the boys engage in with their fathers at the age of three years. RTP is a proximate mechanism that has been theorized to contribute to the development of the father-child activation relationship in preschoolers and to encourage the development of competition skills including aggression [16]. Flanders et al. [39, 40] have shown that the association between the frequency of father-child RTP in the preschool period and the frequency of physical aggression (as evaluated through self-report questionnaires) is moderated by the father's dominance during RTP, that is to say the degree to which the father controls the flow of play or holds the dominant position (evaluated through observation). When fathers are not dominant over their children, RTP frequency is greater, children are more physically aggressive, and have less emotion regulation five years later [39, 40].

What is more surprising is that fathers do not make a greater attempt to stimulate risk taking in boys than in girls. However, they do provide more emotional support and basic care to girls than to boys. Also, the lower the degree of emotional support and basic care provided by the father, the higher the boy's activation score. Paquette and Bigras [18] have suggested that low basic care combined with stimulation of risk taking may promote activation more than stimulation of risk taking alone. The higher proportion of girls in the current sample may also have affected averages.

It is worth taking a closer look at some of the results regarding the father-child attachment relationship. First, as in Paquette and Bigras' [18] study with fathers and mothers, the current sample reveals no significant difference with respect to basic care and emotional support by fathers for the three types of attachment. However, two results do differ. On the one hand, the average sociability score for avoidant children is not significantly different from the score for secure children, while both are higher than the average score for resistant children. This result is just as surprising as that of Youngblade et al. [3] who have demonstrated that children with insecure attachment to their fathers have more positive interactions with their peers. In our opinion, the attachment relationship reflected by the Strange Situation procedure is more meaningful when the father is the child's principal caregiver and comfort provider on a daily basis, which of course represents a minority in the general population. In other words, this result supports the notion that the Strange Situation evaluates something different when used with father-child dyads. If such is the case, it would be important not to interpret the abnormally high level of disorganized attachment (24%) in our sample of father-child dyads as an indication of the presence of adjustment issues. Our results show disorganized attachment to be combined with avoidant attachment in 69.2% of cases, a combination found in only 34% of children in middle-class, nonclinical groups [41]. However, according to a meta-analysis by Van Ijzendoorn et al. [41], resistant children have the most significant association with disorganization (46% of cases of disorganization). Given that Van Ijzendoorn's study provides data on parents that does not distinguish between fathers and mothers, it is impossible to know whether the strong association between avoidance and disorganization is typical of the father-child attachment relationship. On the other hand, the average stimulation of risk taking score is linked to attachment classification: the average stimulation of risk taking score for avoidant children is not significantly different from the average score for secure children, but both are higher than the average score for resistant children. This could mean that resistant children elicit more restrictive and overprotective behavior in their fathers. But it could also mean that fathers activate their children even when they are acting as a secure base, comforting children when the latter are tired, hungry, sick, afraid, or feeling insecure in the presence of novelty. Indeed, it is entirely possible that fathers activate children through the different way in which they carry out the same caretaking tasks (bottle feeding, changing diapers, etc.) especially when they are the secondary attachment figure and primary activation figure. Despite this association between attachment and the stimulation of risk taking, we have been able to show that paternal stimulation of risk taking explains the activation score after controlling for the father-child attachment relationship.

It is important to point out that the results obtained may be related to the study's limitations. The first limitation is that our sample is not representative of the general population. As recruitment was conducted via newspapers and early childhood centers in the city of Montreal, the fathers who responded to our advertisement would be, on average, more affluent and also probably those fathers who consider themselves to be most involved with their children. In spite of this, we obtained sufficient numbers of cases of each of the three types of activation relationships to conduct analyses. In addition, our sample contained a greater number of girls than of boys. Furthermore, child temperament and parental behavior were assessed solely using self-report questionnaires completed by the father rather than through triangulation of the information with the mother's perception. Finally, the internal consistency (alpha) of the model's central variable, the stimulation of risk taking, was acceptable but weak.

A study with a sample comprised entirely of mother-child dyads might perhaps reveal that it is in fact the activation relationship itself that plays this role, independent of the sex of the person who fulfills the paternal function of opening the child up to the outside world. It would be important now to demonstrate that the activation relationship and the attachment relationship are indeed complementary mechanisms fostering different developmental outcomes in children. It is therefore vital that future studies evaluate these two types of relationships with the mother and the father within the family system to accurately predict the socioaffective development of children to adulthood. The activation relationship theory should predict competition and risk taking in children including aggression. Our results show that sex differences in the father-child activation relationship appear prior to the sex difference in physical aggression that generally appears at about three years of age [26]. However, it will be necessary to demonstrate in future longitudinal studies that the father-child activation relationship predicts the frequency of physical aggression and risk taking in preschool-age boys while the father-child attachment relationship does not. Indeed, to date, problems of aggression have been linked more to disorganization [22] than to the ABC types of attachment [23, 42]. The prediction has been made that overactivated children will have a greater tendency to develop externalizing problems while underactivated children will have a greater tendency to develop internalizing problems [18].

Acknowledgment

Researchers thank Dr. Jacinthe Emery for coding the Strange Situation.

References

[1] G. J. Suess, K. E. Grossmann, and L. A. Sroufe, "Effects of infant attachment to mother and father on quality of adaptation in preschool: from dyadic to individual organization of self," *International Journal of Behavioral Development*, vol. 15, pp. 43–65, 1992.

[2] M. H. Van Ijzendoorn, "Adult attachment representations, parental responsiveness, and infant attachment: a meta-analysis on the predictive validity of the adult attachment interview," *Psychological Bulletin*, vol. 117, no. 3, pp. 387–403, 1995.

[3] L. M. Youngblade, K. A. Park, and J. Belsky, "Measurement of young children's close friendship: a comparison of 2 independent assessment systems and their associations with attachment security," *International Journal of Behavioral Development*, vol. 16, pp. 563–587, 1993.

[4] K. E. Grossmann and K. Grossmann, "Développement de l'attachement et adaptation psychologique du berceau au tombeau," *Enfance*, vol. 3, pp. 3–12, 1998.

[5] K. Grossmann, K. E. Grossmann, H. Kindler, and P. Zimmermann, "A wider view of attachment and exploration: the influence of mothers and fathers on the development of psychological security from infancy to young adulthood," in *Handbook of Attachment, Theory, Research, and Clinical Applications*, J. Cassidy and P. R. Shaver, Eds., pp. 857–879, Guildford Press, New York, NY, USA, 2nd edition, 2008.

[6] I. Bretherton, "Fathers in attachment theory and research: a review," *Early Child Development and Care*, vol. 180, no. 1-2, pp. 9–23, 2010.

[7] C. Dumont and D. Paquette, "L'attachement père-enfant et l'engagement paternel: deux concepts centraux pour mieux prédire le développement de l'enfant," *Revue de Psychoéducation*, vol. 37, no. 1, pp. 27–46, 2008.

[8] K. Kazura, "Father's qualitative and quantitative involvement: an investigation of attachment, play, and social interactions," *The Journal of Men's Studies*, vol. 9, no. 1, pp. 41–57, 2000.

[9] L. A. Newland and D. D. Coyl, "Fathers' role as attachment figures: an interview with Sir Richard Bowlby," *Early Child Development and Care*, vol. 180, no. 1-2, pp. 25–32, 2010.

[10] O. N. Saracho and B. Spodek, "Father's: the "invisible" parents," *Early Child Development and Care*, vol. 178, no. 7-8, pp. 821–836, 2008.

[11] S. D. Dixon, M. Yogman, and E. Tronick, "Early infant social interaction with parents and strangers," *Journal of the American Academy of Child Psychiatry*, vol. 20, no. 1, pp. 32–52, 1981.

[12] K. MacDonald and R. D. Parke, "Parent-child physical play: the effects of sex and age of children and parents," *Sex Roles*, vol. 15, no. 7-8, pp. 367–378, 1986.

[13] F. Labrell, "Paternal play with toddlers: recreation and creation," *European Journal of Psychology of Education*, vol. 11, no. 1, pp. 43–54, 1996.

[14] S. Kromelow, C. Harding, and M. Touris, "The role of the father in the development of stranger sociability during the second year," *American Journal of Orthopsychiatry*, vol. 60, no. 4, pp. 521–530, 1990.

[15] K. Grossmann, K. E. Grossmann, E. Fremmer-Bombik, H. Kindler, H. Scheuerer-Englisch, and P. Zimmermann, "The uniqueness of the child-father attachment relationship: fathers' sensitive and challenging play as a pivotal variable in a 16-year longitudinal study," *Social Development*, vol. 11, no. 3, pp. 307–331, 2002.

[16] D. Paquette, "Theorizing the father-child relationship: mechanisms and developmental outcomes," *Human Development*, vol. 47, no. 4, pp. 193–219, 2004.

[17] D. Paquette, "La relation père-enfant et l'ouverture au monde," *Enfance*, vol. 2, pp. 205–225, 2004.

[18] D. Paquette and M. Bigras, "The risky situation: a procedure for assessing the father-child activation relationship," *Early Child Development and Care*, vol. 180, no. 1-2, pp. 33–50, 2010.

[19] M. D. S. Ainsworth, M. C. Blehar, E. Waters, and S. Wall, *Patterns of Attachment: A Psychological Study of the Strange Situation*, Lawrence Erlbaum, Hillsdale, NJ, USA, 1978.

[20] G. Cooper, K. Hoffman, B. Powell, and R. Marvin, "The circle of security intervention," in *Enhancing Early Attachments: Theory, Research, Intervention, and Policy*, L. J. Berlin, Y. Ziv, L. M. Amaya-Jackson, and M. T. Greenberg, Eds., Guilford Press, New York, NY, USA, 2005.

[21] M. Main and J. Solomon, "Procedure for identifying infants as disorganized/disoriented during the Ainsworth strange situation," in *Attachment in the Preschool Years: Theory, Research and Intervention*, M. T. Greenberg, D. Cicchetti, and E. M. Cummings, Eds., pp. 121–160, University of Chicago Press, Chicago, Ill, USA, 1990.

[22] K. Lyons-Ruth and D. Jacobvitz, "Attachment disorganization: genetic factors, parenting contexts, and developmental transformation from infancy to adulthood," in *Handbook of Attachment: Theory, Research, and Clinical Applications*, J. Cassidy and P. R. Shaver, Eds., pp. 666–697, Guilford Press, London, UK, 2nd edition, 2008.

[23] M. DeKlyen and M. T. Greenberg, "Attachment and psychopathology in childhood," in *Handbook of Attachment: Theory, Research, and Clinical Applications*, J. Cassidy and P. R. Shaver, Eds., pp. 637–665, Guilford Press, New York, NY, USA, 2nd edition, 2008.

[24] W. R. Charlesworth, "Resources and resource acquisition during ontogeny," in *Sociobiological Perspective on Human Development*, K. B. MacDonald, Ed., pp. 24–77, Springer, New York, NY, USA, 1988.

[25] R. E. Tremblay, C. Japel, D. Perusse et al., "The search for the age of "onset" of physical aggression: Rousseau and Bandura revisited," *Criminal Behaviour and Mental Health*, vol. 9, no. 1, pp. 8–23, 1999.

[26] J. Archer and S. Côté, "Sex differences in aggressive behaviour: a developmental and evolutionary perspective," in *Developmental Origins of Aggression*, R. E. Tremblay, W. W. Hartup, and J. Archer, Eds., pp. 425–443, Guilford Press, London, UK, 2005.

[27] S. P. Putnam, M. A. Gartstein, and M. K. Rothbart, "Measurement of fine-grained aspects of toddler temperament. The Early Childhood Behavior Questionnaire," *Infant Behavior and Development*, vol. 29, no. 3, pp. 386–401, 2006.

[28] D. Paquette, M. M. Eugène, D. Dubeau, and M.-N. Gagnon, "Les pères ont-ils une influence spécifique sur le développement des enfants?" in *La Paternité Au 21e Siècle*, D. Dubeau, A. Devault, and G. Forget, Eds., pp. 99–122, PUL, Québec, Canada, 2009.

[29] D. Paquette, C. Bolté, G. Turcotte, D. Dubeau, and C. Bouchard, "A new typology of fathering: defining and associated variables," *Infant and Child Development*, vol. 9, no. 4, pp. 213–230, 2000.

[30] M. H. Van Ijzendoorn, G. Moran, J. Belsky, D. Pederson, M. J. Bakermans-Kranenburg, and K. Kneppers, "The similarity of siblings' attachments to their mother," *Child Development*, vol. 71, no. 4, pp. 1086–1098, 2000.

[31] M. Main and E. Hesse, "Parents unresolved traumatic experiences are related to infant disorganized attachment status: is frightened and/or frightening parental behavior the linking mechanism?" in *Attachment in the Preschool Years: Theory, Research and Intervention*, M. T. Greenberg, D. Cicchetti, and E. M. Cummings, Eds., pp. 161–182, University of Chicago Press, Chicago, Ill, USA, 1990.

[32] N. L. Hazen, L. McFarland, D. Jacobvitz, and E. Boyd-Soisson, "Fathers' frightening behaviours and sensitivity with infants: relations with fathers' attachment representations, father-infant attachment, and children's later outcomes," *Early Child Development and Care*, vol. 180, no. 1-2, pp. 51–69, 2010.

[33] N. M. Else-Quest, J. S. Hyde, H. H. Goldsmith, and C. A. Van Hulle, "Gender differences in temperament: a meta-analysis," *Psychological Bulletin*, vol. 132, no. 1, pp. 33–72, 2006.

[34] M. A. Gartstein and M. K. Rothbart, "Studying infant temperament via the Revised Infant Behavior Questionnaire," *Infant Behavior and Development*, vol. 26, no. 1, pp. 64–86, 2003.

[35] H. Lytton and D. M. Romney, "Parents' differential socialization of boys and girls: a meta-analysis," *Psychological Bulletin*, vol. 109, no. 2, pp. 267–296, 1991.

[36] J. P. Byrnes, D. C. Miller, and W. D. Schafer, "Gender differences in risk taking: a meta-analysis," *Psychological Bulletin*, vol. 125, no. 3, pp. 367–383, 1999.

[37] S. R. Jaffee, T. E. Moffitt, A. Caspi, and A. Taylor, "Life with (without) father: the benefits of living with two biological parents depend on the father's antisocial behavior," *Child Development*, vol. 74, no. 1, pp. 109–126, 2003.

[38] D. Paquette and C. Dumont, "Is father-child rough-and-tumble play associated with attachment or activation relationships?" *Early Child Development and Care*, 2012.

[39] J. L. Flanders, V. Leo, D. Paquette, R. O. Pihl, and J. R. Séguin, "Rough-and-tumble play and the regulation of aggression: an observational study of father-child play dyads," *Aggressive Behavior*, vol. 35, no. 4, pp. 285–295, 2009.

[40] J. L. Flanders, M. Simard, D. Paquette et al., "Rough-and-tumble play and the development of physical aggression and emotion regulation: a five-year follow-up study," *Journal of Family Violence*, vol. 25, no. 4, pp. 357–367, 2010.

[41] M. H. Van Ijzendoorn, C. Schuengel, and M. J. Bakermans-Kranenburg, "Disorganized attachment in early childhood: meta-analysis of precursors, concomitants, and sequelae," *Development and Psychopathology*, vol. 11, no. 2, pp. 225–249, 1999.

[42] L. J. Berlin, J. Cassidy, and K. Appleyard, "The influence of early attachments on other relationships," in *Handbook of Attachment: Theory, Research, and Clinical Applications*, J. Cassidy and P. R. Shaver, Eds., pp. 333–347, Guilford Press, London, UK, 2nd edition.

2

Attitudes to Mathematics in Primary School Children

Ann Dowker,[1] Karina Bennett,[2] and Louise Smith[2]

[1] *Department of Experimental Psychology, University of Oxford, South Parks Road, Oxford OX1 3UD, UK*
[2] *St Hilda's College, Cowley Place, Oxford OX4 1DY, UK*

Correspondence should be addressed to Ann Dowker, ann.dowker@psy.ox.ac.uk

Academic Editor: Helga Krinzinger

44 Grade 3 children and 45 Grade 5 children from English primary schools were given the British abilities scales basic number skills subtest, and a Mathematics Attitude and Anxiety Questionnaire, using pictorial rating scales to record their Self-rating for maths, Liking for maths, Anxiety about maths, and Unhappiness about poor performance in mathematics. There were few year group differences in attitudes. Boys rated themselves higher than girls, but did not differ significantly in actual performance. Overall, Anxiety was not related to actual performance, but Self-rating was. This relationship between Self-rating and actual performance seemed to develop between Grade 3 and Grade 5. Implications of the findings are discussed.

1. Introduction

Mathematics depends not only on cognitive abilities but also on emotional factors and attitudes. Several studies have shown that emotional factors may play a large part in mathematical performance, with mathematics anxiety playing a particularly large role [1–3]. One possible reason for the negative association between mathematics anxiety and actual performance is that people who have higher levels of math anxiety are more likely to avoid activities and situations that involve mathematics and, thus, have less practice [4]. Mathematics anxiety might also influence performance more directly, by overloading working memory. For example, Ashcraft and Krause [5] reported that highly math-anxious individuals had significantly lower working memory capacities in mathematics-related tasks than individuals with low levels of mathematics anxiety.

Relationships between mathematics anxiety and performance may also be in the other direction. Poor mathematical attainment may lead to mathematics anxiety, as a result of repeated experiences of failure. Indeed, there is likely to be a vicious circle, where anxiety and performance affect each other negatively. Maloney and Beilock [6] point out that the development of mathematics anxiety is likely to be due both to social factors, such as exposure to teachers who themselves suffer from mathematics anxiety, and to pre-existing difficulties in numerical cognition, and that those with initial mathematical difficulties are also likely to be more vulnerable to the negative social influences.

Although mathematics anxiety is a major focus for research, not all attitudes to mathematics are negative, and some people express a strong liking for mathematics [7]. This seems to be particularly the case for mathematically gifted people [8] but is not restricted to them.

Most studies of attitudes to mathematics have involved older children and adults. It is particularly important to investigate the early development of attitudes to mathematics, if we are to understand the relationships between these and actual performance, and if possible to prevent the development of strongly negative attitudes. The relatively few studies that have looked at younger children's attitudes to mathematics have usually shown positive attitudes, with most children claiming to like mathematics ([9–11]). However, studies suggest that attitudes may deteriorate with age, especially through the secondary school period [9, 12, 13], but also within the primary age group ([10, 13]). One study by Gierl and Bisanz [14] gave somewhat more ambiguous results, indicating an increase in mathematics anxiety but also an increase in liking for maths over the later elementary school years.

Most studies of secondary school children and adults have been consistent in showing actual performance in mathematics tends to be related positively to liking for mathematics and to high self-ratings in mathematics, and negatively to mathematics anxiety (e.g., [2, 5, 15–17] Lam et al., 2000). This is the case not only for advanced mathematics but for basic magnitude comparison skills [18].

Studies of the relationships between attitudes to maths and performance in younger children have not resulted in as clear results as those for older children. Ma and Kishor [17] found that the relationships between attitudes and performance increase with age. Cain-Caston [19] found little relationship between mathematics performance and attitudes in a sample of 8- to 9-year olds. Thomas and Dowker [20] (also see [10]) and Krinzinger et al. [21] found that 6- to 8-year olds' mathematical performance was related to Liking mathematics and to Self-rating of ability in the subject, but not to anxiety. Krinzinger et al. [21] failed to find either longitudinal or concurrent relationships between anxiety and performance in young children. On the other hand, relationships between mathematics anxiety, other attitudes, and actual performance have been found in primary school children in a white South African community [22], in New Zealand [23], and in several studies in the United States ([24–27]).

It is thus possible that the relationships between attitudes and performance become clearer in the later primary years. The present study aimed to examine relationships between mathematical performance, mathematics anxiety, unhappiness over poor performance, liking for mathematics, and self-rating in mathematics in children of midprimary age (Grade 3; age 7-8) and later primary age (Grade 5; age 9 to 10).

On the basis of the earlier studies using a similar method [20, 21], it was predicted that mathematics performance would be related to liking mathematics and to self-rating of ability in the subject, but not to anxiety. It was also predicted, especially on the basis of Thomas and Dowker's [20] results that there would be specific independent relationships between liking mathematics and self-rating, and between anxiety and performance-related unhappiness, and that otherwise there would be little correlation between the attitude variables.

Another aim was to investigate changes between Grade 3 and Grade 5. It was predicted that older children might show more negative attitudes. We also aimed to look at whether the relationships between the different variables might change between Grade 3 and Grade 5. Although any such analysis would have to be tentative due to reduced numbers, it was predicted that the relationships between mathematics performance and other attitude variables, and especially between mathematics performance and self-rating, might not be noticeable at Grade 3 but might become significant at Grade 5. This prediction is based on the assumption that children's experiences of success and failure might influence their attitudes toward and confidence in mathematics, and that such experiences and their effects would become increasingly salient during the later primary school years.

The study also aimed to look at gender differences in mathematics performance and attitudes. Most current studies suggest that females do not perform lower in mathematics than males, but that they do tend to rate themselves lower, and to experience more anxiety [28, 29]. The study aimed to investigate whether such gender differences would already be present in young children.

2. Method

2.1. Participants. The participants were 89 children taken from two state primary schools in Brentwood, Essex and one in Enfield, London. They were selected randomly from the third- and fifth-grade classes in these schools. These were nonselective schools with varied intakes, but situated in predominantly relatively middle-class areas. They included 44 children (21 boys and 23 girls) in Grade 3 and 45 children (21 boys and 24 girls) in Grade 5. The Grade 3 children had a mean age of 90.1 months (s.d. 3.48) and the Grade 5 children had a mean age of 112.39 months (s.d. 6.51).

2.2. Materials and Procedure. In order to measure their attitudes, children completed the Mathematics Attitudes and Anxiety Questionnaire [20, 30]. The attitude questionnaire consists of 28 questions which focused on 7 areas of maths: maths in general, written sums, mental sums, easy maths, difficult maths, maths tests, and understanding the teacher. For each item, children were asked about their Self-rating ("How good are you?") on a scale consisting of ticks and crosses ("very good" to "very bad"); Liking for the items ("How much do you like it?") on a scale consisting of sweets and wasps ("like very much" to "hate very much"); Anxiety about them ("How worried would you feel?") on a scale of facial expressions based on Roger Hargreaves' "Mr. Men" picture-book characters Mr. Happy and Mr. Worry ("very relaxed" to "very worried"); Unhappiness at poor performance ("How unhappy would you feel if you did badly?") on a scale consisting of faces with frowning or happy faces ("very unhappy" to "very happy"). Possible rating scores for each item ranged from 1 to 5, so the total possible scores on each scale ranged from 7 to 35. Scores were calculated so that a higher score represented a more positive attitude. Thus, the Anxiety and Unhappiness scores represent relative *freedom* from Anxiety and Unhappiness. In places where there may be ambiguity, the paper will refer to "(Non-)Anxiety" and "(Non-)Unhappiness".

3. Results

Table 1 shows the BNS standard score and the attitude scores according to gender and school year.

3.1. Effects of Gender and School Year on Mathematical Performance and Attitude Scores. An ANOVA was carried out with Year Group (Grade 3 versus Grader 5) and Gender (Male versus Female) as the grouping factor, and BNS standard score and the attitude scores of Liking, Self-rating, Anxiety, and Unhappiness as the dependent variables. There

Table 1: Maths performance and attitude scores by year group and gender.

Year group	Gender	BAS Basic Number Skills standard score	Self-rating	Liking	(Non-)Anxiety	(Non-)Unhappiness
Year 3	Boys ($n = 21$)	109.14 (13.42)	28.9 (4.31)	25.62 (7.89)	23.19 (7.57)	22.71 (4.36)
	Girls ($n = 23$)	112.65 (12.8)	27.26 (4.46)	24.43 (5.56)	23.0 (6.33)	21.04 (5.23)
Total year 3 ($n = 44$)		110.98 (13.07)	28.04 (4.42)	25.0 (6.72)	23.09 (6.87)	21.84 (4.86)
Year 5	Boys ($n = 21$)	120.52 (13.61)	29.05 (4.76)	24.62 (8.52)	23.05 (4.86)	21.00 (4.86)
	Girls ($n = 24$)	115.71 (16.59)	25.75 (5.56)	24.46 (5.73)	23.46 (6.21)	19.71 (5.7)
Total year 5 ($n = 45$)		117.96 (15.29)	27.29 (5.4)	24.53 (7.08)	23.27 (5.57)	20.31 (5.3)
	Total boys ($n = 42$)	114.83 (14.54)	28.98 (5.56)	25.12 (8.12)	23.11 (6.28)	21.86 (4.64)
	Total girls ($n = 47$)	114.21 (14.78)	26.49 (5.06)	24.45 (5.58)	23.23 (6.21)	20.36 (5.46)
Total ($n = 89$)		114.51 (14.59)	27.66 (4.93)	24.76 (6.87)	23.18 (6.21)	21.07 (5.11)

Means are given with standard deviations in brackets.

was a significant effect of Year Group on basic number skills standard score ($F(1,85) = 5.7$; $P = 0.019$; $\eta P^2 = 0.063$), indicating higher scores by the Grade 5 children. There was a significant effect of Gender on Self-rating ($F(1,85) = 5.93$; $P = 0.018$; $\eta P^2 = 0.064$), indicating higher self-rating by boys. No other effects were significant.

Because there were year group differences in BNS standard score, and because the year groups differed in both chronological age *and* school experience, an ANCOVA was then carried out including BNS standard score and chronological age in months (Age) as covariates. Again, Year Group (Grade 3 versus Grade 5) and Gender (Male versus Female) were the grouping factors, and BNS standard score and the attitude scores of Liking, Self-rating, Anxiety, and Unhappiness were the dependent variables. BNS standard score made a significant independent contribution to the variance in Self-rating ($F(1,83) = 6.58$; $P = 0.012$; $\eta P^2 = 0.073$). Age made a significant independent contribution to Unhappiness ($F(1,83) = 13.79$; $P < 0.001$; $\eta P^2 = 0.143$). After controlling the effects of the covariates, Gender still had a significant effect on Self-rating ($F(1,83) = 5.64$; $P = 0.02$; $\eta P^2 = 0.064$). Year Group now had a significant effect on Unhappiness ($F(1,83) = 16.38$; $P < 0.001$; $\eta P^2 = 0.165$).

3.2. Correlations between Attitudes and Mathematics Performance. Pearson correlation coefficients were obtained between the attitude scores of Liking, Self-rating, Anxiety and Unhappiness, BNS standard score, and age in months. These are shown in Table 2.

3.3. What Attitudes Predict Mathematical Performance? Table 3 shows entry-type linear regressions on each of the test variables, with the other variables as predictors. First, in order to investigate more directly the influence of attitudes on mathematical performance an entry-type linear regression was carried out with *BNS standard score* as the dependent variable, and Liking, Self-rating, (Non-)Anxiety and (Non-)Unhappiness as the predictors. The only significant predictor was Self-rating.

Similar analyses were then carried out for each of the attitude variables, with BNS standard score and the other attitude variables as predictors.

Self-rating was predicted by *all* the other variables except (Non-)Anxiety; BNS standard score, (Non-)Unhappiness, and Liking were all significant independent predictors of Self-rating.

Liking was independently predicted by Self-rating and (Non-)Anxiety.

(Non-)*Anxiety* was independently predicted only by Liking, though (Non-)Unhappiness almost reached significance as a predictor ($P = 0.058$).

(Non-)*Unhappiness* was independently predicted only by Self-rating, though, as expected from the previous analysis, (Non-)Anxiety almost reached significance as a predictor.

The same analyses were then carried out separately for the group of third-grade children (Table 4) and the group of fifth-grade children (Table 5).

The findings for third-grade children are shown in Table 4.

None of the attitude variables predicted BNS standard score. Liking and (Non)-Unhappiness predicted Self-Rating. Self-Rating and (Non-)Anxiety predicted Liking. Self-Rating and Liking predicted (Non-)Anxiety. Self-rating predicted (Non-)Unhappiness.

The findings for fifth-grade children are shown in Table 5.

Self-rating was the only significant predictor of BNS standard score. Similarly, BNS standard score was the only significant predictor of Self-rating, (Non-)Anxiety was the only significant predictor of Liking, and Liking was the only significant predictor of (Non-)Anxiety. No predictor approached significance for (Non-)Unhappiness.

4. Discussion

The results support previous studies with primary age children in suggesting that attitudes to mathematics are generally positive in the primary age group. All attitude scores, except for (Non-)Unhappiness at poor performance, were considerably higher than the notional neutral score of 3, though questions could be raised as to whether such a rating

TABLE 2: Correlations between attitude scores, British abilities scales basic number skills standard score, and age in months.

	Self rating	Liking	(Non-)Anxiety	(Non-)Unhappiness	Basic Number Skills: standard score	Age in months
Self-rating	1					
Liking	0.264*	1				
(Non-)Anxiety	0.191	0.413**	1			
(Non-)Unhappiness	0.329**	0.178	0.268*	1		
Basic Number Skills: Standard score	0.255*	−0.1	−0.069	0.021	1	
Age in months	−0.055	−0.083	0.232	0.075	0.231	1

*$P < 0.05$ **$P < 0.01$.

TABLE 3: Entry-type multiple regressions on British abilities scales basic number skills standard score and the attitude variables: whole group.

	Regression on Basic Number Skills standard score	Regression on Self-rating	Regression on Liking	Regression on (non-)Anxiety	Regression on (non-)Unhappiness
Degrees of freedom	4	4	4	4	4
Residual	84	84	84	84	84
R^2	0.106	0.484	0.226	0.211	0.159
F	2.502	6.414	6.148	5.631	3.96
P	0.048*	0.000**	0.000**	0.000**	0.005**
Predictors:					
Basic number skills	—				
β	—	0.286	−1.415	0.034	−0.047
t	—	2.973	−1.402	−0.333	−0.446
P	—	0.004**	0.164	0.74	0.657
Self-rating					
β	0.333	—	0.236	0.021	0.306
t	2.973	—	2.219	0.191	2.795
P	0.004**	—	0.029*	0.849	0.006**
Liking			—		
β	−0.163	0.234	—	0.368	0.006
t	−1.402	2.219	—	3.591	0.049
P	0.104	0.029*	—	0.001**	0.961
(Non-)Anxiety					
β	0.039	0.021	0.361	—	0.212
t	0.333	0.191	3.591	—	1.919
P	0.74	0.849	0.001**	—	0.058
(Non-)Unhappiness					
β	−0.05	0.278	0.005	0.198	—
t	−0.446	2.973	0.049	1.919	—
P	0.657	0.006**	0.961	0.058	—

*$P < 0.05$ **$P < 0.01$.

really does represent "neutrality". There was little difference in attitude between Grade 3 and Grade 5, contradicting the hypothesis that attitudes might deteriorate during this period.

In this particular group, the standard scores on a standardized arithmetic test were rather higher in Grade 5 than in Grade 3, giving rise to the possibility that group differences in mathematical attainment were masking deterioration in attitudes. However, even after controlling both arithmetic standard score and chronological age, there continued to be little effect of year group on attitude.

The exception was (non-)Unhappiness at poor performance, where the year group effect did become significant. However, this reflected a more positive attitude in Grade 5

Table 4: Entry-type multiple regressions on British abilities scales basic number skills standard score and the attitude variables: Grade 3 alone.

	Regression on Basic Number Skills standard score	Regression on Self-rating	Regression on Liking	Regression on (non-)Anxiety	Regression on (non-)Unhappiness
Degrees of freedom	4	4	4	4	4
Residual	39	39	39	39	39
R^2	0.01	0.318	0.281	0.204	0.264
F	0.095	4.552	3.45	2.503	3.496
P	0.984	0.004**	0.017*	0.058	0.016*
Predictors:					
Basic number skills:					
β	—	0.019	−0.016	−0.011	0.08
t	—	−0.145	−0.112	−0.074	0.583
P	—	0.885	0.911	0.942	0.563
Self-rating					
β	−0.028	—	0.414	−0.054	0.417
t	−0.145	—	2.035	−0.314	2.74
P	0.885	—	0.01*	0.755	0.009**
Liking					
β	−0.021	0.382	—	0.322	−0.121
t	−0.112	2.707	—	2.035	−0.764
P	0.911	0.01*	—	0.049*	0.449
(Non-)Anxiety					
β	−0.013	−0.047	0.298	—	0.288
t	−0.074	−0.314	2.035	—	1.957
P	0.942	0.785	0.049*	—	0.058
(Non-)Unhappiness					
β	0.108	0.387	−0.122	0.311	—
t	0.583	2.74	−0.764	1.957	—
P	0.563	0.009**	0.449	0.058	—

$^*P < 0.05$ $^{**}P < 0.01$.

than Grade 3 children. Age was also separately significant as a covariate, and it correlated negatively with this attitude variable. As Unhappiness was not significantly related to either age or year group when they were considered separately, these results should be taken with caution at this point, but attempts should be made to replicate them in future studies.

It should be noted that there may be more ambiguity about the positive or negative nature of Unhappiness at poor performance than over the other attitudes. Certainly, a high level of unhappiness at poor performance is a negative attitude, but at the end of the scale where children are relatively free of such unhappiness, individual differences in scores may be more reflective of a preference for performing well, arguably a positive attitude. Perhaps the somewhat puzzling results here could reflect this ambiguity.

Correlational analyses indicate little relationship between chronological age and the attitude variables, supporting the findings with regard to year group effects. As predicted, they support the earlier results of [10] and Krinzinger et al. [21], in showing no consistent relationship between mathematics Anxiety and performance among primary school children. There was, however, a significant relationship between Anxiety and Liking for mathematics; not surprisingly, a Liking for mathematics was strongly associated with a freedom from Anxiety.

The only attitude variable that correlated significantly with actual performance was Self-rating. Those who rated themselves higher at maths performed better. Self-rating appeared indeed to be the only variable that was strongly related to all the other variables. As well as being related to actual performance, it was related to Liking for maths and to freedom from Anxiety. After controlling for other variables in regression analyses, it was also related to freedom from performance-related Unhappiness.

Somewhat unexpectedly, there was no significant relationship between Liking for maths and actual performance, though Liking for maths was significantly related to other attitude variables.

It had been predicted that Anxiety and Unhappiness at poor performance might be strongly and independently

TABLE 5: Entry-type multiple regressions on British abilities scales basic number skills standard score and the attitude variables: Grade 5 alone.

	Regression on basic number skills standard score	Regression on self-rating	Regression on liking	Regression on (non)anxiety	Regression on (non)unhappiness
Degrees of freedom	4	4	4	4	4
Residual	40	40	40	40	40
R^2	0.31	0.337	0.275	0.281	0.103
F	4.495	5.084	3.794	3.903	1.154
P	0.004**	0.002**	0.01*	0.009**	0.346
Predictors:					
Basic number skills	—				
β	—	0.522	−0.157	−0.15	−0.05
t	—	3.983	−0.979	−0.939	−0.277
P	—	0.000**	0.334	0.353	0.784
Self-rating					
β	−0.028	—	0.135	0.133	0.243
t	−0.145	—	0.821	0.813	1.354
P	0.885	—	0.416	0.421	0.183
Liking					
β	−0.021	0.123	—	0.436	0.087
t	−0.112	0.821	—	3.082	0.498
P	0.911	0.416	—	0.004**	0.621
(Non)anxiety					
β	−0.013	0.122	0.44	—	0.129
t	−0.074	0.813	3.082	—	0.735
P	0.942	0.421	0.004**	—	0.467
(Non)unhappiness					
β	0.108	0.18	0.021	0.103	—
t	0.583	1.354	0.498	0.735	—
P	0.563	0.183	0.621	0.467	—

*$P < 0.05$ **$P < 0.01$.

correlated with one another but not with the other attitude variables, and that Liking for maths and Self-rating might be strongly and independently correlated with one another but not with the other attitude variables. This prediction was not entirely borne out. Self-rating and Liking for maths did show an independent relationship, but Self-rating was also independently related to the other attitude variables. Liking for maths was correlated with Anxiety as well as Self-rating. There was only a weak relationship between Anxiety and performance Unhappiness, and each correlated more strongly with other factors: Anxiety with Liking for maths, and performance Unhappiness with Self-rating.

The results of separate regression analyses for different year groups suggest that, although there are few age or year group differences in the attitude scores themselves, there may be some differences in the relationships between the variables. A great deal of caution is needed in interpreting these results, because of the reduced sample sizes in these analyses, resulting in relatively low statistical power. It is possible that there were some small effects that would only have become obvious in larger samples. However, the results do support the hypothesis that the relationship between self-rating and actual performance may develop between Grade 3 and Grade 5. There was no relationship between the two variables in Grade 3 children. In Grade 3, none of the attitude variables predicted mathematical performance, and Self-rating was predicted by Liking for maths and freedom from Anxiety, but not by performance. In Grade 5, by contrast, there was a very strong and specific relationship between Self-rating and actual performance. This finding may suggest that children become more aware of their mathematical performance in relation to that of their peers as they become older, either because of generally greater self-awareness, or because of greater experience of tests and teacher assessments. Alternatively, or additionally, it may be that children's self-assessment has an increasing influence on their motivation, and thereby on their performance, as they get older.

The only significant gender difference was in self-rating, where boys rated themselves higher than girls did. There were no gender differences in actual performance or in other attitudes. This supports findings from previous studies that indicate that males tend to rate themselves higher than females in mathematics, although at least in recent studies the genders usually perform similarly. Future research should investigate whether this finding is specific to self-rating in mathematics, where it may reflect existing stereotypes about the subject, or whether it might indicate generally higher self-ratings by boys in other subjects as well.

One key limitation of this study is of course that the sample is relatively small. It is important for future studies to extend both the number and the range of the sample. For example, the children in the sample were attending schools in relatively middle-class catchment areas and, perhaps linked to this fact, were generally performing at somewhat above average levels in mathematics. The mean standard score on the basic number skills test was 114.51, as compared with an assumed population mean standard score of 100. It is possible that a lower-attaining group, or one including a higher proportion of children from low-SES backgrounds, might show more negative attitudes and/or stronger relationships between attitudes and performance.

Also, it is important to carry out cross-cultural comparisons. This study aligns with most similar non-American studies (e.g., [17, 21]), in suggesting that younger children do not show a significant relationship between mathematics anxiety and actual mathematical performance, but, as indicated in the Introduction, most American studies have given contrasting results (e.g., [24–26]). It would be interesting to investigate whether there is some difference in cultural attitudes or in methods of mathematics education that contributes to this disparity. It would also be desirable to investigate young children's attitudes to mathematics in a wider variety of cultures.

It could be argued that a questionnaire measure is not ideal as a sole measure of attitudes in young children, or perhaps in any group. In future studies, it would be desirable to include other measures: for example implicit attitude tests [31], behavioural measures such as children's responses when given a choice between activities with and without mathematical content, and perhaps physiological indicators of anxiety. It would also be desirable to use a wider variety of mathematics tests, in particular, to use tests of mental as well as written arithmetic, as the former is more likely to be affected by the increased load that anxiety may place on working memory ([5, 25]).

Despite such potential limitations, the study yields some important conclusions. Young children appear to show relatively positive attitudes to mathematics, though a larger sample of different ages would be needed to confirm this. They show little relationship between mathematics anxiety and mathematical performance, but they do show a relationship between self-rating and mathematical performance, which seems to develop during the later primary years. There are also significant relationships between self-rating and other attitudes. It is thus arguable that self-rating, rather than mathematics anxiety, is the key factor in the primary school age group, and that perhaps researchers on younger children's attitudes to mathematics should focus more on self-rating.

References

[1] M. Baloğlu and R. Koçak, "A multivariate investigation of the differences in mathematics anxiety," *Personality and Individual Differences*, vol. 40, no. 7, pp. 1325–1335, 2006.

[2] R. Hembree, "The nature, effects, and relief of mathematics anxiety," *Journal For Research in Mathematics Education*, vol. 21, no. 1, pp. 33–46, 1990.

[3] H. Miller and J. Bichsel, "Anxiety, working memory, gender, and math performance," *Personality and Individual Differences*, vol. 37, no. 3, pp. 591–606, 2004.

[4] M. H. Ashcraft, "Math anxiety: personal, educational, and cognitive consequences," *Current Directions in Psychological Science*, vol. 11, no. 5, pp. 181–185, 2002.

[5] M. H. Ashcraft and J. A. Krause, "Working memory, math performance, and math anxiety," *Psychonomic Bulletin and Review*, vol. 14, no. 2, pp. 243–248, 2007.

[6] E. A. Maloney and S. Beilock, "Math anxiety: who has it, why it develops, and how to guard against it," *Trends in Cognitive Sciences*, vol. 16, no. 8, pp. 404–406, 2012.

[7] J. Evans, *Adults' Mathematical Thinking and Emotions: A Study of Numerate Practices*, Routledge, London, UK, 2000.

[8] V. A. Krutetskii, *The Psychology of Mathematical Abilities in Schoolchildren*, University of Chicago Press, London, UK, 1976.

[9] P. Blatchford, "Pupils' views on school work and school from 7 to 16 years," *Research Papers in Education*, vol. 11, no. 3, pp. 263–288, 1996.

[10] A. Dowker, *Individual Differences in Arithmetic: Implications for Psychology, Neuroscience and Education*, Psychology Press, New York, NY, USA, 2005.

[11] B. Tizard, P. Blatchford, J. Burke, C. Farquhar, and I. F. Plewis, *Young Children at School in the Inner City*, Erlbaum, London, UK, 1988.

[12] P. Mortimore, *School Matters: The Junior Years*, Open Books, Wells, UK, 1988.

[13] A. Wigfield and J. L. Meece, "Math anxiety in elementary and secondary school students," *Journal of Educational Psychology*, vol. 80, no. 2, pp. 210–216, 1988.

[14] M. J. Gierl and J. Bisanz, "Anxieties and attitudes related to mathematics in grades 3 and 6," *Journal of Experimental Education*, vol. 63, no. 2, pp. 139–158, 1995.

[15] L. R. Aiken, "Two scale of attitude toward mathematics," *Journal For Research in Mathematics Education*, vol. 5, no. 2, pp. 67–71, 1974.

[16] H. Z. Ho, D. Senturk, A. G. Lam et al., "The affective and cognitive dimensions of math anxiety: a cross-national study," *Journal for Research in Mathematics Education*, vol. 31, no. 3, pp. 362–379, 2000.

[17] X. Ma and N. Kishor, "Assessing the relationship between attitude toward mathematics and achievement in mathematics: a meta-analysis," *Journal for Research in Mathematics Education*, vol. 28, no. 1, pp. 26–47, 1997.

[18] E. A. Maloney, D. Ansari, and J. A. Fugelsang, "The effect of mathematics anxiety on the processing of numerical magnitude," *Quarterly Journal of Experimental Psychology*, vol. 64, no. 1, pp. 10–16, 2011.

[19] M. Cain-Caston, "Parent and student attitudes toward mathematics as they relate to third grade mathematics achievement," *Journal of Instructional Psychology*, vol. 20, no. 2, pp. 96–101, 1993.

[20] G. Thomas and A. Dowker, "Mathematics anxiety and related factors in young children," in *Proceedings of the British Psychological Society Developmental Section Conference*, Bristol, UK, September 2000.

[21] H. Krinzinger, L. Kaufmann, and K. Willmes, "Math anxiety and math ability in early primary school years," *Journal of Psychoeducational Assessment*, vol. 27, no. 3, pp. 206–225, 2009.

[22] K. Newstead, "Aspects of children's mathematics anxiety," *Educational Studies in Mathematics*, vol. 36, no. 1, pp. 53–71, 1998.

[23] J. Young-Loveridge, *The Development of Children's Number Concepts from Ages Five to Nine*, Early Mathematics Learning Project, Education Department, University of Waikato, Hamilton, New Zealand, 1991.

[24] J. A. Dossey, I. V. S. Mullis, M. M. Lindquist, and D. L. Chambers, *The Mathematics Report Card. Are We Measuring up? Trends and Achievement Based on the 1986 National Assessment*, Educational Testing Service, Princeton, NJ, USA, 1988.

[25] G. Ramirez, E. A. Gunderson, S. C. Levine, and S. L. Beilock, "Math anxiety, working memory and math achievement in early elementary school," *Journal of Cognition and Development*. In press.

[26] S. S. Wu, M. Barth, H. Amin, V. Malcarne, and M. Vinod, "Math anxiety in second and third graders and its relation to mathematical achievement," *Frontiers in Developmental Psychology*, vol. 3, p. 162, 2012.

[27] C. B. Young, S. S. Wu, and V. Menod, "The neurodevelopmental basis of math anxiety," *Psychological Science*, vol. 23, pp. 492–501, 2012.

[28] A. Devine, K. Fawcett, D. Szucs, and A. Dowker, "Gender differences in mathematics anxiety and the relation to mathematics performance while controlling for test anxiety," *Behavioral and Brain Functions*, vol. 8, article 33, 2012.

[29] N. M. Else-Quest, J. S. Hyde, and M. C. Linn, "Cross-national patterns of gender differences in mathematics: a meta-analysis," *Psychological Bulletin*, vol. 136, no. 1, pp. 103–127, 2010.

[30] H. Krinzinger, L. Kaufmann, A. Dowker et al., "Deutschsprachige Version des Fragebogens für Rechenangst (FRA) für 6- bis 9-jährige Kinder," *Zeitschrift fur Kinder und Jugendpsychiatrie und Psychotherapie*, vol. 35, no. 5, pp. 341–351, 2007.

[31] O. Rubinsten and R. Tannock, "Mathematics anxiety in children with developmental dyscalculia," *Behavioral and Brain Functions*, vol. 6, article 46, 2010.

3

Developmental Risk: Evidence from Large Nonright-Handed Samples

Filippos Vlachos,[1] Francois Gaillard,[2] Kiriazis Vaitsis,[1] and Argiris Karapetsas[1]

[1] *Department of Special Education, University of Thessaly, Argonafton & Filellinon, 38221 Volos, Greece*
[2] *Institute of Psychology, University of Lausanne, Géopolis, 1015 Lausanne, Switzerland*

Correspondence should be addressed to Filippos Vlachos; fvlachos@uth.gr

Academic Editor: Ross Flom

The aim of the present study is twofold. First, we tested the view that individuals who do not develop a typically strong behavioral laterality are distributed differentially among the two genders across age. Second, we examined whether left handedness and mixed handedness are associated with an elevated risk of some developmental or cognitive deficits. A special recruitment procedure provided norms of the Rey-Osterrieth Complex Figure (ROCF) copy from large samples of left-handed ($N = 420$) and mixed-handed ($N = 72$) compared to right-handed ($N = 420$) schoolchildren and adults ($N = 545$). This graphic task was considered as reflective of the growth of visual-spatial skills and impairment at copying as a developmental risk. Subjects' hand preference was assessed by the Edinburgh Handedness Inventory. Data analysis indicated that (1) the trend towards consistent right handedness is sex related. Girls are clearly ahead of boys in this lateralization process, and boys are overrepresented in mixed-handed subjects. The greater prevalence of mixed-handed boys compared to girls decreases with age. (2) Performance on drawing the ROCF varies according to age and handedness groups. Mixed-handed subjects scored worse in all age groups. The results are discussed in relation to the hormonal-developmental, neuropathological, and learning theories of lateralization.

1. Introduction

Handedness is a significant feature of ontogenetic development. Its consistency and stability provide evidence for brain hemispheric specialization and can be used as an indicator of developmental stages. Lateralization is both cause and consequence of having a brain with two cerebral hemispheres specialized to perform different tasks and work together in order to improve many motor and cognitive tasks. At the first glance, no hand lateralization is observed in young children who have not yet learned to use innate biological asymmetry. However, careful observation of motor behavior in infants already reveals the human specific trend towards dextrality [1, 2].

The study of handedness has been of interest for many years because subtle cognitive and behavioral differences have been demonstrated in relation to various handedness measures [3]. Gender differences in handedness are widely reported. A recent meta-analysis of 144 studies [4] demonstrated that the gender difference in handedness is both significant and robust, indicating that the overall best estimate, albeit not universal, for the male to female odds ratio was 1.23. The purpose of this study is to investigate further the effects of handedness, as a proxy for hemispheric laterality, in terms of gender differences, performance on a cognitive task, and the potential for later cognitive impairment, examining large left-handed and mixed-handed groups of children and adults. Large samples of nonright handers are rare because only 9-10% of the population of schoolchildren is left-handed, and there are even fewer nonlateralized children. In previous studies [5–7], using a special recruitment procedure in order to obtain a large group of left handers (each left-handed child was matched by age and sex to a right-handed child), we have demonstrated differences between left and right handers on the Rey-Osterrieth Complex Figure (ROCF) test, a popular tool used to test visuospatial-constructional functions [8]. In the present study, we complete this observation by including non-lateralized children. We are also adding a group of adults in order to present the whole cognitive development.

A very recent study [9] indicated that there is no single pattern in the development of handedness from 6 to 24 months, and the shift to more robust hand use preferences may be a developmental phenomenon. Inconsistent and unstable handedness has been found in several clinical groups with pathological cognitive development [10, 11]. However, many studies showed no relationship between handedness and cognitive development in samples of normal children [12–16]. These observations show that factors that disrupt cognitive development can also disrupt the development of consistent manual dominance. We can explain this discrepancy between apparently contradictory results by considering progressive handedness to be merely a sign of brain specialization and not a condition of mental development.

However, during the school years, consistent and stable handedness appears as a tool for learning fine motor tasks such as writing and for developing the spatial sense necessary for written language and calculation. Although nonlateralized schoolchildren are not delayed in maturation, they lack the advantage that left and right handers have in their learning. This is why nonlateralized schoolchildren are often at risk of being considered as slow learners or as learning disabled as far as visual-spatial abilities are concerned. In this sense, they are subjected to a true developmental risk.

Progressive hand preference indicates neurophysiological asymmetry which is genetic and biological in origin [17–20]. However, some handedness conditions are pathological. According to the theoretical account of pathological left-handedness syndrome, a subgroup of left handers suffers from a condition that involves an early injury. This syndrome is believed to be caused by a hemispheric lesion that is predominantly left-sided (or bilateral asymmetric), which onsets before the age of 6 and which encroaches upon the critical speech zones of the frontotemporal/frontoparietal cortex [10]. Indeed, the trend towards functional lateralization reveals itself to be sensitive to any cerebral disturbance. The neuropathological hypothesis of handedness would firstly predict that diffused brain injury would result in a lack of hand dominance and, secondly, that lateralized hemispheric damage would produce strong ipsilateral hand dominance.

In the first case, patients present a habitus of mixed handedness characterized by low motor performances on both body sides. Research on prematurity, on risk pregnancy, and on dystocia has shown that very often these conditions are associated with cognitive deficits and an increased frequency of inconsistent right handedness. These studies suggest that the brain might be affected as a whole resulting in mixed handedness and bilateral clumsiness [21–24]. Additionally, several studies consider mixed handedness as a pathological condition [13, 25–27].

In the second case, some of the 100% left handers are suffering from right hand handicap corresponding to left brain damage [1, 10, 28]. The non dominant hand of such strongly lateralized persons actually acts as a symptomatic limb. Obstetricians and pediatricians estimate that 1.5–6% of children are likely to suffer from brain damage early in life [29, 30]. Thus, it is reasonable to expect to have some of these brain damaged patients in a sample of 912 children. Surprisingly there seems to be no literature on pathological 100% right handedness, which is, of course, the reverse possibility. However, the neuropathological hypothesis only accounts for one explanation of the variation in the relationship between handedness and skills. Table 1 presents five hypotheses related to this variation.

The genetic influence on laterality has been proved by comparing parental with child handedness both in normal and adoptive families [31–33]. At present, laterality genetics is far from clear. Some claim that there may be a single gene influencing laterality development with homozygotically and heterozygotically different conditions [17]. Others believe that the inheritance process is polygenetic [19], and the recent molecular studies strongly favor a polygenic model. More specifically, a few years ago Francks et al. [40] identified an imprinted gene, *LRRTM1*, within the 2p12-q11 region, which is expressed during the development of specific forebrain structures. The paternal copy of this gene was associated with both left handedness and schizophrenia, and this was the first potential genetic influence on human handedness identified, and the first putative genetic effect on variability in human brain asymmetry. Other researchers [41] identified the X-linked androgen receptor as a candidate gene for handedness. In another study of genetic influences on handedness [42] researchers after analyzing a large sample of twin and family data for hand preference concluded that the familial aggregation for hand preference was found to be consistent with additive genetic effects, which accounted for about a quarter of the variation in the trait with the remainder accounted for by nonshared environmental influences. All these findings are consistent with the emerging view that handedness is determined by multiple interacting genetic and environmental factors. A recent study [43] showed that human handedness is affected by early lateralised visual experience, thus leading the researchers to the suggestion that a combined gene-environment model could better explain the development of human handedness.

Hormones also influence brain development, as has been demonstrated by comparing female and male brain lateralization and specialization [44, 45]. Female brains show weaker lateralization, but this sex difference only accounts for 1 or 2% of the variance in laterality [46]. Clinically, women suffer less than men from aphasia following brain damage. They also seem to recover better than males when similar aphasic states are observed [47]. There is a slight preponderance of nonright-handed males in child clinical samples where girls appear as more lateralized than boys [34, 48–50]. According to Geschwind and Galaburda's hypothesis [34] there is a fundamental link between abnormal left-hemisphere development, reduced dextrality, various learning disorders, and various immune related and other medical conditions, which is forged by the prenatal influence of testosterone on the developing nervous system. The authors propose that excessive levels of fetal testosterone influence the rate of maturation of the cerebral hemispheres which, in turn, may increase the probability of nonright handedness and learning disorders, affecting males more than females due to the higher rates of testosterone [34]. Two decades ago, a review by

Table 1: Influence on the lateralization process: evidence and implication.

Type of influence	Effect evidenced	Hypothesis for research
Genetic	Children with left-handed parents more often become left handers but not in adopted samples.	Becoming left-handed is as physiological as becoming right-handed. Some people do not inherit the genetic influence, therefore lateralizing themselves by the other influences or even by chance. Healthy genetic left-handed develop an original mind in comparison with right-handed individuals [31–33].
Hormonal/developmental	Greater prevalence of nonright handedness in males. Cerebral lateralization more pronounced in males.	Male's overall maturational gap. Male's overall boost of right-hemispheric functions [34].
Neuropathological	Any brain injury before, during and after birth contradicts the lateralization process.	Results depend on global or focal brain suffering. If global, some ambidextrous subjects suffer bilateral brain damage. If focal, some 100% right-handed and some 100% left-handed suffer hemispheric dysfunction [1, 10, 28].
Neuropsychological	Each hand shows an ability advantage corresponding to the specialization of the direct linked hemisphere.	The right hand is better at communicating, and the left hand is better at visual-spatial tasks [35–37].
Learning	Children take progressively advantage of their lateralization by building body-space relationships and developing constructional abilities.	Lateralized children develop a better spatial sense than nonlateralized ones. Risks for academic learning are lower in lateralized than ambidextrous children. Target: arithmetic, eidetic reading, and writing [38, 39].

Bryden et al. [51] questioned the Geschwind and Galaburda's hypothesis [34] as a cohesive entity. However, this same review did acknowledge an empirical basis for the association of a number of developmental and health problems with hand preference and hormone action. Even though a strong version of the link between handedness with hormone action has been refuted [51], still numerous reports exist to point to some role of hormone action in hand preference. For example, a few years ago [52] pointed out that the length of the index finger relative to that of the ring finger (the 2D : 4D ratio) is a marker of the amount of testosterone that was present in the foetal environment. Recent studies [53, 54] confirmed that the difference between the digit ratios of the right and left hands was a significant predictor of handedness.

There are two more hypotheses that predict a relation between lateralization and neuropsychological development: neuropsychology and learning. Concerning neuropsychology, brain hemispheric specialization directly influences hand specialization. Despite the fact that every human being acts in a bihemispheric manner, the right hand is more effectively used for left-hemispheric functions and the left for right-hemispheric functions. This does not mean that the right hand cannot obey the right hemisphere, but experimental studies have shown that the right hand is simply better than the left hand in performing left hemisphere specialized tasks [35–37]. For our purpose this means that we could predict that the left hand is better than the right in copying the ROCF. Of course, we did not ask our right handers to draw with their left hand in order to check this prediction. However, in a recent study aiming to investigate intermanual differences in copying performance, Yamashita [55] examined the right- and left-hand performance on the ROCF in a nonclinical sample of undergraduates. Yamashita found that hand use had a minimal effect on performance in the copy trial. So the hemispheric specialization theory does not imply that left handers will better succeed in copying the ROCF than right handers. Indeed, a dominant hand for specific tasks is the result of long training which can interfere with hemispheric specialization. This is particularly true for drawing and writing.

As far as learning is concerned, lateralization provides a child with a tool for space behavior, since lateral preference strongly helps the child to build his/her body scheme and organize peri corporal behavior. This boosted training results in a certain advantage in developing visual-spatial abilities, reading, and even calculation in lateralized children [38, 39].

The aim of the study reported here is twofold. First, we tested the view that individuals who do not develop a typically strong behavioral laterality are distributed differentially among the two genders across age. Second, we examined whether left handedness and mixed handedness are associated with an elevated risk of some developmental or cognitive deficits. To this end, we used two popular tools, the Edinburgh Handedness Inventory (EHI) [56] and the Rey-Osterrieth Complex Figure (ROCF) test [57–59] in order to assess handedness and cognitive development, respectively. EHI is a reliable and well-validated instrument and, according to the Citation Index, has been the most widely used handedness inventory in the literature. The ROCF is a popular neuropsychological test designed for adults that has been successfully employed with school-aged children. Its utility with this population stems largely from the fact that it provides such a rich data source, allowing for the assessment of multiple cognitive processes (e.g., perceptual, spatial, metacognitive, and memory). The ROCF has proven useful in the study of normal (Karapetsas and Kantas, 1991 [60];

Waber and Holmes, 1985 [61]) and atypical child development (Brandys and Rourke, 1991 [62]). Children's performance on the ROCF follows a clear developmental trajectory; it is very challenging for early primary school children but becomes more manageable for older children and adults [60, 61].

The five hypotheses concerning the origin and the consequences of handedness in cognitive development mentioned in Table 1 could explain why experimental results often contradict each other depending on case selection and on the handedness characteristics considered. The present study deals with three of them: hormonal-developmental, neuropathological, and learning. In line with the delayed development of the left hemisphere in males proposed by Geschwind and Galaburda [34], we expect to find a preponderance of boys in the nonlateralized group because of their slight delay in brain maturation when compared to girls (*Hypothesis 1*). According to the neuropathological model [1, 10, 28], it was hypothesized that performance on copying the ROCF would be particularly low in mixed-handed and in extremely lateralized persons (*Hypothesis 2*). Finally, the learning model of handedness [38, 39] would predict that the worst scores on ROCF would be found in mixed-handed subjects, because non-lateralized children lack laterality support in the development of their skills (*Hypothesis 3*).

2. Method

2.1. Population. We followed a two-stage process for our case selection. Children were recruited from normal schools using a procedure which aimed at collecting as many left handers as right handers. Teachers were asked to indicate which students wrote with their left hand. Using the Edinburgh Handedness Inventory [56], we subsequently identified 420 children as left-handed and 72 children as nonlateralized. Then, each left-handed child was matched by age and sex to a right-handed child. By the end of this procedure, we collected observations from a total sample of 912 schoolchildren consisting of 420 left handers, 420 right handers, and 72 mixed handers. All of these children were drawn from regular schools and had no history of major medical illness, psychiatric illness, developmental disorder, or significant visual or auditory impairments according to the medical reports of their schools. The 912 children were subdivided into two age groups. The younger age group (5.5 to 9.5 yr.) consisted of 512 subjects, and the older group (aged 9.5 to 12.5 yrs.) consisted of 400 subjects.

The adults were 545 students (199 men and 346 women), aged 17.6 to 32 years ($M = 19.5$, $SD = 1.8$), all drawn from the Engineering Faculty and the Humanities Faculty of the University of Thessaly, Greece. University students in Greece represent 30 percent of the total young adult population, so we selected a subgroup of the total population at the highest academic level. Given the overrepresentation of women in our adult sample and the study's aim to compare the gender ratio of adults with that of children, we calculated a corrective index (dividing the number of men by that of women), in order to represent men and women equally. The corrective index applied was number of women $\times$ 0.575 = corrected number of women compared to men.

2.2. Materials and Procedure

2.2.1. Lateralization Index. In the present study we used a shortened version of the EHI [56] to assess hand preference. Following Bryden and Steenhuis' recommendation [63] we saved the following items from the original version: writing, drawing, use of scissors, striking a match, and opening a box. The five items listed are deemed sufficient to produce reliable and valid results [64] and allow for safe classification of the participants into handedness groups [65]. Numerous studies have confirmed the superior rigour and reliability of the EHI compared to other handedness questionnaires [66–69]. Test-Retest reliability of the EHI as measured by the Pearson r, Kendall τ, and Spearman r_s ranges from 0.95 to 0.98 [68]. The medium to high correlations of the EHI with other behavioral measures of handedness (e.g., the Purdue Pegboard test, a test of manual dexterity) demonstrate the high concurrent validity of the test [70–72].

Procedure. For children aged 5.5 to 7.5, the assessment of hand preference was done through demonstration in order to avoid any interpretational difficulties that could occur with a written questionnaire. For each handedness questionnaire item, children were asked to indicate whether they had used the right hand or the left hand. This type of procedure has been proposed by Coren [65] as the most appropriate means for assessing handedness in younger groups. Further, Steenhuis and Bryden [73] indicated that preference questions are closely related to performance measures concerning similar activities.

Scoring. Children aged 7.5 to 12.5, and adults completed the EHI. The score for the EHI is computed as the difference between the total number of right- or left-handed responses divided by the total number of responses, and the result is multiplied by 100 to produce the Laterality Quotient. Subjects who scored between +91 and +100 were labelled consistent right-handers (CRH), those with scores between +30 and +90 inconsistent right-handers (IRH), those with scores between −29 and +29 mixed-handers (MH), those with scores between −30 and −90 inconsistent left-handers (ILH), and those with scores between −91 and −100 consistent left-handers (CLH).

2.2.2. Visual-Spatial Skills. In order to examine visual-spatial skills, we used the Rey-Osterrieth Complex Figure (ROCF), according to the directions provided by the authors [57–59].

Procedure. The figure was displayed on a piece of white paper measuring 30 cm $\times$ 21 cm so that the base rectangle measured 8.0 $\times$ 5.5 cm. When tested, each participant was provided with a piece of white paper of the same dimensions as the one on which the Rey-Osterrieth figure was presented. Participants were tested in their classroom groups. After the figure had been administered, we asked participants to copy it as best they could without neglecting any of its finer details. There were no time restrictions. When a participant stopped, we asked him/her if he/she had finished. If he/she answered affirmatively, we removed the copying sheet. All the left handers used their left hand for the drawing task, and all the right handers used their right hand. Mixed-handed people were allowed to draw with either hand.

Scoring. To evaluate the data in the manner described by Osterrieth [59], the complex figure was divided into 18 elements, each of which was assigned the same value. Then the number of elements in each figure reproduced by the participants was counted, their positions in relation to the whole figure were noted, and the accuracy of reproduction was noted. The following scoring method was employed. For each element that was correctly placed in its proper position and, moreover, was accurately drawn, a score of 2 was allocated. If the element was correct, but, in the wrong position, a score of 1 was allocated. If the element was distorted or incomplete but recognizable and in the right position a score of 1 was allocated. If the element possessed the same characteristics and was misplaced, a score of 0.5 was allocated. Finally, if an element was not easily recognisable or was absent, the score was zero. The highest possible score for each figure was 36 points. The time required for the completion of the figure was not taken into consideration during scoring, but on average copying took between 3 and 5 minutes. A random sample of 80 figures was scored by two scorers on the basis of the aforementioned criteria, with 94% agreement. This indicated sufficient interrater reliability of the scoring method, and thus the remaining figures were scored by one judge only.

3. Results

3.1. Sex Ratio in Lateralized and Nonlateralized Samples. We found unequal numbers of boys and girls among the mixed-handed children: 27 boys and 7 girls in the younger group (a ratio of 3.6 : 1) and 27 boys and 13 girls in the older group (a ratio of 2.1 : 1). Taking into account the corrected number of women, in order to be able to make comparisons with the data of children, we found a sex ratio of 1.4 men for 1 woman in mixed-handed adults. A Kruskall-Wallis test indicated a significant relationship between sex ratio and age in mixed-handed people ($H = 5.76$, $df = 2$, and $P = .018$). Table 2 recapitulates the frequencies and sex ratio according to handedness and age groups.

Table 2 shows that mixed handedness exists in all age groups. However, there are three times more mixed-handed boys than girls in the younger group. Maturation and learning change the figures. However, mixed handedness is still more frequent in adult males than females.

The right-handedness figures confirm the existence of a relationship between sex and handedness development. Indeed, because left-handers were matched to right-handers for both boys and girls, we would expect to find equivalent frequencies of inconsistent and consistent right-handers regardless of sex. This was held true for younger children where we observed 57 IRH boys compared to 59 IRH girls and 63 CRH boys compared to 61 CRH girls ($\chi^2 = .07$, $df = 1$, ns). However, a developmental trend seems to be observed regarding sex ratio in right-handers since we found 41 IRH boys compared to 28 IRH girls and 49 CRH boys compared to 62 CRH girls in older children ($\chi^2 = 3.97$, $df = 1$, and $P = .046$). To examine whether the older right-handed children were making a transition from the inconsistence use of the right hand to the consistence use and the possible effect of sex a Kruskall-Wallis test was performed. The significance test between younger and older children revealed a main effect for hand consistency ($\chi^2 = 4.16$, $P = .041$) and a main effect for sex ratio ($\chi^2 = 18.01$, $P < .001$). Thus, even when applying a strict recruitment procedure in order to balance left-handed and right-handed boys and girls, we found a tendency for older right-handed girls to become more strongly lateralized than boys with age, and sex-related developmental trends appeared to exist.

To summarize, we observed a sex-related developmental change in handedness distribution. This refers to the hormonal-developmental hypothesis of lateralization. Both the diminishing prevalence of boys in the mixed-handed sample and the stronger lateralization of older right-handed girls compared to boys indicate a relative delay in the lateralization process of boys.

3.2. Age, Sex, and Handedness Differences in Visual-Spatial Skills (Intelligence). ROCF raw scores show systematic changes across ages (see Table 3). Scores were evaluated using a 5 × 3 × 2 (handedness × age × sex) mixed-effect analysis of variance. There were statistically significant main effects for handedness ($F_{4,1427} = 25.26$, $P < .001$) and age ($F_{2,1427} = 182.46$, $P < .001$), which means, respectively, that performance improved with age (as can be seen in Table 3) and that handedness groups differed in their performance. The main effect between males and females was not statistically significant ($F_{1,1427} = 3.19$, ns). There was also a statistically significant age by handedness interaction ($F_{8,1427} = 154.39$, $P < .001$), which indicates that the effect of handedness differed at different ages. No other significant interaction between the factors was found (handedness × sex $F_{4,1427} = 0.59$, ns; age × sex $F_{2,1427} = 1.47$, ns; handedness × age × sex $F_{8,1427} = 0.63$, ns).

In order to identify the differences in ROCF performance by handedness in the various age groups, we applied one-way analysis of variance followed by Duncan tests for post hoc comparisons between the handedness groups. The results of these analyses revealed statistically significant differences between handedness groups in the younger children ($F_{4,507} = 14.99$, $P < .001$). Duncan tests showed that there were significant differences between the mixed-handed group (MH) and all the other groups. The difference in ROCF mean scores regarding handedness was also statistically significant in older children ($F_{4,395} = 20.23$, $P < .001$). The Duncan test showed that the MH group differed significantly from all the other groups. As was previously demonstrated, left handers did not perform as well as right handers [5, 6]. This was true for children in both age groups. In adults, the difference

TABLE 2: Sex ratio (males/females) according to handedness and age groups.

Handedness groups	Lateralization index	Younger children	Older children	Adults
CRH	*+100*	1.0	0.8	0.9
IRH	*+90 to +30*	0.9	1.5	1.1
MH	*+20 to −20*	3.6	2.1	1.4
ILH	*−30 to −90*	1.0	0.9	0.8
CLH	*−100*	1.0	1.1	1.0

Note: CRH: consistent right-handers, IRH: inconsistent right-handers, MH: mixed handers, ILH: inconsistent left handers, CLH: consistent left-handers.

TABLE 3: Rey-Osterrieth Complex Figure scores by handedness and age group.

Handedness group	Younger children		Older children		Adults		Total	
	M	SD	*M*	SD	*M*	SD	*M*	SD
CRH	24.7	8.5	30.3	6.3	30.9	2.9	29.2	6.2
IRH	24.7	8.8	31.9	5.0	31.5	2.5	29.6	6.2
MH	16.1	5.1	22.9	5.6	29.9	2.9	21.9	7.1
ILH	21.6	7.2	27.7	5.1	31.0	2.1	24.9	7.0
CLH	18.8	6.7	27.4	5.4	31.0	2.2	23.2	7.6
Total	22.3	8.2	28.6	6.1	31.1	2.7	27.3	7.1

Note: CRH: consistent right handers, IRH: inconsistent right handers, MH: mixed handers, ILH: inconsistent left-handers, CLH: consistent left-handers.

in ROCF scores between handedness groups was marginally significant ($F_{5,540} = 2.38$, $P = .05$) with the Duncan test showing that the MH group differed significantly only with the IRH group, which was the handedness subgroup which revealed the higher performance. These differences are presented in Figure 1. The limited differences between handedness groups in adults could be attributed to a ceiling effect as the maximum score was 36, with an average score being 31.1 with much less variability than in the children samples (2.7 versus 6.1 and 8.2). A similar ceiling effect for the copy measure of the ROCF has been previously reported in a study of college students [74].

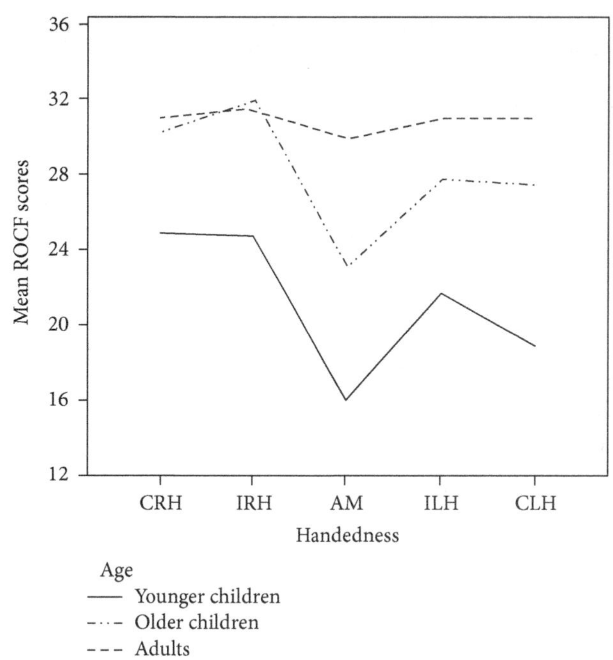

FIGURE 1: Rey-Osterrieth Complex Figure scores by handedness in younger children (—), older children (-···-), and adults (- - -).

4. Discussion

The present study investigated whether individuals who do not develop a typically strong behavioral laterality are distributed differentially among the two genders across age and whether left handedness and mixed handedness are associated with an elevated risk of some developmental or cognitive deficits. Thanks to the vast amount of data collected from nonright-handed samples, the present study revealed developmental and sex-related lateralization effects on a task of visual-spatial skills and evaluated these effects with regard to the hypotheses based on the hormonal-developmental, the neuropathological, and the learning models of handedness.

Firstly, based on the hormonal-developmental hypothesis [34] we predicted sex differences in the distribution of handedness across age groups. Our results confirm that the trend towards consistent right handedness is sex related. Specifically, girls in our sample were more advanced than boys in this lateralization process. Moreover, right-handed girls in the older group of this study had become more strongly lateralized than boys. On the other hand, boys were over represented in the mixed-handed group. This tendency appears in our study to continue into adulthood, albeit to a much lesser extent. However, further longitudinal research is needed in order to substantiate this claim. Such longitudinal studies are vital given the discrepancy that exists between neuropsychological studies suggesting that functional brain asymmetry is more characteristic of the right-handed male population and magnetic resonance imaging (MRI) studies [75] pointing to a greater asymmetry in females, at least for motor functions.

The finding that men are more prone to mixed handedness compared to women is in accordance with that of a recent meta-analysis [4]. Additionally, the same meta-analysis concluded that the magnitude of the difference between sexes was significantly moderated by the way in which handedness was assessed (e.g., by hand writing or by other means). Papadatou-Pastou et al. [4] suggested that, in addition to innate biological differences between the two sexes, handedness is also modulated by psychological influences. This suggestion has been confirmed by the recent study of Dirnberger [76], which examined whether the modulating factors of sex and self-perception (measured as hypochondriac traits) interact and affect handedness in a mixed male and female sample. Their findings suggested that handedness data are influenced by self-perception, attention to action, or inconsistent sensitivity to stimuli from the environment. Nevertheless, the researchers concluded that some modulating psychological or behavioural variables may also underlie genetic influences, which, in turn, might even be sex specific.

The second hypothesis of the present study emanated from the neuropathological model of handedness [1, 10, 28]. According to this hypothesis the prediction was that performance on copying the ROCF would be particularly low in mixed-handed and in extremely lateralized persons. Our results showed that performance on this visual-spatial and graphic task was comparatively low in extremely lateralized persons, who may include symptomatic hemiparesis. The present study complements previous findings [5, 6] concerning the left handers' disadvantage in ROCF copying: extreme left handers performed at a lower level in copying than inconsistent left-handers in the younger children's group. Some pathological cases among left-handers might be responsible for this group trend. It could be postulated that pure left handedness emerged precociously in such cases because of an impaired right hand. We know from developmental neuropsychological studies that when the right hemisphere is required to take over language functions in addition to visual-spatial functions, the latter does not develop completely [77]. This might well be the case happening in some of our extreme left-handed youngsters. It is also interesting to note that in the present study extreme lateralization does not correspond to higher cognitive scores than moderate lateralization. Furthermore, the clear disadvantage of extreme left-handedness gradually dissolves with age and completely vanishes in adults. Thus, either our sampling strategy has prevented us from choosing neuropathological cases in the student population, or the visual-spatial impairment is compensated for or even cured by adulthood.

Our third hypothesis based on the learning model [38, 39] predicted that low scores on ROCF test would be found in mixed-handed subjects, because these persons lack laterality support in the development of their skills. Backwardness in visual-spatial skills as detected by low ROCF scores is confirmed in mixed-handed children from first to sixth grade.

Overall, the results of this study confirm the learning model predictions but are not in agreement with all the predictions of the neuropathological model. Although poor performance among strong dextral has been found for many types of cognitive and educational tests (for a review see [78]), in our study no differences were found in visual-spatial skills between consistent and inconsistent right handers in this age group. It could be suggested that the appropriate brain mechanisms for successful ROCF copying are established earlier in both right-handed groups. Moreover, another study [79] examined the motor skills of young (approximately seven years old) children and discovered that left- and mixed-handed children were inferior to right-handed children in motor performance. The present data seem to fit in with Crow et al.'s findings [25] that the most substantial deficits in ability are close to the point of equal hand skill or hemispheric indecision. Crow and his collaborators [25] claimed that the failure to establish unequivocal hemispheric dominance is indicative of developmental delay. Similar findings are supported by research on giftedness. In children aged 8 to 14, more nongifted than gifted students are distributed in the left- and mixed-handedness categories [80]. Replication of the Crow et al. study [25] by Mayringer and Wimmer [81] was unsuccessful, probably, in our view, for two reasons: firstly the experimental sample involved was relatively modest and biased since the researchers had deliberately brought reading difficulties to the fore (boys only), and, secondly, because hemispheric indecision was less precisely defined. A more recent study [82] using a multiple regression approach, showed that the Mayringer and Wimmer's [81] reanalysis suffered from statistical problems and that the lower scores close to the point of equal hand skill reported by Crow et al. [25] are part of a general monotonic relationship of laterality to cognitive ability, which is independent of overall hand skill. Additionally, our findings are in accordance with recent studies [83, 84] which indicated that mixed handedness compared to right handedness was associated with poorer scholastic performance. Overall from the aforementioned studies [25, 82–84] we could conclude that mixed handedness could aid in the recognition of children who are at risk for academic problems.

In adults, however, all handedness groups performed equally. Only a marginal difference in copying the Rey-Osterrieth Complex Figure was detected between mixed-handed and the inconsistent right-handed university students. Does this mean that such cognitive difficulties in children are only incidental and can be ignored? Indeed, we do not know if time will complete the gap in visual-spatial development, particularly in the most exposed group, that is, the non-lateralized children. Ignoring what appears to be a simple gap and not a permanent handicap would mean paying little attention to the learning disability condition. For example, the fact that dyslexic children can eventually succeed in professional careers should not prevent consideration of their suffering during development.

We think that this gap in development is pathological both from the pediatric and the psychological points of view. Yeo et al. [85] have shown that left or nonright handers and extreme right handers are characterized by some degree of developmental instability, that is, minor physiological abnormalities. They propose that the underpinnings of developmental instability may illuminate the association of handedness with a variety of developmental disorders.

Our results show that delayed learning affects boys three times more than girls in the early school years. Whether they are boys or girls, schoolchildren exhibiting developmental and learning gap deserve our attention in order to prevent academic failure. The sex ratio in mixed-handed schoolchildren reminds us of the prevalence of learning disability which touches two to three times more males than females. The present findings fit in with the epidemiology of learning disabilities.

In sum, even if minority handedness status is not the direct cause of learning disability, as was believed in Orton's time, for example, it nevertheless provides us with an easy means of detecting developmentally "at risk" children. Neuropathological cases are likely to be found in all handedness groups. Some children with mild neurological syndromes are likely to be present among consistent right handers. However, these pathological cases represent a very small percentage of the consistent right-handed group, a larger proportion of consistent left handers, and a much larger proportion of mixed-handed children.

Moreover, recent structural neuroimaging findings [86, 87] have indicated that mixed handedness is associated with neuroanatomical differences, thus offering additional support to the view that individuals who do not develop a typically strong behavioral laterality differ significantly and are at somewhat higher risk of certain disorders and brain abnormalities from consistently left- and right-handed individuals. More specifically, a recent study [86] showed that mixed handedness was associated with increased hippocampal and amygdalar atrophy in ageing. Another study [87] showed that mixed handedness, but not left handedness per se, was associated with corpus callosum thickness, which is indicative of increased interhemispheric interaction. These findings provide evidence for a somewhat different neurobiological background (of either biological or environmental origin) in mixed handers, which might give rise to a number of risk factors leading to certain developmental disabilities.

In conclusion, nonright handedness should not be considered as a risk for cognitive development per se, but the rarity of this condition makes it more likely to count in pathological cases. This has been proven in the present observation by collecting relatively large samples of nonright-handed children. Furthermore, this supports studies [88] that have found (perhaps excessively) neurological pathology in all non-right-handed subjects, suggesting that future research might focus not so much on left handedness itself but rather on those who lack consistent handedness and/or cerebral asymmetry.

References

[1] L. Harris and D. Carlson, "Pathological left-handedness: an analysis of theories and evidence," in *Brain Lateralization in Children: Developmental Implications*, D. L. Molfese and S. J. Segalowitz, Eds., pp. 289–372, Guiford Press, New York, NY, USA, 1988.

[2] J. Liederman and J. Coryell, "The origin of left hand performance: pathological and non-pathological influences," *Neuropsychologia*, vol. 20, no. 6, pp. 721–725, 1982.

[3] D. Johnston, M. Nicholls, M. Shah, and M. Shields, "Handedness, health and cognitive development: evidence from children in the national longitudinal survey of youth," *Journal of the Royal Statistical Society A*, vol. 176, pp. 1–20, 2013.

[4] M. Papadatou-Pastou, M. Martin, M. R. Munafò, and G. V. Jones, "Sex differences in left-handedness: a meta-analysis of 144 studies," *Psychological Bulletin*, vol. 134, no. 5, pp. 677–699, 2008.

[5] A. B. Karapetsas and F. M. Vlachos, "Sex and handedness in development of visuomotor skills," *Perceptual and Motor Skills*, vol. 85, no. 1, pp. 131–140, 1997.

[6] F. Vlachos, *Neuropsychological assessment of visuomotor skills in right and left-handed child [Ph.D. thesis]*, University of Thessaly, Thessaly, Greece, 1997.

[7] F. M. Vlachos and A. B. Karapetsas, "Visual-motor organization and memory in the right-handed and the left-handed child: a comparative neuropsychological approach," *Child Neuropsychology*, vol. 2, no. 3, pp. 204–212, 1996.

[8] M.-S. Shin, S.-Y. Park, S.-R. Park, S.-H. Seol, and J. S. Kwon, "Clinical and empirical applications of the Rey-Osterrieth Complex Figure Test," *Nature Protocols*, vol. 1, no. 2, pp. 892–899, 2006.

[9] E. Nelson, J. Campbell, and G. Michel, "Unimanual to bimanual: tracking the development of handedness from 6 to 24 months," *Infant Behavioral Development*, vol. 36, no. 2, pp. 181–188, 2013.

[10] P. Satz, D. L. Orsini, E. Saslow, and R. Henry, "The pathological left-handedness syndrome," *Brain and Cognition*, vol. 4, no. 1, pp. 27–46, 1985.

[11] H. V. Soper, P. Satz, D. L. Orsini, W. G. Van Gorp, and M. F. Green, "Handedness distribution in a residential population with severe or profound mental retardation," *American Journal of Mental Deficiency*, vol. 92, no. 1, pp. 94–102, 1987.

[12] F. Gaillard and P. Satz, "Handedness and reading disability: a developmental study," *Archives of Clinical Neuropsychology*, vol. 4, no. 1, pp. 63–69, 1989.

[13] D. Bishop, *Handedness and Developmental Disorder*, Blackwell Scientific Publications, Oxford, UK, 1990.

[14] L. Harris, "Left-handedness," in *Handbook of Neuropsychology*, I. Rapin and S. J. Segalowitz, Eds., vol. 6 of *Child Neuropsychology*, pp. 145–208, Elsevier Science Publishers, Amsterdam, The Netherlands, 1992.

[15] D. Natsopoulos, G. Kiosseoglou, and A. Xeromeritou, "Handedness and spatial ability in children: further support for Geschwind's hypothesis of "pathology of superiority" and for Annett's theory of intelligence," *Genetic, Social, and General Psychology Monographs*, vol. 118, pp. 103–126, 1992.

[16] D. Natsopoulos and A. Xeromeritou, "Verbal abilities of left-and right-handed children," *The Journal of Psychology*, vol. 123, pp. 121–132, 1989.

[17] M. Annett, *Left, Right, Hand and Brain: The Right Shift Theory*, Erlbaum, Hillsdale, NJ, USA, 1985.

[18] A. Gessell and L. Ames, "The development of handedness," *Journal of Genetic Psychology*, vol. 70, pp. 155–176, 1947.

[19] I. McManus, *Handedness, Language Dominance and Aphasia: A Genetic Model*, Psychological Medicine, Monograph Supplement #8, Cambridge University Press, 1985.

[20] D. S. Ramsay, "Beginnings of bimanual handedness and speech in infants," *Infant Behavior and Development*, vol. 3, no. 1, pp. 67–77, 1980.

[21] M. J. O'Callaghan, D. I. Tudehope, A. E. Dugdale, H. Mohay, Y. Burns, and F. Cook, "Handedness in children with birthweights below 1000 gr," *The Lancet*, vol. 1, no. 8542, p. 1155, 1987.

[22] G. Ross, E. Lipper, and P. A. Auld, "Hand preference, prematurity and developmental outcome at school age," *Neuropsychologia*, vol. 30, no. 5, pp. 483–494, 1992.

[23] S. Saigal, P. Rosenbaum, P. Szatmari, and L. Hoult, "Non-right handedness among ELBW and term children at eight years in relation to cognitive function and school performance," *Developmental Medicine and Child Neurology*, vol. 34, no. 5, pp. 425–433, 1992.

[24] A. Searleman, C. Porac, and S. Coren, "Relationship between birth order, birth stress, and lateral preferences: a critical review," *Psychological Bulletin*, vol. 105, no. 3, pp. 397–408, 1989.

[25] T. J. Crow, L. R. Crow, D. J. Done, and S. Leask, "Relative hand skill predicts academic ability: global deficits at the point of hemispheric indecision," *Neuropsychologia*, vol. 36, no. 12, pp. 1275–1282, 1998.

[26] M. Kinsbourne, "Sinistrality, brain organization and cognitive defects," in *Brain Lateralization in Children: Developmental Implications*, D. Molfese and S. Segalowitz, Eds., Guilford, New York, NY, USA, 1988.

[27] H. V. Soper and P. Satz, "Pathological left-handedness and ambiguous handedness: a new explanatory model," *Neuropsychologia*, vol. 22, no. 4, pp. 511–515, 1984.

[28] P. Satz, "Pathological left-handedness: an explanatory model," *Cortex*, vol. 8, pp. 121–135, 1972.

[29] M. L. Levene, J. Kornberg, and T. H. Williams, "The incidence and severity of post-asphyxial encephalopathy in full-term infants," *Early Human Development*, vol. 11, no. 1, pp. 21–26, 1985.

[30] J. Volpe, *Neurology of the Newborn*, W.B. Saunders, Philadelphia, Pa, USA, 3rd edition, 1995.

[31] M. Annett, "Handedness in families," *Annals of Human Genetics*, vol. 37, no. 1, pp. 93–105, 1973.

[32] L. Carter-Saltzman, "Biological and sociocultural effects on handedness: comparison between biological and adoptive families," *Science*, vol. 209, pp. 1263–1265, 1980.

[33] J. Levy, "A review of evidence for a genetic component in the determination of handedness," *Behavior Genetics*, vol. 6, no. 4, pp. 429–453, 1976.

[34] N. Geschwind and A. Galaburda, *Cerebral lateralization*, MIT Press, Cambridge, UK, 1987.

[35] J. Levy and C. Trevarthen, "Metacontrol of hemispheric function in human split-brain patients," *Journal of Experimental Psychology: Human Perception and Performance*, vol. 2, no. 3, pp. 299–312, 1976.

[36] J. Levy, C. Trevarthen, and R. W. Sperry, "Reception of bilateral chimeric figures following hemispheric deconnexion," *Brain*, vol. 95, no. 1, pp. 61–78, 1972.

[37] R. Sperry, "Lateral specialization in the surgically separated hemispheres," in *The Neurosciences: Third Study Program*, E. O. Schmitt and F. G. Worden, Eds., pp. 5–19, MIT Press, Cambridge, Mass, USA, 3rd edition, 1974.

[38] B. De Jong, F. Van der Graaf, and A. Paans, "Brain activation related to the representations of external space and body scheme in visuomotor control," *NeuroImage*, vol. 14, no. 5, pp. 1128–1135, 2001.

[39] O. Simon, J.-F. Mangin, L. Cohen, D. Le Bihan, and S. Dehaene, "Topographical layout of hand, eye, calculation, and language-related areas in the human parietal lobe," *Neuron*, vol. 33, no. 3, pp. 475–487, 2002.

[40] C. Francks, S. Maegawa, J. Laurén et al., "LRRTM1 on chromosome 2p12 is a maternally suppressed gene that is associated paternally with handedness and schizophrenia," *Molecular Psychiatry*, vol. 12, no. 12, pp. 1129–1139, 2007.

[41] S. E. Medland, D. L. Duffy, A. B. Spurdle et al., "Opposite effects of androgen receptor CAG repeat length on increased risk of left-handedness in males and females," *Behavior Genetics*, vol. 35, no. 6, pp. 735–744, 2005.

[42] S. E. Medland, D. L. Duffy, M. J. Wright et al., "Genetic influences on handedness: data from 25,732 Australian and Dutch twin families," *Neuropsychologia*, vol. 47, no. 2, pp. 330–337, 2009.

[43] S. Ocklenburg, C. Bürger, C. Westermann, D. Schneider, H. Biedermann, and O. Güntürkün, "Visual experience affects handedness," *Behavioral Brain Research*, vol. 207, pp. 447–451, 2010.

[44] M. Hiscock, R. Inch, J. Hawryluk, P. J. Lyon, and N. Perachio, "Is there a sex difference in human laterality? III. An exhaustive survey of tactile laterality studies from six neuropsychology journals," *Journal of Clinical and Experimental Neuropsychology*, vol. 21, no. 1, pp. 17–28, 1999.

[45] D. Kimura, *Sex and Cognition*, MIT Press, Cambridge, UK, 1999.

[46] M. Hiscock, M. Israelian, R. Inch, C. Jacek, and C. Hiscock-Kalil, "Is there a sex difference in human laterality? II. An exhaustive survey of visual laterality studies from six neuropsychology journals," *Journal of Clinical and Experimental Neuropsychology*, vol. 17, no. 4, pp. 590–610, 1995.

[47] S. F. Cappa and L. A. Vignolo, "Sex differences in the site of brain lesions underlying global aphasia," *Aphasiology*, vol. 2, no. 3-4, pp. 259–264, 1988.

[48] J. Hellige, *Hemispheric Asymmetry: What's Right and What's Left*, Harvard University Press, Cambridge, UK, 1993.

[49] J. Obrzut and M. Atkinson, "Relations among learning disorders, handedness, and immune disease," *Journal of Clinical and Experimental Neuropsychology*, vol. 15, p. 86, 1993.

[50] F. E. Tønnessen, A. Løkken, T. Høien, and I. Lundberg, "Dyslexia, left-handedness, and immune disorders," *Archives of Neurology*, vol. 50, no. 4, pp. 411–416, 1993.

[51] M. P. Bryden, I. C. McManus, and M. B. Bulman-Fleming, "Evaluating the empirical support for the geschwind-behan-galaburda model of cerebral lateralization," *Brain and Cognition*, vol. 26, no. 2, pp. 103–167, 1994.

[52] J. T. Manning, D. Scutt, J. Wilson, and D. I. Lewis-Jones, "The ratio of 2nd to 4th digit length: a predictor of sperm numbers and concentrations of testosterone, luteinizing hormone and oestrogen," *Human Reproduction*, vol. 13, no. 11, pp. 3000–3004, 1998.

[53] J. T. Manning and M. Peters, "Digit ratio (2D : 4D) and hand preference for writing in the BBC Internet Study," *Laterality*, vol. 14, no. 5, pp. 528–540, 2009.

[54] A. A. Beaton, N. Rudling, C. Kissling, R. Taurines, and J. Thome, "Digit ratio (2D:4D), salivary testosterone, and handedness," *Laterality*, vol. 16, no. 2, pp. 136–155, 2011.

[55] H. Yamashita, "Right- and left-hand performance on the rey-osterrieth complex figure: a preliminary study in non-clinical sample of right handed people," *Archives of Clinical Neuropsychology*, vol. 25, no. 4, pp. 314–317, 2010.

[56] R. C. Oldfield, "The assessment and analysis of handedness: the edinburgh inventory," *Neuropsychologia*, vol. 9, no. 1, pp. 97–113, 1971.

[57] A. Rey, "L'examen psychologique dans le cas d'encephalopathie traumatique," *Archives de Psychologie*, vol. 28, pp. 286–340, 1941.

[58] A. Rey, *Manuel: Test de Copie d'une Figure Complexe*, Centre de Psychologie Appliquee, Paris, France, 1959.

[59] P. Osterrieth, "Le teste de copie d'une figure complexe: contribution a l'etude de la perception et de la mémoire," *Archives de Psychologie*, vol. 30, pp. 206–256, 1944.

[60] A. Karapetsas and A. Kantas, "Visuomotor organization in the child: a neuropsychological approach," *Perceptual and Motor Skills*, vol. 72, no. 1, pp. 211–217, 1991.

[61] D. P. Waber and J. M. Holmes, "Assessing children's copy productions of the Rey-Osterrieth Complex Figure," *Journal of Clinical and Experimental Neuropsychology*, vol. 7, no. 3, pp. 264–280, 1985.

[62] C. Brandys and B. Rourke, "Differential memory abilities in reading- and arithmetic-disabled children," in *A Critical Analysis. Neuropsychological Validation of Learning Disability Subtypes*, B. P. Rourke, Ed., pp. 15–44, The Guilford Press, New York, NY, USA, 1991.

[63] M. Bryden and R. Steenhuis, "The assessment of handedness in children," in *Neuropsychological Foundations of Learning Disabilities*, J. Obrzut and G. Hynd, Eds., Academic Press, New York, NY, USA, 1991.

[64] D. Raczkowski, J. W. Kalat, and R. Nebes, "Reliability and validity of some handedness questionnaire items," *Neuropsychologia*, vol. 12, no. 1, pp. 43–47, 1974.

[65] S. Coren, "Measurement of handedness via self-report: the relationship between brief and extended inventories," *Perceptual and Motor Skills*, vol. 76, no. 3, pp. 1035–1042, 1993.

[66] N. J. Dorthe, T. D. Blumenthal, D. R. Jason, and P. E. Lantz, "The use of next-of-kin in assessing handedness," *Perceptual and Motor Skills*, vol. 81, no. 1, pp. 203–208, 1995.

[67] E. McMeekan and W. Lishman, "Retest reliabilities and interrelationship of the annett hand preference questionnaire and the edinburgh handedness inventory," *British Journal of Psychology*, vol. 66, pp. 53–59, 1975.

[68] B. J. Ransil and S. C. Schachter, "Test-retest reliability of the edinburgh handedness inventory and global handedness preference measurements, and their correlation," *Perceptual and Motor Skills*, vol. 79, no. 3, pp. 1355–1372, 1994.

[69] S. M. Williams, "Factor analysis of the edinburgh handedness inventory," *Cortex*, vol. 22, no. 2, pp. 325–326, 1986.

[70] D. Raczkowski, J. W. Kalat, and R. Nebes, "Reliability and validity of some handedness questionnaire items," *Neuropsychologia*, vol. 12, no. 1, pp. 43–47, 1974.

[71] W. J. Triggs, R. Calvanio, M. Levine, R. K. Heaton, and K. M. Heilman, "Predicting hand preference with performance on motor tasks," *Cortex*, vol. 36, no. 5, pp. 679–689, 2000.

[72] M. Verdino and S. Dingman, "Two measures of laterality in handedness: the edinburgh handedness inventory and the purdue pegboard test of manual dexterity," *Perceptual and Motor Skills*, vol. 86, no. 2, pp. 476–478, 1998.

[73] R. Steenhuis and M. Bryden, "Hand preference and performance: right-handers, left-handers and left-handers who are not consistently left-handed," *Journal of Clinical and Experimental Neuropsychology*, vol. 11, p. 37, 1989.

[74] M. B. Casey, E. Winner, I. Hurwitz, and D. DaSilva, "Does processing style affect recall of the rey-osterrieth and taylor complex figures?" *Journal of Clinical and Experimental Neuropsychology*, vol. 13, no. 4, pp. 600–606, 1991.

[75] F. Robichon, K. Giraud, M. Berbon, and M. Habib, "Sexual dimorphism in anterior speech region: an MRI study of cortical asymmetry and callosal size," *Brain and Cognition*, vol. 40, no. 1, pp. 241–246, 1999.

[76] G. Dirnberger, "Handedness is modulated by sex and self-perception, laterality: asymmetries of body," *Brain and Cognition*, vol. 17, pp. 275–186, 2012.

[77] F. Vargha-Khadem, E. Isaacs, S. van der Werf, S. Robb, and J. Wilson, "Development of intelligence and memory in children with hemiplegic cerebral palsy. The deleterious consequences of early seizures," *Brain*, vol. 115, no. 1, pp. 315–329, 1992.

[78] M. Annett, "The right shift theory of a genetic balanced polymorphism for cerebral dominance and cognitive processing," *Current Psychology and Cognition*, vol. 14, pp. 427–480, 1995.

[79] C. Gabbard, S. Hart, and V. Gentry, "General motor proficiency and handedness in children," *Journal of Genetic Psychology*, vol. 156, pp. 411–416, 1995.

[80] J. M. Piro, "Handedness and intelligence: patterns of hand preference in gifted and nongifted children," *Developmental Neuropsychology*, vol. 14, no. 4, pp. 619–630, 1998.

[81] H. Mayringer and H. Wimmer, "No deficits at the point of hemispheric indecision," *Neuropsychologia*, vol. 40, no. 7, pp. 701–704, 2002.

[82] D. Nettle, "Hand laterality and cognitive ability: a multiple regression approach," *Brain and Cognition*, vol. 52, no. 3, pp. 390–398, 2003.

[83] T. Björk, O. Brus, W. Osika, and S. Montgomery, "Laterality, hand control and scholastic performance: a british birth cohort study," *British Medical Journal Open*, vol. 2, no. 2, article e000314, 2012.

[84] A. Rodriguez, M. Kaakinen, I. Moilanen et al., "Mixed-handedness is linked to mental health problems in children and adolescents," *Pediatrics*, vol. 125, no. 2, pp. e340–e348, 2010.

[85] R. A. Yeo, S. W. Gangestad, and W. F. Daniel, "Hand preference and developmental instability," *Psychobiology*, vol. 21, no. 2, pp. 161–168, 1993.

[86] N. Cherbuin, P. Sachdev, and K. Anstey, "Mixed handedness is associated with greater age-related decline in volumes of the hippocampus and amygdala: the PATH through life study," *Brain and Behavior*, vol. 1, pp. 125–134, 2011.

[87] E. Luders, N. Cherbuin, P. M. Thompson et al., "When more is less: associations between corpus callosum size and handedness lateralization," *NeuroImage*, vol. 52, no. 1, pp. 43–49, 2010.

[88] I. Sommer, N. Ramsey, R. Kahn, A. Aleman, and A. Bouma, "Handedness, language lateralisation and anatomical asymmetry in schizophrenia: meta-analysis," *British Journal of Psychiatry*, vol. 178, pp. 344–351, 2001.

4

Primary School Age Students' Spontaneous Comments about Math Reveal Emerging Dispositions Linked to Later Mathematics Achievement

Michèle M. M. Mazzocco,[1,2] Laurie B. Hanich,[3] and Maia M. Noeder[4]

[1] *Institute of Child Development, University of Minnesota, 51 East River Parkway, Minneapolis, MN 55455, USA*
[2] *Johns Hopkins University School of Education Baltimore, MD 21218, USA*
[3] *Department of Educational Foundations, Millersville University of Pennsylvania, P.O. Box 1002, Millersville, PA 17551, USA*
[4] *Department of Psychology, Case Western Reserve University, 10900 Euclid Avenue, Cleveland, OH 44106-7123, USA*

Correspondence should be addressed to Michèle M. M. Mazzocco, mazzocco@umn.edu

Academic Editor: Ann Dowker

To longitudinally explore children's developing beliefs towards mathematics, we asked 207 children to define "math" and "reading" at grades 2 and 3 and coded for spontaneous references to likability or difficulty of math (or reading) in their definitions. We found that children attributed more difficulty to math than to reading despite their relatively neutral comments on the likability of either subject. Children described math and reading with comparable degrees of specificity, but girls' definitions were more specific than boys'. Relative to their peers, children with mathematics learning disability (MLD) provided less specific definitions overall, were more likely to describe math as more difficult than reading, and were more likely to show a decrease in likability ratings of math (but not reading) from grades 2 to 3. Grade 2 ratings predicted math ability at grade 3, more so than predictors from grade 3. These findings, although based on informal analyses not intended to substitute for validated assessments of disposition, support the notions that distinct aspects of dispositions towards math emerge in early childhood, are revealed through casual discourse, and are predictive of later math achievement outcomes. This further supports current interests in developing formal measures of academic disposition in early childhood.

1. Introduction

A productive disposition towards mathematics is an essential component of mathematics proficiency [1]. Like many elements of successful mathematics outcomes, the construct of a "productive disposition" is multifaceted. The National Research Council [1] defines it as "the tendency to see sense in mathematics, to perceive math as both useful and worthwhile, and to believe that steady effort in learning mathematics pays off." At a minimum, this description captures features of positive attitudes about mathematics, seeing sense in mathematics, the belief that effort is needed to support math learning, and a perspective that math is useful within and beyond school experiences—regardless of whether it is liked or disliked or achieved with minimal or great effort. Associations between these and other distinct features of a productive disposition are likely to be dynamic, but the nature and emergence of the elements themselves are not yet fully understood, particularly in early childhood. Here we report on a brief, exploratory study of whether second and third graders' definitions of mathematics shed light on their emerging dispositions and are related to their later mathematics achievement.

The recent interest in measuring beliefs about mathematics in early childhood (e.g., [2, 3]) has yielded evidence of a reciprocal relationship between math interest or beliefs and math ability, even in preschoolers [4]. Accordingly, in this study we ask whether children's spontaneous conversations about math reveal tendencies in their beliefs. Specifically, we ask if children's definitions of "math" reveal children's beliefs about whether math is easy or difficult, liked or disliked, or useful. We ask whether these potential disposition features apply to math specifically or to school subjects in general by asking our participants to also define "reading." By comparing definitions of math (and reading) among children with a wide range of math achievement levels (including children with mathematics learning disability (MLD)), we test the plausibility that early indicators of children's beliefs about math contribute to predicting their future mathematics outcomes. We base this hypothesis on prior research demonstrating that elementary school students' beliefs about their ability and subjective task values in mathematics predict their current and future activity choices [5, 6].

Until recently, dispositions towards math and related constructs, such as math anxiety, were often not evaluated before middle school [7] or high school [8]. This is troubling in light of evidence of age-related changes in children's motivational patterns. Whereas most students begin schooling enthusiastically [1], a shift from intrinsic to extrinsic motivational orientations emerges at about grade 3 (approximately 8 years of age) [9, 10]. This type of progression has been reported for measures of attitudes and curiosity [11, 12], perceived competence [13–15], and beliefs about intelligence [16], and suggests that early childhood (prior to and up to grade 3) may be an essential period for establishing, maintaining, or at least initiating the foundation of a positive disposition towards mathematics. Moreover, while developing productive dispositions is important for children across a wide range of achievement levels, this may be especially important for students at risk for low mathematics achievement and/or MLD.

To explore how productive learning dispositions are cultivated in early childhood, we utilized an expectancy-value model of achievement motivation [17] which asserts a proportional relationship between task engagement, expectations for success, and subjective task values. Specifically, the amount of effort children invest in an activity (e.g., mathematics engagement) is a product of their expectations for success and the extent to which they value the task. These components are influenced by children's perceptions of competence, task difficulty, and affect, and have been shown to directly affect achievement-related behaviors (as reviewed elsewhere [17]). In the present study, we did not objectively measure students' efforts nor did we rely on self-report measures related to subjective task value. Rather, we used open-ended questioning to specifically test whether indicators of beliefs and values related to mathematics emerge from spontaneous conversations with young children. In particular, we focused on the extent to which children's responses reflect affect (likability), perceived task difficulty, and values reflected in the specificity with which their responses relate to the usefulness of mathematics. The expectancy-value model provided a useful framework for considering the types of beliefs on which to focus in coding children's responses, and for interpreting our findings given the similarities between our variables of interest and those proposed as part of this theoretical model.

What is the relevance of spontaneous conversations of this type in the context of evaluating children's beliefs about math? First, early conversations about math provide a mechanism by which adults can deliberately attend to the potential influences they have on their children's or students' math-oriented beliefs. Second, in addition to using conversations to nurture the development of a healthy math disposition, conversations can be monitored for indicators of a child's emerging beliefs. In other words, early conversations are useful as a platform for adults' messages to children, but also for attending to children's comments—spontaneous or structured.

Why are children's early comments about math potentially important? In view of emerging evidence that early beliefs about mathematics are related to later achievement outcomes, efforts to steer children from paths towards negative outcomes should begin in early childhood, when children's beliefs may be more malleable rather than deeply rooted. Consequences of negative beliefs towards math are frequently described in terms of secondary-school behaviors, such as avoidance of elective mathematics courses after grade 10 (age 15 years) [18]. But the antecedents of such avoidance likely occur much earlier. For example, a negative relationship between math anxiety and math achievement has been observed among elementary school aged children with high working memory capacity [19, 20], and among elementary aged students who believe math-gender stereotypes with female students showing weaker identification with mathematics than their male counterparts despite similar levels of achievement [21, 22]. Gender stereotypes have been shown to influence mathematics achievement gains in first or second grade (ages 6 and 7 years), at least among young girls who conform to the belief that females underperform in math relative to males, and particularly among girls who receive instruction from a teacher with elevated levels of anxiety about mathematics [2]. These early associations warrant attention; information from informal conversation may be among the earliest indicators to direct adults' attention to students' emerging dispositions.

Children's math ability self-perceptions become well established in elementary school (e.g., [6]), but parent expectancies and attributions may influence children's math beliefs [23, 24] before and after the onset of formal schooling. Parents who believe that math and science are male-oriented domains tend to overestimate their sons' math and science performance and underestimate their daughters' performance in math and science at least in mid- to late-elementary school [25]. In middle school students, this underestimation may impact self-concepts and self-underestimation of math ability [26, 27]. These findings suggest that teacher and parent behaviors *can* and *do* play a major role in student learning, and that efforts to counter such effects on negative beliefs about math and achievement-related perceptions should begin in early childhood [23]. Listening to children's dialogues about math may contribute to these efforts and provide opportunity for intercession.

There are a number of ways to evaluate math beliefs. Ratings of children's math self-perception and their enjoyment of mathematics are objectively measureable in elementary school aged children [13–15, 28] and earlier [4]. Here, we propose that discourse may serve not only as a means for parents and teachers of young children to help shape a positive disposition towards math through adult-initiated "math talk," but also as a means for adults to glean information about a child's emerging disposition, despite the fact that dialogues are no substitute for formal screening and diagnostic assessments of risk for poor math outcomes.

What aspects of children's early dispositions towards mathematics are revealed during open-ended discussions, and are these beliefs related to formal math outcomes? To address these questions, in the present study we used a simple and straightforward approach to elicit children's spontaneous comments about math. Importantly, we avoided explicit prompting for information about beliefs about math in order to focus on children's spontaneous comments. Although findings to emerge from this approach do not reveal causal pathways to successful mathematics, evidence of the mere presence of relevant information from spontaneous speech has implications for the role of early conversations about mathematics among children and their parents, teachers, and care providers in shaping or supporting a child's disposition towards mathematics.

2. Method

2.1. Participants. Participants were drawn from a larger longitudinal study of mathematics achievement and mathematics learning disabilities during the primary school aged years, described elsewhere in more detail [29]. Briefly, the participants from the larger study were recruited from 23 kindergarten classrooms across seven schools in one large metropolitan public school district. The participating schools were selected based on their relatively low rates of mobility and free or reduced lunch participation, to diminish attrition and decrease the likelihood that poor math performance observed among participants was linked to low socioeconomic status. Of the 445 kindergartners from these classrooms invited to participate, 249 enrolled (129 girls). Participation in the present study was limited to the 207 children (107 girls) who completed annual assessments during both grades 2 and 3. Of the 207 included, most (86.5%) participants were white, 8% were black, 3% were Asian, and the remaining 2.5% represented other or mixed ethnicities.

2.2. Materials and Procedures. During each year of the study, children were tested individually by one of five female examiners. Testing occurred during two or three sessions up to 45 minutes each, in a room separate from the classroom or other distracting activities. The testing battery included a range of standardized and experimental assessments. The measures relevant to the present report are two measures of mathematical ability, and a vocabulary probe administered to glean information about each participant's beliefs about mathematics.

2.2.1. Test of Early Math Ability-Second Edition (TEMA-2, [30]). The TEMA-2 is a standardized measure of formal and informal mathematical ability normed for use with children ages 2 to 8 years, 11 months. Items from the TEMA-2 include basic knowledge items such as counting principles, calculation and fact retrieval items, and items testing place value concepts or word problem solving. Total correct scores are converted to age-referenced standard scores for which test-retest reliability is 0.94 [30].

We administered the TEMA-2 to participants in the longitudinal study, from kindergarten through grade 3. In the present study, we used the standard scores from all four grades to assign children to one of three groups: children with mathematical learning disability (MLD), children with low mathematics achievement (LA), and children with age appropriate math achievement (typically achieving or TA). For the participants who exceeded the upper age level for the TEMA-2 ceiling at grade 3, we calculated prorated standard scores using regression-models to predict age 9 years and age 9.5 years outcomes, based on data from over 200 children who completed the TEMA-2 during all four years of the study. The criteria for these participant groups, described elsewhere in detail [31], reflect the growing consensus that MLD classification is strengthened by considering scores over time, rather than one score at a single assessment. Children with TEMA-2 scores below the 10th percentile of the study sample were classified as having MLD ($n = 18$) and children with scores between the 11th to 25th percentile were classified as having low achievement in mathematics (LA; $n = 26$). These criteria were met during at least two of the four grades tested, provided that scores during any remaining years fell within the 95th percentile confidence interval of the 10th or 25th percentile cut off, respectively. Children who did not meet these criteria and who scored above the 25th percentile (or within the 95th percentile confidence interval for this range) were classified as typically achieving (TA; $n = 163$).

2.2.2. Woodcock Johnson—Revised Calculations (WJ-R Calc). The Woodcock Johnson Psycho-Educational Battery-Revised [32] is a widely used standardized test of formal academic skills and is normed for use with children ages 2 to 21 years. The WJ-R Calculation subtest, normed for ages 6 and older, is an untimed paper-and-pencil test that includes a range of arithmetic problems presented in order of increasing difficulty. We administered this subtest at grades 1 and 3. Due to floor effects, we did not administer the test at kindergarten; due to time constraints, it was not administered at grade 2. Internal consistency reliability for the WJ-R Calc subtest ranges from $r = .89$ to $r = .93$ across ages 6–9 years [33]. In the present study, we used the standard scores from the WJ-R Calc subtest at grade 3 as the dependent variable in select analyses, controlling for earlier math performance (WJ-R Calc performance at grade 1).

2.2.3. Defining "Mathematics." During select years of the longitudinal study, the test battery included a standardized expressive vocabulary test from the Stanford Binet Fourth Edition [34] (at grades K to 2) or the Wechsler Abbreviated Scale of Intelligence [35] (at grade 3). These subtests involved asking children to define a word presented orally by the examiner, beginning and ending at standardized basals and ceilings based on the examinee's age. In accordance with these standardized protocols, we asked each participant, "what is math?" followed by, "what is reading?" without any prompting for any specific or additional information. Only if a child responded with the equivalent of, "I do not know," we added the following prompt: "Just tell me what you think (math/reading) is." These definitions were elicited after a child reached a performance ceiling on the standardized vocabulary subtest, so that the point at which a definition was requested occurred at comparable levels of performance fatigue for all participants. This procedure also avoided unintentional alteration of the standardized vocabulary subtest. Also, by requesting a definition of math at the end of the expressive vocabulary test, we implicitly established expectations for the amount of information expected in response, and could indirectly convey comparable expectations about length of definitions for both "math" and "reading." Definitions of math and reading were obtained during grades 2 and 3.

Children's responses were recorded verbatim and transcribed into a central database with child identifiers removed. This ensured that coders were blind to the children's identity, gender, or math achievement status. Each response was coded independently by two trained coders. Coding responses were compared, and discrepancies were resolved in a coding meeting with the study PI and both coders present. Therefore, all definitions were double coded and, if there was disagreement, by three coders. Coding reliability is reported subsequently.

2.3. Coding Variables and Guidelines. Each definition was coded separately for three attributes: the extent to which the child's definition spontaneously reflected a like or dislike for math or reading (*likability* code), whether the child's definition made reference to ease or difficulty associated with math or reading (*difficulty* code), and how specifically math or reading concepts, procedures, or uses were described (*specificity* code). One set of scoring criteria was developed for each of the likability and difficulty coding protocols (Tables 1 and 2, resp.), each of which was applied to definitions of math and reading. Two parallel sets of criteria were established for coding the specificity of math (Table 3) and reading (Table 4) definitions.

The full range of possible *likability* codes was −2 (extremely dislikes math or reading) to 2 (extremely likes math or reading), with a code of 0 reflecting a neutral response (Table 1). Children's responses were assigned codes based on whether they were moderate (1) to strong or exaggerated (2) statements; these were further coded as positive (1 or 2) or negative (−1 or −2). Neutral responses included either no negative or positive comments, or included both (e.g., "it is kind of fun, but sometimes it is boring"). Of the four sets of 207 valence codes assigned, there were 2 disagreements among the 2 coders (99.9% agreement), which were resolved with a third coder/arbitrator. No child received a likability code of "2" for math at either grade, although at both grades, codes of "2" were assigned for reading.

The full range of possible *difficulty* codes was −2 (very difficult) to 2 (very easy), with a code of 0 reflecting no reference to either the difficulty or ease associated with mathematics or reading (Table 2). Of the four sets of 207 difficulty codes, there were 19 disagreements among the 2 coders (99.97% agreement), which were all resolved with a third coder/arbitrator. No child received a code of "2" (very easy) for either math or reading, at either grade.

Specificity codes ranged from 1 to 5, reflecting irrelevant or otherwise uninformative responses (1) to responses reflecting mathematics (or reading) as a useful tool (5). A summary of these coding criteria and sample responses appears in Tables 3 and 4. Of the four sets of 207 specificity codes, there were 58 disagreements among the 2 coders (93.0% agreement), which were resolved with a third coder/arbitrator.

All data were double entered into two excel spreadsheets, subtracted, and reviewed for discrepancies that were then corrected until the subtraction comparisons yielded no errors.

3. Results

3.1. Defining Math and Reading. First we asked whether qualitative features of children's definitions of math and reading differ as a function of gender or MLD status. We carried out three analyses of variance (ANOVAs), each based on a 2 (subject area: math versus reading) × 2 (grades: 2 and 3) × 2 (gender) × 3 (MLD status: TA, LA, and MLD) design, with repeated measures of the first two factors. The outcome variables were likability codes, difficulty codes, or specificity codes from children's spontaneous definitions of math and reading. Note that the means reported in the text are marginal estimated means whereas means reported in the figures are observed means.

3.1.1. Children's Likability for Math and Reading Definitions. We found no main effects of grade, MLD status, or gender on likability codes, $P > .437$. Although mean codes for reading were slightly more positive than those for math, the effect of subject area was not statistically significant, $F(1, 201) = 3.86$, $P = .051$, partial $\eta^2 = 0.019$. Group means for likability codes were essentially neutral for math (−0.011) and reading (0.048) when collapsed across grade and MLD status.

Two-way interactions emerged for grade × MLD status, $F(2, 201) = 3.86$, $P < .03$, partial $\eta^2 = 0.037$; and grade × subject area, $F(1, 201) = 6.67$, $P < 0.02$, partial $\eta^2 = 0.032$, but these effects were also very small. From grade 2 to 3, valence codes did not change among children from the TA group (estimated marginal means = 0.032 and 0.023, resp.), became slightly more positive among children in the LA group (means = −0.017 and 0.095, resp.), and slightly more negative among children with MLD (means = 0.013 and −0.036, resp.). From grade 2 to 3, valance codes did not change as much for math (means = 0.013 and −0.035, resp.) as they did for reading (means = 0.006 and 0.090,

Table 1: Likability scores: coding criteria and real examples of math and reading definitions.

Score	Definition	Math examples	Reading examples
−2	Extremely disliked, hated, or dreaded. Includes reference to words such as hate, worst, awful, and so forth.	n/a[a]	"When you sit and read a book bored out of your mind."
−1	Disliked or avoided. Includes reference to words such as do not like, not fun, boring, bad, and so on.	"Math is something I do not like."	"Something you do only when you need to do it, you have to read to figure out information."
0	Neutral feeling or tolerated. Includes no reference to an emotion.	"When you learn math problems."	"Like when you read a book in school or at home."
1	Liked or enjoyed. Includes reference to words such as play, fun, like, good, and so forth.	"Math is fun, you could do math at school—you could do it anywhere!"	"You can read for information or just for the fun of it."
2	Extremely liked, loved, or favored. Includes reference to words such as love, favorite, best, and so forth.	n/a[a]	"Oh I love to read."

Note: [a]No responses were coded at this value.

Table 2: Difficulty scores: coding criteria and real examples of math and reading definitions.

Score	Definition	Math examples	Reading examples
−2	Really hard. Includes reference to words such as *difficult*, *hard*, or *complex*.	"Something you do in school. Something that's very, very hard."	"Like you are reading and you are bad at reading and you read something like hard words."
−1	Kind of hard. Includes reference to words such as the noun form of *work*, words like *learn*, phrases that imply exertion zero, or implicit or explicit reference to cognitive processes.	"It is like problems that you have to solve."	"It is when there is like lots of sentences and you read it to get information."
0	Neutral difficulty. Includes no reference to difficulty, refers to verbs such as work, do, use, teach, or "work with" without implying exertion.	"Like math projects. Doing math homework."	"You have a book and you read the words."
1	Kind of easy. Includes reference to words such as "not hard" or words implying ease.	"It is easy and you have to do it in your homework."	"To just lay back and read a book."
2	Really easy. Includes reference to words such as simple, effortless, or speed.	n/a[a]	n/a[a]

Note: [a]No responses were coded at this value.

resp.), but the direction of these changes differed with math scores becoming slightly more negative, and reading scores becoming slightly more positive (Figure 1).

Even the strongest interaction to emerge from this analysis was associated with a small effect size, for a three-way interaction between subject area, grade, and MLD status, $F(2, 201) = 5.53$, $P < .01$, partial $\eta^2 = 0.052$. Pairwise comparisons indicated that children in the TA group made relatively neutral references to both math and reading at both grades (means = 0.012 for math at grades 2 and 3; and means = .051 and .034 for reading at grades 2 and 3, resp.), with little change from grades 2 to 3. Among children in the LA group, valence codes for definitions of math became slightly more negative over time (means = .000 to −0.045 at grades 2 to 3, resp.), and slightly more positive for reading during the same time period (means = −0.033 to 0.236). Children with MLD made neutral references when defining reading at both grades (both means = 0.000), whereas the

TABLE 3: Specificity scores: coding criteria and real examples of math definitions.

Score	Definition	Examples
1	No response, a circular response, a response unrelated to math, or another uninformative response.	"You do your math." "I cannot explain it." "I do not know."
2	Response is unspecific or only indirectly related to math as a primary school subject. The response may include references to activities performed in relation to math or in a math class but with no discernible reference to math concepts or procedures.	"You play games and stuff." "Science." "Like you do something. . .and you have pennies and money."
3	Unelaborated basic concepts or mechanics of math. Includes reference to real numbers, operations, math problems, or learning math.	"It has to do with numbers and sizes and fractions." "It means taking away, subtracting, and multiplication." "When you do all sorts of problems like divide, multiply, fractions, decimals." "In my class we do like a drill so it like refreshes our memory from the other day."
4	Elaborated concepts of math.	"Like if you have a word problem, like Jim has 18 apples and eats 3, you use math to solve it."
5	Concept of math as a useful tool.	"Math is something that people do and they have to know math to be able to get a job and do other stuff."

largest difference over time was the shift towards more negative ratings of math among the MLD group (means = 0.026 to −.071 from grades 2 to 3, a difference of −0.097).

In summary, at grades 2 and 3, boys and girls do not spontaneously make reference to extremely positive or negative sentiments about math or reading when defining either term, but there is a slight tendency for more negative comments about math (versus reading) among children with MLD, and, to a lesser degree, among children with low achievement in math.

3.1.2. Children's Reference to the Difficulty of Math and Reading. We also evaluated spontaneous comments about the difficulty versus easiness of math or reading in our second set of repeated measures ANOVAs. Here, the main effect of subject area was significant, $F(1, 201) = 16.02$, $P < .0001$, partial $\eta^2 = 0.074$. Children's definitions of math included more references to difficulty (mean code = −0.347) than did their definitions of reading (mean code = −0.171). The main effect of MLD status reflected significantly more negative references (i.e., more ratings reflecting difficulty) to math *and* reading in the MLD group (mean rating across subject areas = −0.378), relative to the LA and TA groups (whose means ratings were −0.174 and −0.225, resp.), $F(2, 201) = 3.40$, $P < .05$. Still, the effect was small, partial $\eta^2 = 0.033$. Pairwise comparisons showed that math and reading ratings combined were significantly more negative among the MLD versus LA or TA groups, $P < .03$, but did not differ between the TA and LA groups, $P = .361$.

There was no main effect of grade or gender on difficulty ratings, $P > .87$. No interactions were significant, with the exception of a weak three-way interaction between subject area × grade × gender, $F(1, 201) = 4.26$, $P < .05$, partial $\eta^2 = .021$. Here, both boys and girls reported slightly greater difficulty for math than reading at both grades. This difference was more pronounced for girls than for boys at grade 2 but not at grade 3. Over time, boys showed a slight shift towards reporting greater difficulty from grades 2 to 3, for both math and reading; among girls, there was a slight shift towards reporting less difficulty for math (and no change in reports of difficulty for reading) from grades 2 to 3 (Figure 2).

In sum, at both grades 2 and 3, both boys and girls make references to math or reading as difficult (or as requiring "work" or exertion), but there is a tendency for math to be described as slightly more difficult than reading, and a tendency for children with MLD to rate both math and reading as more difficult compared to ratings assigned by their non-MLD peers.

3.1.3. Likability and Difficulty as Distinct Constructs. It is possible that likability and difficulty ratings simply represent

TABLE 4: Specificity scores: coding criteria and real examples of reading definitions.

Score	Definitions	Examples
1	No response, a circular response, or a response unrelated to reading or otherwise uninformative.	"Reading means you read a lot." "I do not know that one."
2	Response related to unspecific reading activities, or indirectly related to reading activities. Includes reference to activities that may be performed in relation to reading or for a reading class but without a clear reference to the concept of reading.	"It means that you do reading projects." "It is if you have a book report you can report."
3	Unelaborated basic principles or mechanics of reading. Includes reference to sounding out and/or to reading materials or to learning to read.	"To like sound out something." "You read a book, you read a piece of paper." "When you like read words and books and sound out letters." "Something you do to get smarter at knowing words and learning what the words mean and how to pronounce the words and how to say them. That is why you have teachers to help you pronounce, read, and spell the words."
4	Elaborated concepts of reading. Includes reference to the extraction of meaning from written material through the act of reading.	"Like if you have a book, it has words, and you read the words not to just look and say, but to know what the words say and what the story is about."
5	Concept of reading as a useful tool. Must demonstrate usage of reading or usage of meaning derived from reading.	"To like look at books and some books help you make things and repair your house and some people just read for fun."

TABLE 5: Observed means or definition codes among total study sample (n = 207).

	Math		Reading	
	Mean (SD)	Range	Mean (SD)	Range
Grade 2				
Likability	0.01 (0.14)	−1 to 1	0.03 (0.30)	−2 to 2
Difficulty	−0.29 (0.52)	−2 to 0	−0.11 (0.33)	−2 to 0
Specificity	2.85 (0.473)	1 to 4	2.96 (0.63)	1 to 5
Grade 3				
Likability	0.00 (0.14)	−1 to 1	0.06 (0.39)	−2 to 2
Difficulty	−0.32 (0.50)	−2 to 0	−0.21 (0.43)	−2 to 1
Specificity	3.03 (0.66)	1 to 5	2.97 (0.61)	1 to 5

Note: Standard deviations shown in parentheses.

a general reporting tendency, rather than specific constructs. For example, each measure may reflect a positive or negative disposition towards academic subjects in general, in which case likability codes for math and reading should be positively correlated, and difficulty codes for math and reading should also be correlated. Alternatively, the measures may reflect an even broader tendency for positive or negative reporting in general, in which case likability and difficulty codes should be correlated with each other. Finally, if the codes represent stable, subject-domain sentiments, then math (or reading) likability scores should be correlated across grades.

To explore which of these alternatives is supported, we ran three sets of four correlations, using 12 Spearman rank tests, with alpha adjusted to 0.004 based on multiple correlations (.05/12). With respect to the three alternatives posed above, we found only weak, partial support for the notion of a general academic valence bias, based on the weak positive correlation between likability codes for math and reading observed at grade 2 (Spearman *Rho* = .150,

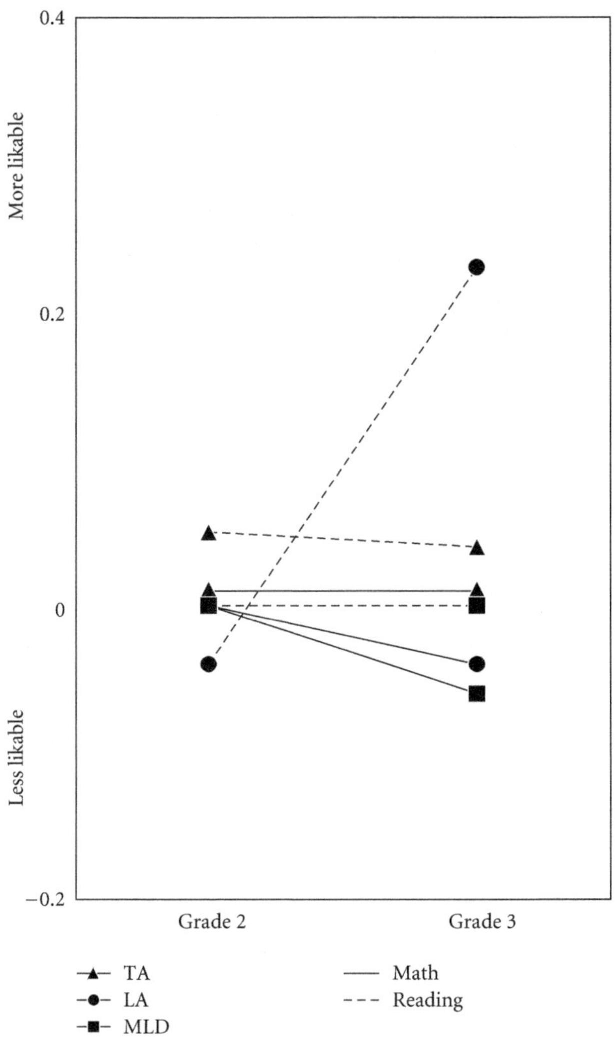

FIGURE 1: Observed means for likability scores, from grades 2 and 3, depict the three following interactions: grade × MLD status, grade × subject area, and grade × MLD status × subject area.

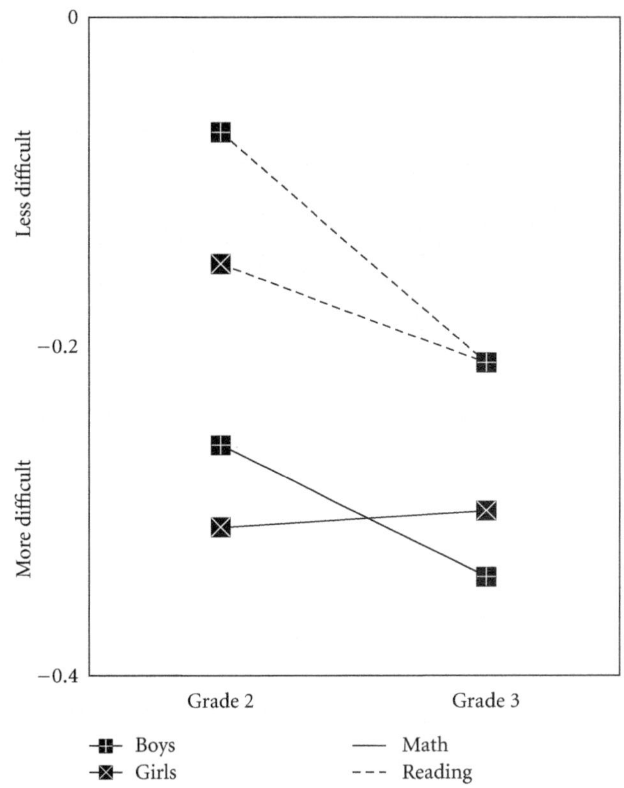

FIGURE 2: Observed means for difficulty scores in grades 2 and 3 depict the significant main effects of subject area and MLD status, and the significant three way interaction between grade, gender, and subject area.

$P = .031$) but not at grade 3 (Spearman *Rho* = .0, $P = 1.0$); and positive correlations between difficulty codes for math and reading at Grades 2 (Spearman *Rho* = .160, $P = .022$) and 3 (Spearman *Rho* = .311, $P = .0001$). Only the latter correlation at grade 3 met our adjusted significance criteria for multiple correlations.

There was less support for a broad reporting disposition bias, because likability and difficulty codes were not correlated with each other, P ranging from .096 to .594, with the exception of the association between math likability and difficulty at grade 3 only, −.148, $P = .033$, which did not meet criteria adjusted for multiple correlations.

There was far more support for subject-specific likability (or difficulty) over time, suggesting that our codes are indicative of stable, and subject-domain beliefs, at least over the short term (from grade 2 to 3): reading likability at grade 2 was correlated with reading likability at grade 3 (Spearman *Rho* = .239, $P = .001$), and reading difficulty at grades 2 and 3 were also correlated with each other (Spearman *Rho* = .210, $P = .002$). Likewise, math likability at grades 2 and 3 were correlated with each other, (Spearman *Rho* = .251, $P < .0003$), although math difficulty scores were not correlated across grades ($P = .816$). All three of the significant results met our criteria adjusted for multiple correlations. Grade level means are reported in Table 5.

3.1.4. Subject-Area Specificity of Children's Definitions of Math and Reading. The third set of repeated measures ANOVAs concerned the specificity of children's descriptions of math or reading, with codes reflecting noninformative to elaborate descriptions (exemplified in Tables 3 and 4). There was no main effect of subject area on this aspect of children's definitions, $P = .49$. Responses ranged from 1 to 5 for both math and reading, with estimated marginal mean ratings of 2.86 for math and 2.90 for reading, collapsed across all other variables. There was no effect of grade on the specificity of definitions (means = 2.85 to 2.91, at grades 2 and 3, resp.), $P = .29$.

Gender and MLD status each contributed significantly to variance in the specificity of definitions. Girls gave slightly more specific definitions of mathematics or reading (mean = 3.00) than did boys (mean = 2.75), $F(1, 201) = 10.53$, $P = .001$, partial $\eta^2 = 0.050$. The main effect of MLD status, $F(2, 201) = 4.30$, $P < .02$, partial $\eta^2 = 0.041$, reflected more specific definitions of math or reading by children in the TA

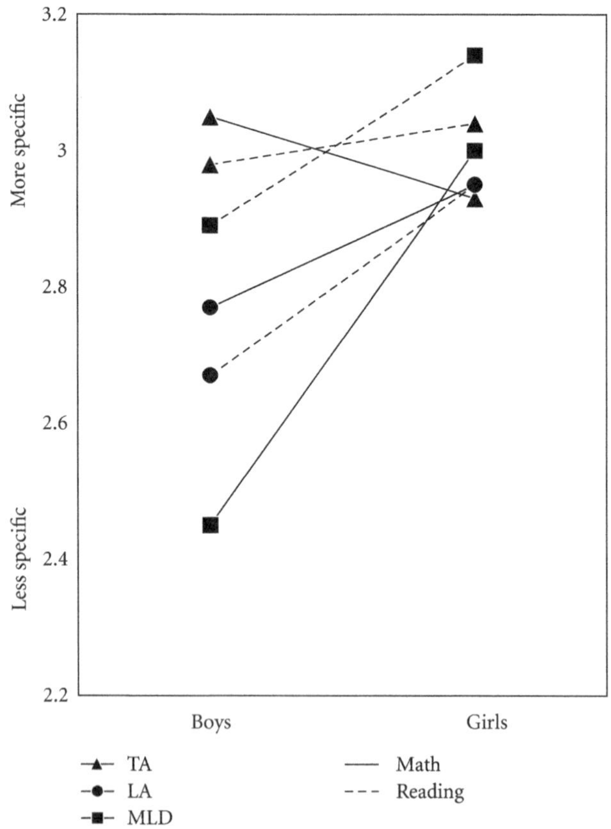

FIGURE 3: Observed means for specificity scores depict significant main effects of MLD status and gender, and the significant MLD status × gender interaction. Subject area is not significant.

group (mean = 3.00), relative to the MLD or LA groups ($P <$ .02), which did not differ from each other, $P = .68$ (means = 2.84 and 2.80, resp.).

The only interaction to reach statistical significance was a two way interaction between MLD status and gender, $F(2, 201) = 5.96$, $P < .004$, partial $\eta^2 = 0.056$. This interaction reflects that girls' ratings did not differ across MLD groups (with estimated marginal mean ratings of 2.99, 2.96, and 3.07 across the TA, LA, and MLD groups, resp.), whereas boys' ratings did (means = 3.02, 2.72, and 2.52, resp.; Figure 3).

3.2. Predicting Mathematics Achievement. Do these exploratory measures predict future or concurrent math performance? We carried out two regression models, each comprised of three predictors of grade 3 WJ-R math Calculation score as the outcome variable of interest. These models were based on predictors obtained at grade 2 or grade 3 (grade level predictors examined separately). When combined, grade 2 likability, difficulty, and specificity codes accounted for approximately 5% of the variance in WJ-R Calculation scores obtained at grade 3, $F(3, 206) = 5.03$, $P < .003$, adjusted $r^2 = .055$. However, likability and difficulty codes did not contribute significantly to the model, $P > .12$, whereas specificity codes did, $t(206) = 3.11$, $beta = .212$, $P < .01$.

Model strength improved significantly when grade WJ-R Calculation score was included as a predictor, $F(4, 206) = 32.47$, $P < .0001$, adjusted $r^2 = .379$. Still, the small contribution made by the specificity score remained significant, $t(206) = 2.40$, $beta = .134$, $P < .02$.

To examine whether *concurrent* predictors would be stronger than predictors obtained one year prior, the analysis was repeated using grade 3 likability, difficulty, and specificity codes to predict grade 3 WJ-R Calculation scores. The model strength for the grade 3 predictor model was weaker than the aforementioned grade 2 predictor model, $F(3, 206) = 3.00$, $P < .04$, adjusted $r^2 = .028$. Here, both the specificity and likability codes predicted grade 3 WJ-R Calculation scores, but effects were small ($t(206)s$ ($beta$) = 2.12 (.147), and 1.99 (.138), resp., $P < .05$), and these effects disappeared when the grade 2 WJ-R Calculation scores were added to the model, $P > .31$

To evaluate whether the effect to emerge from grade 2 predictors was specific to math disposition, we carried out parallel regression models using grade 2 or grade 3 likability, difficulty, and specificity codes from *reading* definitions, to predict WJ-R Calculation scores. Neither model accounted for significant variation in grade 3 WJ-R Calculation scores, adjusted $r^2 < .02$, $P > .10$.

4. Discussion

Our research questions examined primary school aged students' spontaneous comments about mathematics and specifically tested whether these comments reveal emerging dispositions linked to students' later mathematics achievement. Additionally, we tested the notion that beliefs about math may differ among children with versus without MLD. For comparative purposes, children's spontaneous comments about reading were also obtained. Our approach involved a straightforward design to elicit spontaneous comments of the kind that may emerge during casual verbal dialogue between young children and their parents or teachers. Finally, by repeating this procedure during two consecutive grades, we were able to test short term stability or reliability of the codes we collected.

Despite the subtlety of our approach, our findings indicate that children's spontaneous comments about math are informative even if they are no substitute for a structured and validated assessment of disposition. Specifically, we found that subject-specific comments about likability (or difficulty) appear to be stable beliefs, at least from grade 2 to 3. Lower likability ratings (i.e., more negative comments) were evident in definitions of math (versus reading) among children with MLD, and, to a lesser degree, among children with LA in math; but overall, reference to liking or disliking mathematics was absent from most of the participants' spontaneous comments of math and variability was greater among definitions of reading.

With regard to *difficulty*, children made more references to difficulty in definitions of math versus reading, collapsed across grades, groups, and gender. Children rarely, if ever, spontaneously remarked that math was easy but this was also true of reading. Children with MLD were more likely to make references to difficulty of math than their peers, but they also made more references to reading as difficult. This finding is consistent with reports of high co-occurrence of math and reading difficulties [36] and with reports that children with MLD recognize their academic weakness in mathematics, as determined by ratings on self-perception measures [37]. However, Hanich and Jordan [37] found that, on measures of reading, children with math difficulties and normal reading achievement do not rate their competence lower than children without math difficulties, although children with co-morbid math and reading difficulty do. They hypothesized that children in the math and reading difficulty group in their study were more accurate at evaluating their reading performance than math performance given that many of the children in this group were receiving special education services for reading related problems, which may have contributed to the formation of children's achievement-related beliefs.

Analyses related to *specificity* of children's definitions of math and reading showed that, in general, children report unelaborated conceptions regarding the usefulness or importance of both math and reading as a tool. The only contributions of MLD status to the *specificity* rating from children's definitions of math concerned slightly less specific definitions by the MLD and LA groups, relative to the TA group, more so for boys versus girls; but this finding also emerged from definitions of reading. Greater specificity in definitions for math and reading were also observed among girls versus boys, which may simply reflect girls' superior expressive vocabulary during the school age years.

Of the four main predictor variables examined across these analyses—MLD status, subject area, gender, and grade—the only variable to account for variability in all three outcome variables was MLD status. Main effects or interactions involving MLD status emerged for likability, difficulty, and specificity. Although it is erroneous to infer that brief, open-ended questions like the ones used in our study are appropriate for diagnosis of MLD, future and ongoing work is needed to address the dynamic role(s) of a productive disposition and long term math achievement outcomes.

There were no gender differences in likability ratings for math or reading, but boys and girls reported slightly greater difficulty for math than reading at both grades. From grades 2 to 3, boys shifted towards reporting slightly greater difficulty for both math and reading over time, whereas girls shifted towards reporting slightly less difficulty for math over time. This may reflect differences in shift towards behavioral compliance rather than a specific shift in beliefs about mathematics, but neither explanation is supported by our data. The effect was small and warrants more in depth evaluation, especially in light of research that has found primary school aged boys identify more strongly with mathematics and have higher self-concepts than girls despite similar levels of mathematics achievement [22]. Other research conducted with eighth graders found an absence of gender differences in attitudes towards mathematics and achievement, although boys were more likely to attribute their math achievement to their intellectual abilities than girls [38].

It is quite clear that the effects that emerged in this exploratory study are small. Yet the fact that *any* such findings would emerge given the simplistic nature of our questioning is somewhat intriguing. Our ratings were based on children's unstructured responses to brief, open-ended questions, "what is math?" and "what is reading?" and their definitions hint at potentially distinct elements of a productive disposition towards math, evident at second and third grades. This finding is consistent with factors to emerge from formal assessments based research. For instance, Adelson and McCoach [28, 39] found evidence of two factors from their math attitudes survey given to upper elementary students (grades 3 to 5), reflecting an "enjoyment of math" construct (similar to our "likability" codes) and a "math self-perceptions" construct (similar to both our "difficulty" and "specificity" codes). Their development of a structured survey supports the notion that individual differences in dispositions towards math exist and can be measured at grade 3 and above; we add that this work can likely be extended downward to grade 2 and below. As our work and that of others indicates, some dispositional factors may be math-specific ("math is difficult") whereas others may generalize to academic subjects.

4.1. Implications for Further Studies. Although our findings do not indicate causal pathways, they are consistent with evidence that primary school aged students' interests or beliefs about mathematics affect their achievement level or reflect risk status for future math outcome [2, 4]. The predictive contribution of grade 2 specificity ratings to math scores at grade 3 suggests associations emerging in early childhood. One possibility is that *opinions* about the importance or challenges of math precede and direct learning or performance success, as has been implicated in work with adults [40]; alternatively, earlier ability levels may influence emerging opinions, such that these features operate dynamically throughout schooling. There is some evidence that students' perceived competence ratings and ratings of enjoyment of mathematics are independent of achievement in the early years, but are related to math performance at the end of elementary school [41]. Our findings run counter to this conclusion, and thus support the contention that research on dispositional contributions to mathematics achievement must include studies of early childhood.

These findings in early childhood have implications for teachers, parents, and care providers of young children. In general, children in our study expressed relative flat affect with regard to their enjoyment of mathematics, did not hold very elaborate conceptions regarding the usefulness of mathematics, and attributed more difficulty to mathematic than reading. Despite the small effect size that emerged from these findings, these suggest potential negative outcomes when considered in the context of expectancy-value theory. According to the model, these dispositions run counter to facilitating engagement in mathematics activities given the proportional relationship among components of the model (i.e., engagement = success expectancies × task value). However, the "neutral" codes for likability were based on spontaneous comments, and children may have responded very differently to prompts eliciting remarks about liking or disliking mathematics. To foster adaptive motivational behaviors, parents and teachers should provide feedback to young children about the task values associated with mathematics, help students develop positive but accurate perceptions of their abilities, and teach children to effectively appraise learning to modify their achievement behaviors.

4.2. Limitations and Conclusions. There are several limitations to our exploratory study. Although our sample size was large and data collection over time was longitudinal, the time period over which we examined definitions of math and reading was limited to two consecutive years, and the number of students with MLD and LA was limited by the defining criteria of these constructs (e.g., MLD occurring in only ~6–10% of the population, as it was in our study). The deliberately simplistic nature of our data collection was consistent with our goal to evaluate more naturalistic and spontaneous versus prompted comments about mathematics likability, difficulty, and specificity, but children's comments could be elaborated upon through structured probes and conversations. For instance, most children's definitions received "neutral" codes for likability, but this does not mean that children did not have beliefs about liking or disliking mathematics.

Our research question did not concern the strength of children's beliefs about math so much as the likelihood of their emergence during conversation. In addition to expressing (or not expressing) beliefs about math and reading, the children in this study remind us of the importance of listening to what they say, even during casual discourse. That is, adult-child discourse provides a means for parents and teachers to both nurture a child's positive disposition towards math, and monitor the child's emerging disposition.

Acknowledgments

This work was supported by a Grant from the Spencer Foundation awarded to M. M. M. Mazzocco and L. B. Hanich, based on data collected from a study supported by NIH Grant HD R01 34061 awarded to M. M. M. Mazzocco. The views expressed are solely those of the authors. They would like to thank the children who participated in the study, their parents and teachers, the staff at participating Baltimore County Public School elementary schools; and an anonymous reviewer of an earlier version of this paper. They also acknowledge the outstanding contributions of Gwen F. Myers, Project Manager for the longitudinal study, to this work and to the overall longitudinal research program.

References

[1] National Research Council, *Adding It Up: Helping Children Learn Mathematics*, Mathematics Learning Study Committee, Center for Education, Division of Behavioral and Social Sciences and Education, National Academy Press, Washington, DC, USA, 2001.

[2] S. L. Beilock, E. A. Gunderson, G. Ramirez, and S. C. Levine, "Female teachers' math anxiety affects girls' math achievement," *Proceedings of the National Academy of Sciences of the United States of America*, vol. 107, no. 5, pp. 1860–1863, 2010.

[3] T. Kutaka, C. P. Edwards, and W. M. Smith, "The relationship between math competence beliefs and math ability scores in the early primary years," in *Proceedings of the Annual Meeting of the American Education Research Association*, Vancouver, Canada, April 2012.

[4] P. H. Fisher, J. Dobbs-Oates, G. L. Doctoroff, and D. H. Arnold, "Early math interest and the development of math skills," *Journal of Educational Psychology*, vol. 104, no. 3, pp. 673–681, 2012.

[5] J. S. Eccles and A. Wigfield, "In the mind of the actor: the structure of adolescents' achievement tasks values and expectancy-related beliefs," *Personality and Social Psychology Bulletin*, vol. 21, pp. 215–225, 1995.

[6] A. Wigfield, "Expectancy-value theory of achievement motivation: a developmental perspective," *Educational Psychology Review*, vol. 6, no. 1, pp. 49–78, 1994.

[7] J. Garofalo, "Beliefs and their influence on mathematical performance," *Mathematics Teacher*, vol. 82, pp. 502–505, 1989.

[8] A. H. Schoenfeld, "Explorations of students' mathematical beliefs and behavior," *Journal for Research in Mathematics Education*, vol. 20, pp. 238–355, 1989.

[9] J. S. Eccles and C. Midgley, "Changes in academic motivation and self-perceptions during early adolescence," in *Advances in Adolescent Development: From Childhood to Adolescence*, R. Montemayor, G. R. Adams, and T. P. Gullotta, Eds., pp. 134–155, Sage, Thousand Oaks, Calif, USA, 1990.

[10] S. Harter, "A new self-report scale of intrinsic versus extrinsic orientation in the classroom: motivational and informational components," *Developmental Psychology*, vol. 17, no. 3, pp. 300–312, 1981.

[11] J. H. Corpus, M. S. McClintic-Gilbert, and A. O. Hayenga, "Within-year changes in children's intrinsic and extrinsic motivational orientations: contextual predictors and academic outcomes," *Contemporary Educational Psychology*, vol. 34, no. 2, pp. 154–166, 2009.

[12] A. E. Gottfried, J. S. Fleming, and A. W. Gottfried, "Continuity of academic intrinsic motivation from childhood through late adolescence: a longitudinal study," *Journal of Educational Psychology*, vol. 93, no. 1, pp. 3–13, 2001.

[13] J. Eccles, A. Wigfield, R. D. Harold, and P. Blumenfeld, "Age and gender differences in children's self- and task perceptions during elementary school," *Child Development*, vol. 64, no. 3, pp. 830–847, 1993.

[14] J. E. Jacobs, S. Lanza, D. W. Osgood, J. S. Eccles, and A. Wigfield, "Changes in children's self-competence and values: gender and domain differences across grades one through twelve," *Child Development*, vol. 73, no. 2, pp. 509–527, 2002.

[15] A. Wigfield, R. D. Harold, C. Freedman-Doan et al., "Changes in children's competence beliefs and subjective task values across the elementary school years: a three year study," *Journal of Educational Psychology*, vol. 89, no. 3, pp. 451–469, 1997.

[16] D. J. Stipek and D. MacIver, "Developmental changes in children's assessment of intellectual competence," *Child Development*, vol. 60, pp. 521–538, 1989.

[17] A. Wigfield and J. S. Eccles, "Expectancy-value theory of achievement motivation," *Contemporary Educational Psychology*, vol. 25, no. 1, pp. 68–81, 2000.

[18] M. C. Steffens, P. Jelenec, and P. Noack, "On the leaky math pipeline: comparing implicit math-gender stereotypes and math withdrawal in female and male children and adolescents," *Journal of Educational Psychology*, vol. 102, no. 4, pp. 947–963, 2010.

[19] S. Lau, A. D. Liem, and Y. Nie, "Task- and self-related pathways to deep learning: the mediating role of achievement goals, classroom attentiveness, and group participation," *British Journal of Educational Psychology*, vol. 78, no. 4, pp. 639–662, 2008.

[20] G. Ramirez, E. A. Gunderson, S. C. Levine, and S. L. Beilock, "Math anxiety, working memory and math achievement in early elementary school," *Journal of Cognition and Development*. In press.

[21] A. G. Greenwald, D. E. McGhee, and J. L. K. Schwartz, "Measuring individual differences in implicit cognition: the implicit association test," *Journal of Personality and Social Psychology*, vol. 74, no. 6, pp. 1464–1480, 1998.

[22] D. Cvencek, A. N. Meltzoff, and A. G. Greenwald, "Math-gender stereotypes in elementary school children," *Child Development*, vol. 82, no. 3, pp. 766–779, 2011.

[23] E. A. Gunderson, G. Ramirez, S. C. Levine, and S. L. Beilock, "The role of parents and teachers in the development of gender-related math attitudes," *Sex Roles*, vol. 66, pp. 153–166, 2012.

[24] M. P. Levpušček and M. Zupančič, "Math achievement in early adolescence: the role of parental involvement, teachers' behavior, and students' motivational beliefs about math," *Journal of Early Adolescence*, vol. 29, no. 4, pp. 541–570, 2009.

[25] J. Tiedemann, "Parents' gender stereotypes and teachers' beliefs as predictors of children's concept of their mathematical ability in elementary school," *Journal of Educational Psychology*, vol. 92, no. 1, pp. 144–151, 2000.

[26] R. Bhanot and J. Jovanovic, "Do parents' academic gender stereotypes influence whether they intrude on their children's homework?" *Sex Roles*, vol. 52, no. 9-10, pp. 597–607, 2005.

[27] P. M. Frome and J. S. Eccles, "Parents' influence on children's achievement-related perceptions," *Journal of Personality and Social Psychology*, vol. 74, no. 2, pp. 435–452, 1998.

[28] J. L. Adelson and D. B. McCoach, "Development and psychometric properties of the Math and Me survey: measuring third through sixth graders' attitudes towards mathematics," *Measurement and Evaluation in Counseling and Development*, vol. 44, pp. 225–247, 2011.

[29] M. M. M. Mazzocco and G. F. Myers, "Complexities in identifying and defining mathematics learning disability in the primary school-age years," *Annals of Dyslexia*, vol. 53, pp. 218–253, 2003.

[30] H. Ginsburg and A. Baroody, *Test of Early Mathematics Ability*, PRO-ED, Austin, Tex, USA, 2nd edition, 1990.

[31] M. M. Murphy, M. M. M. Mazzocco, L. B. Hanich, and M. C. Early, "Cognitive characteristics of children with Mathematics Learning Disability (MLD) vary as a function of the cutoff criterion used to define MLD," *Journal of Learning Disabilities*, vol. 40, pp. 467–487, 2007.

[32] R. W. Woodcock and M. B. Johnson, *Woodcock-Johnson PsychoEducational Battery-Revised. Tests of Achievement*, Riverside, Itasca, Ill, USA, 1989.

[33] R. W. Woodcock and N. Mather, *Woodcock Johnson Psycho-Educational Battery Revised, Tests of Achievement, Examiner's Manual*, Riverside, Chicago, Ill, USA, 1990.

[34] R. L. Thorndike, E. P. Hagen, and J. M. Sattler, *Guide for Administering and Scoring the Fourth Edition Standford Binet Intelligence Scale*, Riverside, Chicago, Ill, USA, 1986.

[35] D. Wechsler, *Wechsler Abbreviated Scale of Intelligence (WASI)*, The Psychological, San Antonio, Tex, USA, 1999.

[36] L. B. Hanich, N. C. Jordan, D. Kaplan, and J. Dick, "Performance across different areas of mathematical cognition in children with learning difficulties," *Journal of Educational Psychology*, vol. 93, no. 3, pp. 615–626, 2001.

[37] L. B. Hanich and N. C. Jordan, "Achievement-related beliefs of third-grade children with mathematics and reading difficulties," *Journal of Educational Research*, vol. 97, no. 5, pp. 227–233, 2004.

[38] S. N. Geogiou, P. Stavrinides, and T. Kalavana, "Is Victor better than Victoria at maths?" *Educational Psychology Review in Practice*, vol. 23, pp. 329–342, 2007.

[39] J. L. Adelson and D. B. McCoach, "Measuring the mathematical attitudes of elementary students: the effects of a 4-point or 5-point likert-type scale," *Educational and Psychological Measurement*, vol. 70, no. 5, pp. 796–807, 2010.

[40] M. Cadinu, A. Maass, A. Rosabianca, and J. Kiesner, "Why do women underperform under stereotype threat? Evidence for the role of negative thinking," *Psychological Science*, vol. 16, no. 7, pp. 572–578, 2005.

[41] P. Kloosterman and M. C. Cougan, "Students' beliefs about learning mathematics," *The Elementary School Journal*, vol. 94, pp. 375–388, 1994.

Linking Early Adversity, Emotion Dysregulation, and Psychopathology: The Case of Extremely Low Birth Weight Infants

Lauren A. Drvaric,[1] Ryan J. Van Lieshout,[2] and Louis A. Schmidt[1]

[1] *Department of Psychology, Neuroscience & Behaviour, McMaster University, Hamilton, ON, Canada*
[2] *Department of Psychiatry & Behavioural Neurosciences, McMaster University, Hamilton, ON, Canada*

Correspondence should be addressed to Lauren A. Drvaric; drvaril@mcmaster.ca

Academic Editor: Annie Vinter

The ability to regulate emotion is a crucial process that humans utilize in order to adapt to the demands of environmental constraints. Individuals exposed to early adverse life events such as being born at an extremely low birth weight (ELBW, 501–1000 g) are known to have problems regulating emotion which have been linked to the development of psychopathology in this population. Recent studies have used psychophysiological measures, such as electroencephalogram (EEG) and cardiac vagal tone, to index emotion regulatory processes. The purpose of this paper was three-fold: (1) to investigate the relation between ELBW and emotion regulation issues (pathway 1), (2) to review studies investigating the relation between early emotion regulation and later internalizing problems (pathway 2); and (3) to provide a model in which two psychophysiological measures (i.e., frontal EEG asymmetry and cardiac vagal tone) are suggested to understand the proposed conceptual pathways in the relation between ELBW and psychopathology.

1. General Introduction

Emotions are complex processes that humans use to evaluate the environment, recognize environmental changes, and adjust behaviors according to environmental demands [1]. They are an integral part of human life and have important inter- and intrapersonal functions [2]. Interpersonally, emotions function as signals to others about our internal states and intentions. The intrapersonal functions of emotions give us pertinent information, which we use to make decisions about environmental stressors.

Emotions and their regulation involve cognitive, behavioral, and physiological components. Interactions among these provide one with emotion-specific action tendencies and eventually facilitate explicit action, which can be adaptive or maladaptive [3]. How emotions can be effectively regulated is the topic of significant debate. Of particular interest has been how their dysregulation can lead to problems with adaptive behaviour, and how emotion dysregulatory processes affect the risk for adverse mental and physical health outcomes [3].

Normal development of emotion regulation leads to successful adaptations to the demands of environmental constraints. What is less known is how pervasive problems with emotional regulation, as indexed by psychophysiological measures, can contribute to the development of mental health problems and how early experience shapes these processes.

Early adversity has been defined as early exposure to environmental conditions that negatively impact normative human development [4]. In particular, these adverse exposures are thought to have the capacity to negatively affect the development of emotion regulatory processes. Much research has documented the fact that such adversity affects not only cognitive but also social-emotional development and functioning [1, 4]. Some special types of early adversity that are particularly deleterious to the development of emotion regulation include childhood maltreatment (i.e., physical, emotional, and sexual abuse, and neglect) [1, 5, 6], rearing in poorly staffed orphanages [5, 7], being exposed to recreational and certain prescribed drugs in utero [8], and being born prematurely and/or at low birth weight [9–15].

Some researchers have proposed that these aberrant experiences can affect adult mental health by (1) causing successive damage to the self over time, and/or (2) affecting the individual during sensitive developmental periods [16]. In many cases, these mechanisms may act in concert to affect the risk of the development of psychiatric impairment.

While a multitude of studies have been published on (1) later internalizing problems seen in groups seen exposed to early forms of adversity, (2) early adversity and emotion regulation, and (3) early emotion regulation, and later internalizing problems, relatively few reviews have been conducted on investigating the associations among early adversity, emotion dysregulation and psychopathology. The purpose of this paper was to provide evidence that those exposed to a specific, rare type of early adversity, namely, being born at extremely low birth weight (ELBW, i.e., <1000 grams), represent an adverse circumstance. ELBW individuals have problems with emotion regulation and are at a heightened risk for the development of later internalizing problems.

In this paper, we will (1) discuss how ELBW represents an adverse event, (2) review studies relating ELBW, with emotional regulation issues (pathway 1), (3) review studies relating early emotional regulation with later internalizing problems (pathway 2), (4) propose a model hypothesizing the association between early adversity (ELBW as the adverse circumstance), emotion dysregulation, and psychopathology, and (5) provide some perspectives in which measures of frontal EEG asymmetry and cardiac vagal tone should be considered as means to investigate the conceptual pathways 1 and 2 described in this paper.

2. How Extremely Low Birth Weight (ELBW) Represents an Adverse Circumstance

Infants born preterm are among the most vulnerable groups exposed to early adversity. Not only is their small and underdeveloped size at birth suggestive of exposure to prior physiological stresses, but they are also more vulnerable than normal birth weight infants to postnatal environmental risks. Infants born preterm may experience similar risks to those exposed to other types of early adversity, such as problems with emotion dysregulation and increased risk for developing psychopathology [13, 17].

It is, however, important to make a distinction here between infants born prematurely and those born low birth weight. Those born prematurely are not born full term, meaning that they were born preterm and are subject to underdevelopment. Infants born at low, very low, or extremely low birth weight do not necessarily imply preterm birth. It is possible for those born low birth weight are born full-term but low birth weight and thus subject to similar adversities as preterm infants. These similar early adverse experiences shared by both groups contribute to difficulties in emotional regulation. Thus, it is reasonable to suggest that studies investigating the negative effects of preterm birth on development of emotion regulation can be extrapolated to the case of early adversities experienced by those born ELBW in the development of emotion regulation [18, 19].

In this section, we will (1) provide an overview of the adverse environmental and biological factors that ELBW infants face in the early stages of development, and (2) demonstrate how these adverse environmental and biological factors have strong implications for negative impact on the early stages of the developing brain, specifically in the development of important processes such as self-regulation.

ELBW infants are especially vulnerable to environmental risk factors. Infants born ELBW are extremely underdeveloped in size and weight (<1000 g) and arrive usually preterm between 23 and 28 gestation weeks. ELBW infants first enter the world subjected to the neonatal intensive care unit (NICU) where neonatal interventions, therapies, and procedures are imposed on the infant in order to increase their chances of survival. Some interventions, therapies, and procedures include surfactant therapy, intravenous fluid therapy, umbilical artery catheter placement to monitor oxygenation, neonatal monitoring of cardiac and respiratory functioning, and phototherapy in the treatment of jaundice [20]. Although the medical procedures are designed to reduce mortality rates of ELBWs, of those who survive, there are a small percentages (~15%) of ELBWs who experience severe developmental outcomes, such as cerebral palsy (CP) [20, 21] and about half develop cognitive and behavioral deficits [21]. Furthermore, ELBW infants receiving intensive care are highly susceptible to neonatal infections—imposing more biological stress on the infant in terms of early developmental growth and increased risk of death [21]. In order to treat neonatal infection, a number of medical procedures are put into place. Some of these include antenatal antibiotics and steroid use, which on their own have significant biological effects on neurodevelopment.

During the early days and weeks of postnatal life in the NICU, neonatal pain exposure due to various medical procedures and susceptibility to neonatal infection (putting ELBW infants at a heightened risk for mortality) are not the only stressful environmental exposures to which ELBW survivors are subjected. ELBW infants are also deprived of immediate primary caregiver attachment. At this sensitive and crucial time where an infant needs to rely on maternal support, there is very little and often none available because of the neonatal interventions imposed on the infant. In the early stages of infant development, the infant relies heavily on caregiver support and feedback in order to self regulate [22–25]. In circumstances of ELBW, the infant is unable to rely on this crucial support for self regulation purposes. Moreover, while intensive care is necessary in order to reduce the risk of morbidity in the ELBW infant, this event not only is stress inducing for the infant, but also becomes a stressful time period for primary caregivers.

There is an extensive literature published demonstrating the importance of the transactional nature/reciprocal relationship between caregiver and infant on the development and acquisition of self-regulation (for a comprehensive review, see Walker et al., 2004). The psychological impact of having an infant born ELBW can be extremely taxing on parents, and even more so, if there is only one parent support system [23, 25]. The untimely birth of the infant is a stressful event, especially when the infant born ELBW and is subjected to NICU procedures. How caregivers adjust to this distress, behave toward the infant (i.e., maternal touch), and how they go about parenting the infant, all represent important factors in infant regulation. When the caregivers are unable to make positive adjustments to cope with the distressing series of events, the unavailability can result in symptoms of depression and even posttraumatic stress disorder (PTSD).

There are a number of studies published on the negative influence of maternal depression as well as PTSD on the developing infant [24, 26–29]. Depression and PTSD are related to the difficulty in emotion regulation. Consequently, caregiver-infant interaction may be biased by the caregivers' difficulty to regulate emotions and may influence the development of early self regulation.

Neonatal pain exposure via NICU, primary caregiver detachment, and exposure to maternal depression and/or PTSD, all have deleterious effects on the ELBW infant. These environmental factors strongly influence high levels of biological stress. Biological stress in the form of increased glucocorticoids (GCs) exposure, which have damaging effects on the development of brain systems [20, 22, 23]. These brain systems (specifically, the hypothalamic-pituitary-adrenal axis (HPA), amygdala, hippocampus, and prefrontal cortex (PFC)) are highly susceptible to programming in early development [25].

The HPA is part of stress-response activation of which one needs to respond and cope with the demands of the environment. Responses of the HPA axis are programmed by early experiences (e.g., in the ELBW infant, extreme NICU procedures, maternal separation, and maternal psychopathology). The production of high levels of basal cortisol in ELBWs suggests reprogramming of stress physiology [20, 22, 23], where it is thought that the ELBW neonatal reprogramming of stress systems has taken place and has been proposed as the mechanism in altered behavior, cognitive, and emotion processes [23, 25]. In ELBW infants, stress exposure related to unexpected medical procedures, separation from parents, and the impact of primary caregiver psychopathology can have a negative impact on the development of many brain systems involved in regulation of stress.

3. Studies Relating ELBW with Emotional Regulation Issues (Pathway 1)

The emotion regulatory resources one utilizes change across developmental periods and individuals, but individuals become more effective in the ways they regulate emotion across the lifespan. The development of early emotion regulatory processes begins with transactional exchange between caregiver and infant [25]. Feedback and support from the caregiver to infant (i.e., maternal touch, maternal-infant bond) set the fundamental building blocks for important brain systems involved in emotion regulation and dictate behavioral responses from the infant [30]. Successive interaction with primary caregivers, as well as other factors, such as age-related brain maturation, environmental influences, and the refinement of cognitive and behavioral processes, contribute to the development of emotion regulation [30]. As one moves from the early stages of development, the individual becomes less dependent on others, resulting in a greater dependence on self-regulatory processes by the time children attend school [31]. As individuals progress to adolescence, they develop even more self-sufficient mechanisms of emotion regulation, which become more complex and involve higher cognitive processes. These developmental changes arise with frontal lobe maturation and further augmentation of executive control, allowing more complex cognitive strategies (i.e., self-talk, decision making) and behavioral responses (e.g., such as ability to remove oneself from stress inducing situations) to play a larger role in the regulation of emotion.

Neural processes underlying emotion regulation cannot be defined as independent processes, but rather the regulation of emotion requires synchronization of several brain systems, whereby different systems (i.e., PFC, amygdala, HPA, and hippocampus) work in coordination to regulate each other [32]. In brief, the brainstem mediates arousal and behavioral activation; the limbic system mediates perception, memory, learning, and affective feeling; the cerebral cortex mediates higher order perceptual processes, voluntary control, and executive functioning (i.e., attention, working memory, cognitive control) (for a comprehensive review of the emotional brain, see Dalgleish [33], and Lewis and Stieben [32]). The synchronization of these brain systems underlies emotion and its regulation, including psychological features of "specific action readiness, a restricted attentional focus, a stable cognitive appraisal, and a distinct emotional feeling," [32]. The activation and coordination of these brain systems does not occur in a top-down or bottom-up fashion to produce this psychological series of functions, but rather the systems coevolve at a rapid rate, coordinating with each other [32].

As previously mentioned, infants born preterm are among the most vulnerable groups exposed to early adversity. Not only is their small and underdeveloped size at birth suggestive of exposure to prior physiological stresses, but they are also more vulnerable than normal birth weight infants to postnatal environmental risks. Infants born preterm may experience similar risks to those exposed to other types of early adversity, such as difficulties with emotion regulation [13, 17]. It is well known that early adversities can alter the development of prefrontal brain regions. By altering the development of prefrontal brain regions, which is a foundational component in self-regulatory processes, and specifically, emotion regulatory processes, this can potentially affect how one regulates emotion in order to combat environmental stresses.

It is also important to point out that, as mentioned above, not all ELBW infants were born preterm, but most were. Here we review studies involving preterm as well as low birth weight given the limited research on low birth weight infants versus those born prematurely.

Conrad et al. (2010) provided evidence that there are deficits in neuromotor and intellectual functioning in children born preterm [14]. Consistent with other research published on infants born preterm, Conrad et al. (2010) found that in the childhood and adolescent years, survivors of premature birth demonstrated lower IQ and higher rates of emotional and behavioural problems (e.g., internalizing, externalizing, hyperactivity/inattention problems). Similar findings were reported by Lowe et al. (2005), demonstrating that infant behavioral characteristics had an adverse effect on developmental outcome from 8 to 18–22 months of age in ELBW infants. Lowe et al. (2005) concluded that the majority of children whose cognitive scores significantly decreased from time 1 (8 months) and time 2 (18–22 months) demonstrated low emotional regulation subscale scores on a behavior rating scale. This finding by Lowe et al. (2005) further suggests that the neural mechanisms underlying emotion regulation may also support cognitive processes [34].

Pollak (2008) [1] argued that the earlier the exposure to adversity, the more severe the impact on development. Various studies examining children born at a VLBW and ELBW report that the lower the birth weight and gestational age of these individuals, the more severe the later effects [14]. These findings are supported by other results by Bohnert and Breslau (2008) who reported a greater risk of externalizing and internalizing problems within children of very low birth weight (≤1500 g) compared to heavier children (1501–2500 g) [35].

Attentional and processing biases fall under the umbrella of lack of control over emotion regulatory processes. A lack of cognitive control over emotion regulatory processes may lead to poor adaptive functioning [34]. This idea is in line with findings from studies that document high levels of poor adaptive functioning in children born at ELBW [12, 36, 37]. Finally, problems with emotion regulation in infants born prematurely may be due to a natural inclination for this population to engage in emotional over control, either by using avoidance-type behaviors or the use of suppression of emotion [19]. This vulnerable population shows relatively fewer externalizing problems than internalizing problems as they get older, which is evident in studies that demonstrate that personality traits of infants born preterm are shy, inhibited, and/or avoidant into young adulthood [38].

Conversely, there are various studies published reporting no significant problems in cognitive and behavioral functioning in premature and ELBW infants compared to their normal birth weight counterparts [39, 40]. Weisglas-Kuperus et al. (1993) report that VLBW children at high biological risk were able to catch up on their cognitive delay in a highly stimulating home environment, and that VLBW children who were both low and high biological risk in a less stimulating home environment demonstrated a decline in cognitive development. This outcome highlights the influence of environmental factors on the biology of the infant. Despite exposure to the negative impact of adverse circumstance, these studies suggest that there is an avenue to intervene and reverse the damaging effects premature and ELBW can have on cognitive and emotional development [39]. To support this claim, various intervention studies assessing the effects of different therapy interventions on the cognitive development and the development of attachment patterns (i.e., the nature of the relationship between primary caregiver-infant) in premature and ELBW infants have demonstrated that cognitive level and behavioral levels to be notably higher in the intervention group compared to control [41, 42].

There are a number of other studies that report those born preterm/very low birth weight to have more emotional and behavioral problems and less competence compared to normative children/adolescents as given by parent reports and other various measures [11, 15, 43]. Thus, the increasing reports of attentional problems and emotional overcontrol in children born preterm may be a partial explanation of emotion dysregulation in populations born prematurely and in turn may be a possible explanation to the increasing rates of psychopathology and its stability into childhood, adolescent, and young adult years [13, 17]. This notion is evident in findings by Saigal et al. [10, 44, 45], where data suggest that the nature of the problems ELBWs experience may change over time; however, what does remain stable is that there are an increasing number of problems.

4. Studies Relating Early Emotional Regulation with Later Internalizing Problems (Pathway 2)

Many negative outcomes are associated with the failure to develop successful emotional regulation, ranging from problems with self-esteem to shyness and impairment in interpersonal relationships. On the more severe end of the spectrum is a heightened risk of developing psychopathology. Indeed, Werner and Gross (2010) suggest that 75% of the diagnostic categories of psychopathology in the Diagnostic and Statistical Manual of Mental disorders (DSM-IV) are based on problems associated with emotion and emotion regulation [46].

Throughout this paper, we have discussed and reviewed the development of emotion regulation and both the environmental and biological factors that may play a role in the early stages of its development. Here, we will review studies relating early emotion regulation with later psychopathology, namely, the development of internalizing disorders (i.e., depression and anxiety).

A significant number of studies investigating the role of emotion regulation in psychopathology illustrate that less effective means of emotional regulation strategies/techniques are at the core of internalizing disorders, such as in depression and anxiety disorders (for a review of studies, see, Aldao et al., 2010) [47]. Gross (1998, 1999) has proposed a process model of emotion regulation strategies, where the individual appraises both external and internal events that then necessitate expressive emotion (see Gross, 1998) [48, 49]. Gross' model demonstrates how the individual's capacity to regulate emotion depends on the ability to tolerate and experience emotion, the frequency to which one regulates emotion, and the timing of emotion regulatory strategies, all impact how effective the strategy will be [50]. Emotion regulation strategies include acceptance, avoidance, problem solving, reappraisal, rumination, and suppression. These emotion regulation strategies may be viewed as having adaptive or maladaptive value. They are responses that can be effective or ineffective depending on their function, context, and timing [51]. When emotion regulation strategies are used in a maladaptive manner, they can be both emotionally and cognitively demanding and can result in adverse mental health outcomes [50].

Emotion regulation strategies help one to cope and manage unwanted feelings of negative emotion. In the face of adversity, to combat the stressful impact of negative emotions, one identifies the emotion and chooses how to respond to that emotion utilizing an emotion regulation strategy. Studies examining emotion regulation and optimal mental health have investigated how psychological resiliency and positive emotions influence the experience of negative emotions in the time of stress. These studies have demonstrated that positive emotion and psychological resiliency serve to moderate stress reactivity and mediate stress recovery, which suggest that adaptive emotion regulation strategies may be at play [52, 53]. Successful adaptation to stress over time has implications for psychological resiliency and successful emotion regulation.

Conversely, when emotion regulation is compromised early in development, there may be difficulties in the ability to regulate emotion adaptively, making one more vulnerable to the development of internalizing disorders. Studies exploring emotion regulation in depression demonstrate that the ability to regulate emotional responses to negative events may help further understand the disabling nature of the disorder [54]. Depression has been associated with difficulties in the disengagement from negative stimuli, memory biases, and deficits in cognitive control which may explain the use of maladaptive emotion regulation strategies, such as excessive use of emotion suppression and rumination [55]. The dominant use of emotion suppression and rumination and less frequent use of other emotion regulation strategies have been related to symptoms of depression [55, 56].

Emotion regulation and anxiety disorders have also been explored, and studies examining this relation have found that anxiety disorders are associated with the inability to regulate emotion effectively where increasing levels of anxiety are highly associated with emotion dysregulation [57, 58]. Orgeta (2011) found that adults experiencing increasing levels of anxiety reported greater difficulty in regulating emotional responses. Experiencing anxiety symptoms affects the ability to regulate emotional experiences [59], which has also been demonstrated in other studies [57, 58].

The relation between cognition and emotion in emotional regulation is highly interconnected, as is evident with the use of various different emotion regulation strategies to assess the way in which one processes emotion and determines how to respond to emotion. Thus, optimal development of brain systems in emotion regulation as well as the acquisition of adaptive emotion regulation strategies is crucial for successful emotion regulation. When these brain systems are disrupted in the early years of development due to adverse circumstances (as given by the case of the ELBW infant), it can affect the way in how one acquires effective emotion regulation strategies, stressing the importance of cognitive, emotional, and behavioral functioning in early development.

5. Model

5.1. *Linking Extremely Low Birth Weight, Emotion Dysregulation, and Psychiatric Impairment*

5.1.1. A Possible Hypothesis. Using the material reviewed to this point, we next provide a model (see Figure 1) that interfaces these sections particularly as it relates to pathways 1 and 2 discussed earlier. As shown in Figure 1, our model illustrates that being exposed to an adverse circumstance, using the case of being born ELBW, leads to difficulties in the development of emotion regulation (pathway 1). Exposure to adversity early in life impacts the individual both physiologically and psychologically, contributing to poor ability in regulating emotion throughout core developmental periods. Less optimal development of emotion regulation may have a significant impact on human development, such that the individual is unable to regulate emotion effectively. There is an association relating early emotion regulation with later development of psychopathology in adulthood (pathway 2), where unsuccessful means of regulating emotion are evident in internalizing disorders (i.e., anxiety and depression).

Additionally, there are other factors beyond atypical development of emotion regulatory processes that may mediate the link between exposure to early adversity and the development of psychopathology, which has been accounted for in our proposed model (as provided by the growing literature demonstrating a direct relation between exposure to adverse circumstances and later development of psychopathology in adulthood). It is important to highlight the bidirectional relation between atypical development of emotion regulatory processes and the development of psychopathology in adulthood. Here this bidirectional relation represents the growing literature demonstrating emotion dysregulation as a fundamental feature of various psychopathologies. Finally, we provide perspectives that measures of resting frontal EEG asymmetry and cardiac vagal tone should be considered as means to investigate pathways, for examples of pathways 1 and 2. Overall, our theoretical process model illustrates the mediating and moderating roles of atypical development of emotion regulation on understanding the relation between being born at ELBW and the development of psychopathology.

6. Perspectives on Putative Measures in the Model: Frontal EEG Asymmetry and Cardiac Vagal Tone in Pathways 1 and 2

6.1. Frontal EEG Asymmetry: Linking Early Adversity, Emotion Dysregulation, and Psychopathology. Over the past few decades, numerous studies have examined how early adversity affects the developing brain, the development of emotion regulation, and the risk of psychopathology. Here we will provide frontal EEG asymmetry as a means to investigate pathways, for example emotion regulation between early adversity and the risk to developing psychopathology by reviewing studies of infant and child deprivation.

Davidson and colleagues (2003) postulate that high levels of relative left frontal activity are associated with

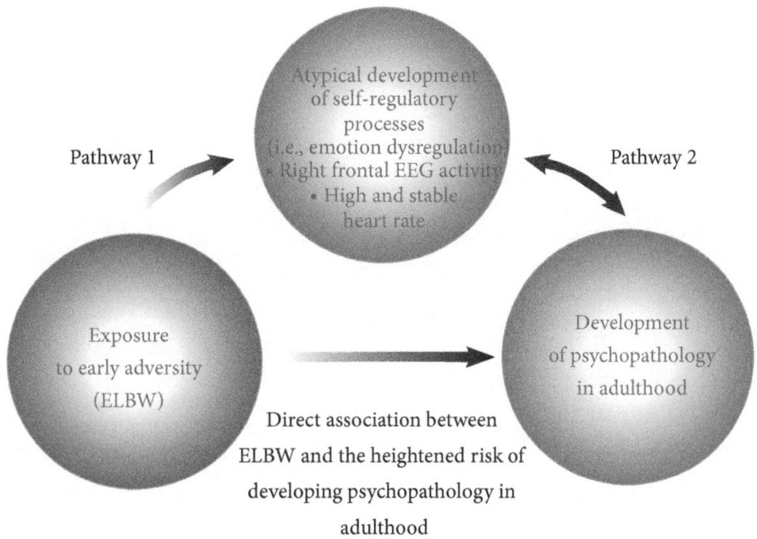

FIGURE 1: Hypothesized associations between early adversity (ELBW representing the adverse circumstance), emotion dysregulation, and later internalizing psychopathology.

the expression and experience of positive, approach-related emotions [60], whereas high levels of relative right frontal activity are associated with the experience and expression of negative, withdrawal-related emotions. Interestingly, this pattern of asymmetry has also been linked to various forms of psychopathology, specifically, anxiety and depression [5, 61–66]. This pattern raises the possibility that right frontal EEG asymmetry provides a means to investigate a pathway, for examples of being born ELBW and the development of psychopathology later in life.

Schmidt et al. (2010) conducted a study examining the development of psychopathology in a group of ELBW survivors in early adulthood. The authors found that ELBWs exhibited greater relative right frontal EEG asymmetry compared to NBW, implicating a tendency for individuals born at ELBW to have difficulties in regulating physical and mental stress [9].

Overall, previous research published on the detrimental effects of premature birth on emotion regulation functioning indicates that problems in neurocognitive functioning persist beyond the postnatal years into young adulthood. Schmidt et al. (2010) demonstrated that frontal EEG asymmetry (as an index of emotion regulation) may mediate the link between ELBW and psychopathology during a young adulthood visit. The authors found that ELBWs exhibited more internalizing behaviour problems than NBW at young adulthood. The authors suggested that greater relative right frontal EEG asymmetry in ELBWs may reflect a predisposition for this population to have difficulties in regulating physical and mental stress. This pattern of right frontal EEG asymmetry observed in survivors of ELBW may be due to early adverse life experiences (such as being born preterm).

6.2. Cardiac Vagal Tone: Linking Early Adversity, Emotion Dysregulation, and Psychopathology. Autonomic nervous system (ANS) measures have been used to specifically index self-regulation of emotion. Basic cardiac function can be determined by measuring heart rate. Variation in heart rate, also known as heart rate variability (HRV), is generally (or usually/often) measured as the standard deviation of heart rate. An important source of this variation, the parasympathetic component of heart rate variability, is often assessed using a metric known as cardiac vagal tone (CVT) [67]. Cardiac vagal tone at rest is considered a primary index of ANS regulatory capacity. High vagal tone indicates greater variability in heart rate over time (i.e., healthy cardiac control). Another metric, respiratory sinus arrhythmia (RSA), a natural irregularity in the cardiac signal that occurs in conjunction with the respiratory cycle, is also often used to index parasympathetic ANS function.

Hae-Kyung, (2009) used CVT as an indicator of autonomic nervous system functioning (specifically, emotion self-regulatory functioning) in healthy and premature infants. Hae-Kyung discovered that healthy newborns exhibited significantly greater CVT than premature infants [68]. Similar findings were reported by Doussard-Roosevelt et al. (1997) who examined HR and RSA as indexes of developmental outcomes in VLBW infants (<1,500 g). The authors found that high RSA was associated with better social functioning and greater RSA maturation was associated with better cognitive and executive functioning [69]. Lower HR was associated with better behavioral regulation, social skills, and greater maturational decreases associated with better motor skills. Extremely low birth weight infants (birth weight <1000 g) also demonstrated less positive functioning than heavier infants, exposing them to more deleterious developmental effects, meaning that infants born of a lower weight compared to other VLBWs demonstrated poorer outcome (i.e., poorer behavioral regulation, social skills, and motor skills) [68].

HRV has been associated with emotion regulation processes, where high HRV is associated with emotion adaptability and regulation and low HRV associated with emotion maladaptability and dysregulation. The ability to regulate emotion involves a cognitive component, where cognitive tasks (e.g., such as executive functioning) are predominantly associated with prefrontal cortical activity. As noted previously, the prefrontal cortex functions to tonically inhibit amygdala output. This relation is important because deficits in executive functioning, such as inability to inhibit behavior or inability for the prefrontal cortex to inhibit emotion activation of the amygdala, are present in negative emotional states and dispositions of varying psychopathologies (i.e., depression and anxiety disorders) [70]. It is also important to note that stress can also impair cognitive functioning; the authors suggest that impairment in cognitive functioning may contribute to the cognitive deficits seen in varying mental health disorders. Thus, the authors conclude that when the prefrontal cortex is unable to tonically inhibit control over the amygdala (and sympathetic neural circuits), it may be the explanatory link between psychosomatics and psychopathology.

7. Concluding Remarks

The main objective of this paper was to provide evidence that individuals exposed to a specific, rare type of early adversity, namely, being born at extremely low birth weight (ELBW; i.e., <1000 grams), represent an adverse event. We provided evidence that individuals born ELBW exhibit problems with emotion regulation and are at an increased risk for the development of psychopathology in adulthood (i.e., development of internalizing disorders). In order to demonstrate this connection, we discussed (1) how ELBW represents an adverse event; (2) studies relating ELBW with emotional regulation issues (presented as pathway 1); (3) studies relating early emotional regulation with later internalizing problems (presented as pathway 2); (4) a model in which we hypothesized an association between early adversity (ELBW as the adverse circumstance), emotion dysregulation, and psychopathology; and (5) some perspectives in which measures of frontal EEG asymmetry and cardiac vagal tone might be as putative measures to investigate the conceptual pathways 1 and 2 described in this paper. Given that these psychophysiological measures are open to change, future research might want to consider targeting interventions at this level in order to effectively manage mental health problems in some survivors of ELBW.

References

[1] S. D. Pollak, "Mechanisms linking early experience and the emergence of emotions: illustrations from the study of maltreated children," *Current Directions in Psychological Science*, vol. 17, no. 6, pp. 370–375, 2008.

[2] J. Denollet, I. Nyklícek, and A. J. J. M. Vingerhoets, "Introduction: emotions, emotion regulation, and health," in *Emotion Regulation Conceptual and Clinical Issues*, J. Denollet, I. Nyklícek, and A. J. J. M. Vingerhoets, Eds., pp. 3–11, Springer, New York, NY, USA, 2008.

[3] J. J. Gross and R. F. Munoz, "Emotion regulation and mental health," *Clinical Psychology*, vol. 2, no. 2, pp. 151–164, 1995.

[4] S. D. Pollack, "Early social experience and the ontogenesis of emotion regulatory behavior in children," in *Origins of Altruism and Cooperation*, R. W. Sussman and R. C. Cloninger, Eds., pp. 333–344, Springer, New York, NY, USA, 2011.

[5] K. A. McLaughlin, N. A. Fox, C. H. Zeanah, and C. A. Nelson, "Adverse rearing environments and neural development in children: the development of frontal electroencephalogram asymmetry," *Biological Psychiatry*, vol. 70, no. 11, pp. 1015–1008, 2011.

[6] V. Miskovic, L. A. Schmidt, K. Georgiades, M. Boyle, and H. L. MacMillan, "Stability of resting frontal electroencephalogram (EEG) asymmetry and cardiac vagal tone in adolescent females exposed to child maltreatment," *Developmental Psychobiology*, vol. 51, no. 6, pp. 474–487, 2009.

[7] N. Tottenham, T. A. Hare, B. T. Quinn et al., "Prolonged institutional rearing is associated with atypically large amygdala volume and difficulties in emotion regulation," *Developmental Science*, vol. 13, no. 1, pp. 46–61, 2010.

[8] S. J. Sheinkopf, L. L. Lagasse, B. M. Lester et al., "Vagal tone as a resilience factor in children with prenatal cocaine exposure," *Development and Psychopathology*, vol. 19, no. 3, pp. 649–673, 2007.

[9] L. A. Schmidt, V. Miskovic, M. Boyle, and S. Saigal, "Frontal electroencephalogram asymmetry, salivary cortisol, and internalizing behavior problems in young adults who were born at extremely low birth weight," *Child Development*, vol. 81, no. 1, pp. 183–199, 2010.

[10] S. Saigal, J. Pinelli, L. Hoult, M. M. Kim, and M. Boyle, "Psychopathology and social competencies of adolescents who were extremely low birth weight," *Pediatrics*, vol. 111, no. 5, pp. 969–975, 2003.

[11] S. A. Reijneveld, M. J. K. De Kleine, A. L. Van Baar et al., "Behavioural and emotional problems in very preterm and very low birthweight infants at age 5 years," *Archives of Disease in Childhood*, vol. 91, no. 6, pp. F423–F428, 2006.

[12] K. Mikkola, N. Ritari, V. Tommiska et al., "Neurodevelopmental outcome at 5 years of age of a national cohort of extremely low birth weight infants who were born in 1996–1997," *Pediatrics*, vol. 116, no. 6, pp. 1391–1400, 2005.

[13] S. Johnson, C. Hollis, P. Kochhar, E. Hennessy, D. Wolke, and N. Marlow, "Psychiatric disorders in extremely preterm children: longitudinal finding at age 11 years in the EPICure Study," *Journal of the American Academy of Child and Adolescent Psychiatry*, vol. 49, no. 5, pp. 453.e1–463.e1, 2010.

[14] A. L. Conrad, L. Richman, S. Lindgren, and P. Nopoulos, "Biological and environmental predictors of behavioral sequelae in children born preterm," *Pediatrics*, vol. 125, no. 1, pp. e83–e89, 2010.

[15] L. B. Dahl, P. I. Kaaresen, J. Tunby, B. H. Handegård, S. Kvernmo, and J. A. Rønning, "Emotional, behavioral, social, and academic outcomes in adolescents born with very low birth weight," *Pediatrics*, vol. 118, no. 2, pp. e449–e459, 2006.

[16] J. P. Shonkoff, W. T. Boyce, and B. S. McEwen, "Neuroscience, molecular biology, and the childhood roots of health disparities: building a new framework for health promotion and disease prevention," *Journal of the American Medical Association*, vol. 301, no. 21, pp. 2252–2259, 2009.

[17] D. Vanderbilt and M. M. Gleason, "Mental health concerns of the premature infant through the lifespan," *Pediatric Clinics of North America*, vol. 58, no. 4, pp. 815–832, 2011.

[18] M. L. Chapieski and K. D. Evankovich, "Behavioral effects of prematurity," *Seminars in Perinatology*, vol. 21, no. 3, pp. 221–239, 1997.

[19] C. A. C. Clark, L. J. Woodward, L. J. Horwood, and S. Moor, "Development of emotional and behavioral regulation in children born extremely preterm and very preterm: biological and social influences," *Child Development*, vol. 79, no. 5, pp. 1444–1462, 2008.

[20] R. P. Martin and S. C. Dombrowski, "Low birth weight and prematurity: effects on child developmental outcomes," in *Prenatal Exposures: Psychological and Educational Consequences for Children*, pp. 29–45, Springer, New York, NY, USA, 2008.

[21] B. J. Stoll, N. I. Hansen, I. Adams-Chapman et al., "Neurodevelopmental and growth impairment among extremely low-birth-weight infants with neonatal infection," *Journal of the American Medical Association*, vol. 292, no. 19, pp. 2357–2365, 2004.

[22] R. E. Grunau, D. W. Haley, M. F. Whitfield, J. Weinberg, W. Yu, and P. Thiessen, "Altered basal cortisol levels at 3, 6, 8 and 18 months in infants born at extremely low gestational age," *The Journal of Pediatrics*, vol. 150, no. 2, pp. 151–156, 2007.

[23] R. E. Grunau and M. T. Tu, "Long-term consequences of pain in human neonates," in *Pain in Neonates and Infants*, K. J. S. Anand, B. J. Stevens, and P. J. McGrath, Eds., pp. 45–55, Elsevier B.V., Philadelphia, Pa, USA, 2007.

[24] R. P. Martin and S. C. Dombrowski, "Maternal stress," in *Prenatal Exposures: Psychological and Educational Consequences for Children*, pp. 113–127, Springer, New York, NY, USA, 2008.

[25] C. D. Walker, S. Deschamps, K. Proulx et al., "Mother to infant or infant to mother? Reciprocal regulation of responsiveness to stress in rodents and the implications for humans," *Journal of Psychiatry and Neuroscience*, vol. 29, no. 5, pp. 364–382, 2004.

[26] T. Field, "Prenatal depression effects on the fetus and the newborn," *Infant Behavior and Development*, vol. 27, no. 2, pp. 216–229, 2004.

[27] B. Pierrehumbert, A. Nicole, C. Muller-Nix, M. Forcada-Guex, and F. Ansermet, "Parental post-traumatic reactions after premature birth: implications for sleeping and eating problems in the infant," *Archives of Disease in Childhood*, vol. 88, no. 5, pp. F400–F404, 2003.

[28] N. M. Talge, C. Neal, and V. Glover, "Antenatal maternal stress and long-term effects on child neurodevelopment: how and why?" *Journal of Child Psychology and Psychiatry and Allied Disciplines*, vol. 48, no. 3-4, pp. 245–261, 2007.

[29] M. Forcada-Guex, A. Borghini, B. Pierrehumbert, F. Ansermet, and C. Muller-Nix, "Prematurity, maternal posttraumatic stress and consequences on the mother-infant relationship," *Early Human Development*, vol. 87, no. 1, pp. 21–26, 2011.

[30] N. B. Pitskel, D. Z. Bolling, M. D. Kaiser, M. J. Crowley, and K. A. Pelphrey, "How grossed out are you? The neural bases of emotion regulation from childhood to adolescence," *Developmental Cognitive Neuroscience*, vol. 1, no. 3, pp. 324–337, 2011.

[31] S. B. Perlman and K. A. Pelphrey, "Regulatory brain development: balancing emotion and cognitiont," *Social Neuroscience*, vol. 5, no. 5, pp. 533–542, 2010.

[32] M. D. Lewis and J. Stieben, "Emotion regulation in the brain: conceptual issues and directions for developmental research," *Child Development*, vol. 75, no. 2, pp. 371–376, 2004.

[33] T. Dalgleish, "The emotional brain," *Nature Reviews Neuro-Science*, vol. 5, no. 7, pp. 583–589, 2004.

[34] J. Lowe, B. Woodward, and L.-A. Papile, "Emotional regulation and its impact on development in extremely low birth weight infants," *Journal of Developmental and Behavioral Pediatrics*, vol. 26, no. 3, pp. 209–213, 2005.

[35] K. M. Bohnert and N. Breslau, "Stability of psychiatric outcomes of low birth weight: a longitudinal investigation," *Archives of General Psychiatry*, vol. 65, no. 9, pp. 1080–1086, 2008.

[36] M. Hack, H. G. Taylor, D. Drotar et al., "Chronic conditions, functional limitations, and special health care needs of school-aged children born with extremely low-birth-weight in the 1990s," *Journal of the American Medical Association*, vol. 294, no. 3, pp. 318–325, 2005.

[37] H. G. Taylor, N. Klein, D. Drotar, M. Schluchter, and M. Hack, "Consequences and risks of ¡1000-g birth weight for neuropsychological skills, achievement, and adaptive functioning," *Journal of Developmental and Behavioral Pediatrics*, vol. 27, no. 6, pp. 459–469, 2006.

[38] A. K. Pesonen, K. Räikkönen, K. Heinonen et al., "Personality of young adults born prematurely: the Helsinki study of very low birth weight adults," *Journal of Child Psychology and Psychiatry, and Allied Disciplines*, vol. 49, no. 6, pp. 609–617, 2008.

[39] N. Weisglas-Kuperus, W. Baerts, M. Smrkovsky, and P. J. J. Sauer, "Effects of biological and social factors on the cognitive development of very low birth weight children," *Pediatrics*, vol. 92, no. 5, pp. 658–665, 1993.

[40] R. E. Grunau, M. F. Whitfield, and T. B. Fay, "Psychosocial and academic characteristics of extremely low birth weight (≤800 g) adolescents who are free of major impairment compared with term-born control subjects," *Pediatrics*, vol. 114, no. 6, pp. e725–e732, 2004.

[41] N. Sajaniemi, J. Mäkelä, T. Salokorpi, L. Von Wendt, T. Hämäläinen, and L. Hakamies-Blomqvist, "Cognitive performance and attachment patterns at four years of age in extremely low birth weight infants after early intervention," *European Child and Adolescent Psychiatry*, vol. 10, no. 2, pp. 122–129, 2001.

[42] A. J. Spittle, J. Orton, L. W. Doyle, and R. Boyd, "Early developmental intervention programs post hospital discharge to prevent motor and cognitive impairments in preterm infants," *Cochrane Database of Systematic Reviews*, no. 2, Article ID CD005495, 2007.

[43] J. G. Zwicker and S. R. Harris, "Quality of life of formerly preterm and very low birth weight infants from preschool age to adulthood: a systematic review," *Pediatrics*, vol. 121, no. 2, pp. e366–e376, 2008.

[44] S. Saigal, P. Szatmari, P. Rosenbaum, D. Campbell, and S. King, "Cognitive abilities and school performance of extremely low birth weight children and matched term regional children at age 8 years: a regional study," *The Journal of Pediatrics*, vol. 118, no. 5, pp. 751–760, 1991.

[45] S. Saigal, L. A. Hoult, D. L. Streiner, B. L. Stoskopf, and P. L. Rosenbaum, "School difficulties at adolescence in a regional cohort of children who were extremely low birth weight," *Pediatrics*, vol. 105, no. 2, pp. 325–331, 2000.

[46] K. Werner and J. J. Gross, "Emotion regulation and psychopathology: a conceptual framework," in *Emotion Regulation and Psychopathology: A Transdiagnostic Approach to Etiology and Treatment*, A. M. Kring and D. M. Sloan, Eds., pp. 13–37, Guilford Publications, New York, NY, USA, 2010.

[47] A. Aldao, S. Nolen-Hoeksema, and S. Schweizer, "Emotion-regulation strategies across psychopathology: a meta-analytic review," *Clinical Psychology Review*, vol. 30, no. 2, pp. 217–237, 2010.

[48] J. J. Gross, "The emerging field of emotion regulation: an integrative review," *Review of General Psychology*, vol. 2, no. 3, pp. 271–299, 1998.

[49] J. J. Gross, "Emotion and emotion regulation," in *Handbook of Personality: Theory and Research*, L. A. Pervin and O. P. John, Eds., pp. 525–552, Guildford Press, New York, NY, USA, 1999.

[50] A. Eftekhari, L. A. Zoellner, and S. A. Vigil, "Patterns of emotion regulation and psychopathology," *Anxiety, Stress and Coping*, vol. 22, no. 5, pp. 571–586, 2009.

[51] J. J. Gross, "Emotion regulation in adulthood: timing is everything," *Current Directions in Psychological Science*, vol. 10, no. 6, pp. 214–219, 2001.

[52] A. D. Ong, C. S. Bergeman, T. L. Bisconti, and K. A. Wallace, "Psychological resilience, positive emotions, and successful adaptation to stress in later life," *Journal of Personality and Social Psychology*, vol. 91, no. 4, pp. 730–749, 2006.

[53] M. Rutter, "Implications of resilience concepts for scientific understanding," *Annals of the New York Academy of Sciences*, vol. 1094, pp. 1–12, 2006.

[54] J. Joormann and C. D'Avanzato, "Emotion regulation in depression: examining the role of cognitive processes," *Cognition and Emotion*, vol. 24, no. 6, pp. 913–939, 2010.

[55] J. J. Gross and O. P. John, "Individual differences in two emotion regulation processes: implications for affect, relationships, and well-being," *Journal of Personality and Social Psychology*, vol. 85, no. 2, pp. 348–362, 2003.

[56] N. Garnefski and V. Kraaij, "Relationships between cognitive emotion regulation strategies and depressive symptoms: a comparative study of five specific samples," *Personality and Individual Differences*, vol. 40, no. 8, pp. 1659–1669, 2006.

[57] A. Amstadter, "Emotion regulation and anxiety disorders," *Journal of Anxiety Disorders*, vol. 22, no. 2, pp. 211–221, 2008.

[58] K. Salters-Pedneault, L. Roemer, M. T. Tull, L. Rucker, and D. S. Mennin, "Evidence of broad deficits in emotion regulation associated with chronic worry and generalized anxiety disorder," *Cognitive Therapy and Research*, vol. 30, no. 4, pp. 469–480, 2006.

[59] V. Orgeta, "Emotion dysregulation and anxiety in late adulthood," *Journal of Anxiety Disorders*, vol. 25, no. 8, pp. 11019–11023, 2011.

[60] R. J. Davidson, D. Pizzagalli, J. B. Nitschke, and N. H. Kalin, "Parsing the subcomponents of emotion and disorders of emotion: perspectives from affective neuroscience," in *Handbook of Affective Sciences*, R. J. Davidson, K. R. Scherer, and H. H. Goldsmith, Eds., pp. 8–24, Oxford University Press, New York, NY, USA, 2003.

[61] G. C. Blackhart, J. A. Minnix, and J. P. Kline, "Can EEG asymmetry patterns predict future development of anxiety and depression? A preliminary study," *Biological Psychology*, vol. 72, no. 1, pp. 46–50, 2006.

[62] J. A. Coan and J. J. B. Allen, "Frontal EEG asymmetry as a moderator and mediator of emotion," *Biological Psychology*, vol. 67, no. 1-2, pp. 7–49, 2004.

[63] X. Feng, E. E. Forbes, M. Kovacs et al., "Children's depressive symptoms in relation to EEG frontal asymmetry and maternal depression," *Journal of Abnormal Child Psychology*, vol. 40, no. 2, pp. 265–276, 2012.

[64] R. Thibodeau, R. S. Jorgensen, and S. Kim, "Depression, anxiety, and resting frontal EEG asymmetry: a meta-analytic review," *Journal of Abnormal Psychology*, vol. 115, no. 4, pp. 715–729, 2006.

[65] D. J. A. Smit, D. Posthuma, D. I. Boomsma, and E. J. C. De Geus, "The relation between frontal EEG asymmetry and the risk for anxiety and depression," *Biological Psychology*, vol. 74, no. 1, pp. 26–33, 2007.

[66] D. K. Hannesdóttir, J. Doxie, M. A. Bell, T. H. Ollendick, and C. D. Wolfe, "A longitudinal study of emotion regulation and anxiety in middle childhood: associations with frontal EEG asymmetry in early childhood," *Developmental Psychobiology*, vol. 52, no. 2, pp. 197–204, 2010.

[67] S. W. Porges, "The polyvagal persepctive," *Biological Psychology*, vol. 74, no. 2, pp. 116–143, 2007.

[68] L. Hae-Kyung, "Cardiac vagal tone as an index of autonomic nervous function in healthy newborn and premature infants," *Journal of Korean Academy of Child Health Nursing*, vol. 15, no. 3, pp. 299–305, 2009.

[69] J. A. Doussard-Roosevelt, S. W. Porges, J. W. Scanlon, B. Alemi, and K. B. Scanlon, "Vagal regulation of heart rate in the prediction of developmental outcome for very low birth weight preterm infants," *Child Development*, vol. 68, no. 2, pp. 173–186, 1997.

[70] J. F. Thayer and J. F. Brosschot, "Psychosomatics and psychopathology: looking up and down from the brain," *Psychoneuroendocrinology*, vol. 30, no. 10, pp. 1050–1058, 2005.

"Getting Ready for School:" A Preliminary Evaluation of a Parent-Focused School-Readiness Program

Kimberly G. Noble,[1] Helena Duch,[2] Maria Eugenia Darvique,[2] Alexandra Grundleger,[2] Carmen Rodriguez,[2] and Cassie Landers[2]

[1] *Department of Pediatrics and GH Sergievsky Center, College of Physicians and Surgeons, Columbia University Medical Center, Columbia University New York, NY 10032, USA*
[2] *Department of Population and Family Health, Mailman School of Public Health, Columbia University Medical Center, Columbia University New York, NY 10032, USA*

Correspondence should be addressed to Helena Duch, hd90@columbia.edu

Academic Editor: Susan A. Gelman

Children from disadvantaged backgrounds tend to start school with fewer school readiness skills than their more advantaged peers. Emergent literacy and math skills play an important role in this gap. The family is essential in helping children build these skills, and the active involvement of families is crucial to the success of any intervention for young children. The Getting Ready for School (GRS) program is a parent-focused curriculum designed to help parents equip their children with the skills and enthusiasm necessary for learning when they start school. Parents meet in weekly workshops led by a trained facilitator and implement the curriculum at home with their children. The objective of this pilot study was to assess the promise of the GRS intervention in children participating in an urban Head Start program and to explore parents' responses to the intervention. We hypothesized that participation in GRS would improve school readiness in literacy and math skills, relative to participation in business-as-usual Head Start. Four Head Start classrooms (two randomly selected "intervention" and two "comparison" classrooms) participated in this study. Preliminary analyses suggest that GRS improves school readiness over and above a Head Start-as-usual experience. Implications for early childhood programs and policies are discussed.

1. Introduction

School readiness, or the development of the cognitive, social, and emotional skills necessary for children to enter school ready to learn, creates the foundation for academic success, physical and mental health, and general well-being [1]. Unfortunately, socioeconomic disadvantage tends to lead to large gaps in the development of both the cognitive [2–5] and socioemotional skills [6–8] underlying school readiness [9, 10].

By the time children enter school, disadvantaged children tend to score between one-half and one-full standard deviation lower than other children on reading and math achievement tests [8]. Additionally, socioeconomic disadvantage is associated with problems in children's self-regulation, including difficulties controlling impulses and regulating emotions [3, 4, 7, 8]. Disparities in cognitive and socioemotional development are not ameliorated during the early elementary years. Indeed, gaps in achievement tend to increase with age [10, 11], having vast implications for future life achievement [12–15]. Disadvantaged children of Latino descent are at particular risk for poor school readiness [16–18] and subsequent school failure [19]. Quality preschool programs can reduce the school-readiness gap to some extent [20, 21], although individual interventions tend to have small effect sizes [22] and do not close the achievement gap.

Head Start was founded on the principle that child development is the product of multiple levels of interaction, with both parents and teachers playing unique and important roles [23]. Traditionally, add-on interventions to promote school readiness tend to be classroom based [20]. When considered separately, center-based programs tend to show stronger effects than home-based programs [12]. On one hand, this underscores the importance of the classroom environment. However, parents and teachers independently influence child development [23], with parenting skills directly related to children's later cognitive development and academic achievement [12, 13, 24].

Bioecological theory predicts that parents play a particularly important role in promoting early childhood school readiness [25]. In particular, this theory states that "proximal processes" are a key factor in child development [26–28]. Proximal processes are defined as enduring, complex, reciprocal interactions between a child and the people in his or her immediate environment [28]. Parents may be the most proximal (and therefore most powerful) external influences in children's lives. To the extent that this theory is accurate, we would predict that an intervention which successfully and positively influences parenting may wield particularly strong effects on child development and school readiness.

In the following, two key domains of school readiness are outlined. Evidence regarding the means by which parents contribute to each is discussed.

1.1. Emergent Literacy and Parents. Emergent literacy refers to the skills and reading-like behaviors that are developmental precursors to their more advanced counterparts [29]. It is a key component of school readiness, and early disparities in emergent literacy in preschool tend to be exacerbated through the elementary years [30]. Effective teaching of these skills requires active involvement of the child. For instance, shared book reading benefits oral language development most substantially when the adult actively engages the child in "dialogic reading," in which the adult asks questions and prompts the child to "become the storyteller" [31–33]. Similarly, explicit teaching about print increases letter knowledge and later reading ability, while informal print exposure does not [29, 34, 35].

The degree to which parents actively engage children in explicit practice with letters and sounds is related to children's understanding of printed words [35] controlling for children's independent pursuit of these activities [36]. Randomized trials suggest that when disadvantaged parents are taught strategies to actively engage children in reading, children's emergent literacy skills improve [5, 33, 37]. Further, greater improvements are seen when children are engaged in such strategies both at home and school, relative to school alone [5, 33].

1.2. Emergent Mathematics Skills and Parents. As with emergent literacy, disadvantaged children are less likely to exhibit well-developed mathematics skills and knowledge than their more advantaged counterparts [38–40]. This achievement gap is measurable by preschool and continues throughout the school years [41, 42].

Prior to starting school, young children use math concepts in their play and daily lives [43, 44], and a general learning path for the acquisition of these concepts has been identified for preschoolers [45, 46]. As with language development, passive exposure to math is not enough; structured educational experiences are necessary. While children's everyday activities and play can be excellent vehicles, these activities may not suffice without scaffolding and guidance [46].

Exposure to math concepts in the home can have a positive impact on school readiness [47]. However, low-income homes tend to provide less support for mathematical development relative to their middle-income counterparts [48, 49]. Disadvantaged families are more likely to focus on simpler topics such as counting and shape recognition, rather than on more complex processes such as numerical or geometric reasoning [50]. Further, low-income parents frequently have different expectations about their role in teaching mathematics to their children [49]. One program designed to address these disparities, the Family Mathematics Curriculum (FMC), provides low-income families with a structured mathematical intervention in which parents and children attend family mathematics classes and also have access to math materials for use at home [51]. In two small evaluations with Head Start families, researchers found that children who participated in FMC with their parents had significantly higher scores in the areas of enumeration, numerical reasoning, and an overall math composite relative to children in a control group [51]. This supports the premise that, with adequate supports and materials, parents can have a significant impact on young children's mathematical skills, enhancing overall school readiness.

1.3. The Getting Ready for School Intervention. The Getting Ready for School (GRS) curriculum was originally designed as an intervention for parents in Central and Eastern Europe with limited or no access to preschool. The goal was to teach parents to create more effective home learning environments for their preschool-aged children, by supporting and expanding parents' ability to promote the literacy and math skills children need for success in school.

Subsequently, the GRS curriculum has been implemented in parent groups in a small number of Head Start centers in the US. Translation of the materials into Spanish was completed by a team of bilingual, bicultural staff members at the Head Start where the present study took place, led by one of the lead authors on this study (H. Duch). The GRS curriculum recently received national attention when it was selected by the National Head Start Family Literacy Center as part of their training for 96 Head Start programs participating in the SPARC (Strengthening Partnerships and Resources in Communities for Literacy) program. In addition, the materials were made available to any interested Head Start program. Since May 2010, over 600 Head Start programs around the country have requested the GRS materials and training. As wide dissemination of the materials began to take place, research examining the potential feasibility and efficacy of this intervention became critical.

1.3.1. Structure of the Intervention. GRS is a nine-unit curriculum of activities, available in both English and Spanish, designed to help parents promote young children's school-readiness skills in reading and math. Parents are shown how to use the activities through weekly group sessions led by a Parent Facilitator. The content of the curriculum is described in detail below. Briefly, the materials include the following.

(a) Parent Activity Guide. This guide is a written set of activity suggestions that parents can use with their children. Activities explain how to use the children's materials, provide additional literacy and math activities, and suggest ways to modify or enrich the activities depending upon their child's needs. The Parent Activity Guide is written with pictorial demonstrations of activities, with text requiring only a minimal literacy level.

(b) Children's Activity Sets. These are nine sets of materials focusing on literacy and math designed for use in the above activities. Each set includes pictures, games, and other materials. These materials are distributed in children's backpacks, containing the book of activities as well as crayons, scissors, and paper.

(c) Facilitator's Guide. This Guide provides a set of lesson plans for the Parent Facilitator in running the weekly parent sessions. A written set of activity suggestions is provided that explains how to teach parents to use the children's materials. The Facilitator's Guide also provides suggestions on ways to modify or enrich the activities depending upon the child's needs. Finally, the Facilitator's Guide provides Parent Facilitators with guidance on soliciting reports of parent experiences with the activity sets.

(d) Train-the-Trainer Guide. This guide teaches Parent Facilitators how to run effective parent meetings. It includes a review of early math and literacy development, as well as exercises to help Facilitators develop problem-solving skills around common issues that parents may describe.

1.3.2. Parent Workshops. Through weekly two-hour workshops, Parent Facilitators disseminate and explore the materials with parents, facilitating a parent-teaching process. The materials are designed to be open-ended and help parents tailor activities to their children's interests and abilities. For example, to encourage children's math development, parents are shown how to teach number concepts using games such as counting when cooking. Similarly, to teach important skills that are critical for emergent literacy, parents are shown how to teach children to focus on the first sounds of words used around the house, and their corresponding letters. The Parent Facilitators provide parents with advice—reiterated in the Parent Activity Guide—on how to make activities easier or more challenging, depending on the child's level of development. In the weekly meetings, parents are also encouraged to share stories involving how their children interacted with the materials, and examine any important questions that might have emerged while working with the material at home. During workshops, parents practice math and literacy activities included in the next activity set and explore ways to adapt the activities to address individual learning styles.

1.3.3. Parent Facilitator Training. Prior to teaching the parents, the Parent Facilitators are provided with a detailed series of training activities to help trainers prepare parents to teach their children. Using active and participatory methods, this training includes a review of basic child development con-cepts with an emphasis on early math and literacy hands-on exploration of parents' and children's games and activities, and practice techniques for running effective parent group sessions.

1.3.4. Content of the Intervention: Literacy and Mathematics. Each of the nine units contains approximately ten activities, of which five focus on literacy and five focus on math. The content progression of GRS for each of the 9 units is summarized in Table 1.

Following the model originally constructed by Whitehurst and Lonigan [31], GRS targets emergent literacy through the development of both "outside-in" and "inside-out" skills. "Outside-in" skills represent children's understanding of the linguistic context and include the semantic and conceptual knowledge that comprises oral language, knowledge of narrative structure and narrative-building skills, and print conventions (e.g., left-to-right, front to back). "Inside-out" skills comprise children's knowledge of the rules for translating the particular writing they are trying to read into sounds and include knowledge of graphemes, phonological awareness, phoneme-grapheme correspondence, and emergent writing. Experience with "outside-in" skills fosters the development of oral language and vocabulary, whereas experience with "inside-out" skills fosters the development of early reading skills [52, 53]. These emergent literacy goals and objectives by unit are summarized in Table 2.

In the area of mathematics, GRS follows the guidelines provided by the National Council of Teachers and Mathematics (NCTM) [46] for the acquisition of math concepts in the following areas: numbers and operations, geometry and spatial sense, measurement, algebra, and data analysis [45, 46]. To support the acquisition of these skills, educators have promoted five main processes: problem solving, reasoning, communicating, connecting, and representing [46]. GRS targets early math readiness through the development of these skills and processes, closely matching the math goals and objectives of NCTM (see Table 2).

Both literacy and math activities in GRS teach parents to use everyday interactions in the home and the community as the vehicles for learning. For instance, math activities include using familiar objects (e.g., buttons, laundry, cookware) to solve math problems, learning how math connects with real life (e.g., while cooking, during community walks or trips to the store), estimating numbers and sizes, and exploring shapes. Literacy activities involve learning through songs and poems, making up and telling stories, making books and reading together, building sight vocabulary, reading, drawing, and talking about ideas together, and exploring

Table 1: Content Progression of the "Getting Ready for School" Intervention.

	Literacy	Math
Activity Set 1	Learn letters in their name, sounds associated with those letters, and how to write their name. Words are made up of groups of letters; letters represent sounds; words begin with the letter on the left and ends with the last letter on the right. Learn to recognize words to familiar songs and poems.	Understand that a number represents a set of objects; practice counting, ordering, and comparing groups of objects. Learn to count, write, identify, and represent numbers 1 to 5.
Activity Set 2	Learn the sound associated with certain letters. Emphasize the sound letters make as words are written. Help children make sense of print by talking with them while writing. Help children listen for and repeat the initial sound in his/her name.	Count a set of objects to 10 and identify the numerals 1 through 10. Sort groups of objects and practice observing, describing, and making distinctions between the characteristics of objects. Practice counting to 10.
Activity Set 3	Listen to and discuss family stories. Through interesting discussions children will understand how "stories" work.	Order sets of objects and learn how to compare the relative differences between them—longest to shortest, lightest to darkest, more to less, lightest to heaviest.
Activity Set 4	By conducting interviews children learn how to ask questions to gather information. Use information to create books and stories to share with family and friends.	Recognize, create, and extend patterns. Understand that a pattern is a form of ordering that eventually repeats itself. Make predictions about what happens next based on an understanding of the pattern.
Activity Set 5	Practice making letter-sound connections. Pronounce words as they are written. Emphasize sounds at the beginning, middle, and end of each word.	Understand that geometry is the study of shapes and spatial relationships. Provide children opportunities to relate math to the real world by looking for and naming different shapes.
Activity Set 6	Understand all the reasons why we read and write. For example, to remember information (make a list), communicate information (write a letter), learn new information (read a paper).	Explore numbers one through 20. Understand that the number 12 is represented by one group of 10 plus 2 ones, 15 is presented by one group of 10 plus 5 ones.
Activity Set 7	Learn new words and understand how words are organized into complete sentences. Learn to organize thoughts and make themselves understood. Learn to express their ideas and stories as well as understand the ideas and stories of others.	Add two sets of numbers together to get a total. Play with sets of objects and counting to find the total number.
Activity Set 8	Recall events, retell stories, and speak in complete sentences. Help children master prerequisites for learning to read.	Practice adding to and taking away from sets of objects.
Activity Set 9	Review all the skills learned during the previous 8 sets. Think about and discuss how to identify and discuss children's questions about Kindergarten.	Review math activities from the previous eight sets. Observe the ways children's approaches differ now from when they did the task earlier. Make up number riddles to challenge children to think about numbers one to twenty.

sound-symbol relationships in everyday life. Each unit builds on the previous unit with content becoming increasingly more complex as the child moves from unit to unit.

1.4. Objectives of the Present Study. We conducted a mixed-methods study to obtain quantitative and qualitative information on the preliminary effectiveness and usability of the GRS intervention. Both quantitative and qualitative data addressed our primary objective: to assess whether the Getting Ready for School parent-focused intervention improves school-readiness skills. A small, quasi-experimental pilot study was conducted with a group of urban Latino preschool children participating in Head Start. We hypothesized that participation in the GRS curriculum would improve school readiness in literacy and math skills, relative to participation in business-as-usual Head Start. Additionally, qualitative data from parent focus groups addressed parental perceptions of children's improvements in these skills. Qualitative data also addressed our secondary objective: to assess parental perceptions of day-to-day use of the GRS intervention.

2. Method

2.1. Participants. Four classrooms in an urban Head Start program were targeted to participate in the study. Two classrooms were randomized to serve as the intervention classrooms, and two served as comparison classrooms. Randomization occurred at the classroom level in an attempt to reduce contamination between participants. Of the 56 children served by these classrooms who participated in this study,

Table 2: Emergent literacy and math objectives by unit.

	GRS Literacy Objectives	GRS Activity Set
"Outside-In Skills"	*Language*—Semantic and conceptual knowledge	1, 2, 3, 4, 5, 6, 7, 8, 9
	Narrative—Understanding and producing narrative	1, 2, 3, 4, 5, 6, 7, 8, 9
	Conventions of print—Knowledge of standard print format	1, 2, 3, 4, 5, 6, 7, 8, 9
	Emergent reading—Pretending to read	1, 2, 3, 5, 6, 7, 8, 9
"Inside-Out Skills"	*Knowledge of graphemes*—letter name knowledge	1, 2, 3, 4, 5, 6, 7, 8
	Phonological awareness—detection of rhyme, manipulation of syllables, manipulation of individual phonemes	1, 2, 3, 5, 6, 7, 8
	Syntactic awareness—repair grammatical errors	3
	Phoneme-grapheme correspondence—letter-sound knowledge, pseudoword decoding	1, 2, 3, 4, 5, 6, 7, 8
	Emergent writing—phonetic spelling	2, 4, 6, 7, 8, 9
	GRS Math Objectives	**GRS Activity Set**
	Numbers and operations	1, 2, 3, 4, 5, 6, 7, 8, 9
	Geometry and spatial sense	4, 5, 9
	Measurement	1, 2, 3, 4, 5, 6, 7, 9
	Algebra	1, 2, 3, 4, 5, 6, 7, 8, 9
	Data analysis	1, 2, 3, 4, 5, 6, 7, 8, 9

Table 3: Demographics by group.

		Intervention ($n = 26$)	Comparison ($n = 30$)	P
Mean age in months at pretest (SD)		46.9 (6.2)	45.6 (7.1)	0.48
Ethnicity (%)	Hispanic or Latino	25 (96%)	28 (93%)	0.24
	Asian	0	2 (7%)	
	Other	1 (4%)	0	
Primary language spoken at home (%)	Spanish	25 (96%)	26 (87%)	0.19
	English	0	3 (10%)	
	Other	1 (4%)	1 (3%)	
Maternal education (%)	Less than high school	14 (54%)	12 (40%)	0.32
	GED or high school	3 (12%)	9 (30%)	
	Some postsecondary school	1 (4%)	4 (13%)	
	Associate degree	1 (4%)	1 (3%)	
	BS or advanced degree	5 (19%)	3 (10%)	
	Other/did not respond	2 (8%)	1 (3%)	

There were no significant demographic differences between groups.

26 were in the GRS intervention classrooms, and 30 participated in Head Start-as-usual classrooms.

Children were 3 to 4 years old at the start of the study (mean age at pretest = 46.2 months, s.d. 6.7). Demographic information was obtained from Head Start records. Ninety-five percent of all participants self-identified as Hispanic or Latino, 91% spoke primarily Spanish at home, and 70% of parents had a high school education or less. Table 3 shows that there were no demographic differences between groups.

Fifty-six children provided pretest data, before the start of the intervention. There were 7 children (1 intervention, 6 comparison) from whom posttest data were not available following completion of the intervention. Of these children, 4 were no longer in the Head Start program and 3 (including the 1 intervention child) did not attend posttest assessments. These children did not significantly differ in terms of age, ethnicity, language spoken at home, or parent education from the remaining children (all P's > 0.6). The remaining 49 children on whom both pre- and posttest data are available constitute the participants in the analyses below.

2.2. Materials and Procedure. The GRS intervention was implemented in an urban Head Start program in Northern Manhattan in sequential Spring and Fall semesters. Prior to the present study, the program had previously implemented GRS in one classroom per semester for two years. This Head Start program operates as a combination model where children and their parents/caregivers participate in biweekly 3.5-hour classroom experiences and receive a monthly home visit. While children are in the preschool classroom, parents/caregivers participate in various educational and vocational workshops. At the time of the study, two GRS-naïve classrooms were randomly selected to receive the GRS intervention. Two additional GRS-naïve classrooms in the Head Start program were randomly selected as comparison groups and offered the intervention at a later date.

Before the GRS implementation began, all parents in the intervention and comparison classrooms were informed of the procedures of the study and were invited to allow their children to participate in the collection of behavioral data before and after the study. GRS was implemented at the classroom level regardless of parents' consent to participate in the study. Additionally, parents in the intervention classrooms were invited to attend a focus group following completion of the study. Informed consent was obtained according to the policies of the Columbia University Institutional Review Board.

2.2.1. Facilitator Training. Parents from both intervention classrooms received workshops led by a bilingual, bicultural Parent Facilitator who had previously been trained by the curriculum developer following the activities in the Train-the-Trainer Manual.

2.2.2. Parent Workshops. Families in the GRS intervention group participated in a weekly 2-hour workshop for 15 weeks focusing on promoting young children's school-readiness skills in reading and math. A trained, bilingual, bicultural facilitator led the parent workshops according to lessons in the Parent Facilitator Guide.

2.2.3. Child Cognitive Testing. Prior to the start of the intervention, participating children from both the intervention and comparison groups were pulled out of their regular classroom by a bilingual, trained research assistant for 20–30 minutes to participate in a brief assessment of early literacy, oral language, and early mathematics skills. This procedure was repeated at the end of the intervention period, approximately 5 months after the pretest (mean = 157 days between testing sessions, s.d. 15 days, with no difference in latency between groups (t (46) = −1.71; P = 0.1). Children's language dominance was established by classroom teacher reports based on teacher's ongoing language assessment conducted in the Head Start program using the Work Sampling System method. Children were tested in their dominant language accordingly.

Language and Emergent Literacy Skills were tested using the following subtests from the Woodcock-Johnson Test of Academic Achievement (WJ III)/*Batería III Woodcock-Muñoz* [54]: *Letter-Word Identification, Passage Comprehension, Understanding Directions,* and *Picture Vocabulary Subscales.* The Letter-Word Identification test involves asking the child to identify printed letters and later to read printed words aloud. The Understanding Directions subtest tests measures of oral language comprehension by asking the child to follow increasingly commands of increasing linguistic complexity. The Spelling subtest assesses children's ability to print letters and words. The Picture Vocabulary subtest assesses oral language and lexical knowledge.

Math Skills were tested using the *Applied Problems* and *Quantitative Concepts* Subscales of the WJIII/Bateria Woodcock-Munoz. Applied Problems measures the child's ability to analyze and solve math problems. Initial items involve counting and identifying the number of objects in a picture, progressing to more complex calculations. Quantitative Concepts measures knowledge of mathematical concepts, including counting, identifying numbers, shapes, and sequences.

2.2.4. Parent Focus Groups. At the end of the intervention session, parents were invited to participate in a focus group to share their experiences with the GRS curriculum. Grounded theory [55] guided the design and analysis of focus groups. The aim was to generate a general explanation/description of the perceived effectiveness and user-friendliness of the intervention based on the views and opinions of participating parents. While our quantitative analyses were hypothesis driven, we used an inductive approach to analyze data from focus groups, responding to two general research questions: (1) What are families' perceptions of the efficacy of the intervention and how well it works? And (2) what are families' perceptions of the day-to-day use of the GRS intervention? [56].

Following Strauss and Corbin's analytic procedures [57], focus group data were transcribed and later analyzed using open and selective coding [57]. During open coding, data were broken into categories representing emergent themes about the GRS intervention. Selective coding was utilized to determine core categories and describe relationships among the categories.

3. Results

To test the short-term impact of the GRS intervention in this small pilot study, several analyses were conducted. First, scores on standardized tests of language, emergent literacy, and math skills were analyzed to determine whether participation in the intervention led to increased improvement over time, relative to business-as-usual Head Start. Second, data from focus groups were analyzed to understand parents' responses to the GRS intervention, including their initial perceptions of its effectiveness and user-friendliness.

3.1. Literacy and Math Testing. Means and standard deviations of raw scores on each task for children in the intervention and comparison groups are shown in Table 4. At pretest, one child in the intervention group did not complete the Spelling subtest, and one child in the comparison group did not complete the Picture Vocabulary or Quantitative Concepts subtest. All children remaining at the study at the time of the posttest completed all subtests.

There were no significant differences between groups in any of the pretest scores (independent samples t-tests; all P's > 0.1). In all the following analyses, raw scores are used, with age in months entered as a covariate.

TABLE 4: Language and math performance by group, before and after the intervention period[a].

Subtest	Time	Intervention			Comparison		
		N	Mean	Standard Deviation	*N*	Mean	Standard Deviation
Letter-word identification	Pre	26	3.8	2.9	30	3.8	3.2
	Post	25	6.4	3.7	24	5.6	4.0
Understanding directions	Pre	26	7.4	3.8	30	6.6	2.9
	Post	25	11.0	5.9	24	10.2	4.4
Spelling	Pre	25	4.2	2.4	30	3.4	2.2
	Post	25	7.2	3.0	24	5.6	2.1
Applied problems	Pre	26	6.8	3.2	30	6.5	3.3
	Post	25	10.5	3.9	24	8.3	4.0
Picture vocabulary	Pre	26	13.5	4.4	29	12.1	3.6
	Post	25	15.8	3.2	24	13.7	3.7
Quantitative concepts	Pre	26	5.1	2.6	29	4.2	2.1
	Post	25	6.9	2.2	24	6.2	2.0

[a]Means and standard deviations of raw scores for each task for the intervention and comparison groups. There were no significant differences between groups in any of the pretest scores (all P's > 0.1).

TABLE 5: Multivariate General Linear Model showing the hypothesized overall time ∗ group interaction[a].

Effect		*F*	Partial Eta squared	Sig.
Between subjects	Intercept	5.600	0.463	0.000
	Age	17.056	0.724	0.000
	Group (GRS versus Comparison)	1.409	0.178	0.236
Within subjects	Time (pre versus post)	2.055	0.240	0.081
	Time ∗ age	1.518	0.189	0.198
	Time ∗ group	**2.515**	**0.279**	**0.037**

[a]To test the hypothesis that children whose parents received the GRS intervention would improve more over time relative to children whose parents received business-as-usual involvement at Head Start, a multivariate repeated measures General Linear Model was run, with scores on all six pre- and posttests entered as the dependent variables, with time entered as the within-group variable (2 levels: pre and post), with intervention group entered as the between-group variable (2 levels: intervention and comparison), and with age at pretest entered as a covariate. As predicted, a significant time ∗ group interaction was found, suggesting that, overall, children in the intervention group improved more than children in the comparison group (F (6, 39) = 2.5; $P < 0.037$).

To test the hypothesis that children whose parents received the GRS intervention would improve more over time relative to children whose parents received business-as-usual involvement at Head Start, a multivariate repeated measures General Linear Model (GLM) was performed, with time as the within-group variable (2 levels: pre and post), intervention as the between-group variable (2 levels: intervention and comparison), and age in months at pretest entered as a covariate. As would be expected, there was a main effect on raw score of age at pretest (F (6, 39) = 17.1; $P < .000$). There was no main effect of time or group. However, as predicted, a significant time ∗ group interaction was found (F (6, 39) = 2.5; $P < 0.037$), confirming that Head Start children whose parents received GRS showed more overall growth in skills relative to children who were enrolled in Head Start-as-usual (see Table 5).

Pos thoc tests of individual subtests revealed that Applied Problems demonstrated a significant time ∗ group interaction (F (1, 46) = 5.9; $P < 0.019$), such that the intervention group improved significantly more than the comparison group (see Table 6). Additionally, Figure 1 illustrates that the change from pretest to posttest is in the predicted direction for most subtests, with a more positive slope in the intervention group in four out of the six tests. Thus, preliminary short-term evidence from a small sample suggests that GRS may improvecertain school-readiness skills over and above a Head Start-as-usual experience.

3.2. Focus Groups. Based on grounded theory [55], focus groups elicited open-ended responses from families in response to their participation in the intervention. Qualitative data were assessed according to our two study objectives: (1) our primary objective of assessing GRS' effectiveness and (2) our secondary objective of assessing parents' impressions of day-to-day usability of the GRS intervention. Regarding the first objective, parents reported positive gains in children's literacy and mathematics skills. In addition, the central and most prevalent theme related to the effectiveness of the intervention was parents' report of "learning about learning," providing a preliminary hypothesis about a possible mechanism of change. Regarding the second objective, several themes emerged, as summarized in the following.

TABLE 6: General Linear Models for Individual Literacy and Math Subtests[a].

Subtest	Factor	F	Sig
Letter-Word ID	Time (Pre versus Post)	0.079	0.780
	Group (Intervention versus Comparison)	0.038	0.846
	Age at Pretest	1.725	0.196
	Time ∗ Age	0.237	0.629
	Time ∗ Group	1.072	0.306
Understanding Directions	Time (Pre versus Post)	0.106	0.746
	Group (Intervention versus Comparison)	0.300	0.587
	Age at Pretest	7.104	0.011
	Time ∗ Age	0.175	0.678
	Time ∗ Group	0.005	0.947
Spelling	Time (Pre versus Post)	1.501	0.227
	Group (Intervention versus Comparison)	4.103	0.049
	Age at Pretest	17.503	0.000
	Time ∗ Age	0.010	0.919
	Time ∗ Group	2.400	0.128
Applied Problems	Time (Pre versus Post)	0.304	0.584
	Group (Intervention versus Comparison)	1.129	0.294
	Age at Pretest	44.827	0.000
	Time ∗ Age	3.100	0.085
	Time ∗ Group	**5.915**	**0.019**
Picture Vocabulary	Time (Pre versus Post)	1.828	0.183
	Group (Intervention versus Comparison)	3.535	0.067
	Age at Pretest	35.075	0.000
	Time ∗ Age	0.792	0.378
	Time ∗ Group	0.834	0.366
Quantitative Concepts	Time (Pre versus Post)	5.856	0.020
	Group (Intervention versus Comparison)	2.395	0.129
	Age at Pretest	27.063	0.000
	Time ∗ Age	2.041	0.160
	Time ∗ Group	0.734	0.396

[a]Separate General Linear Models show that the Applied Problems subtest demonstrated a significant Time ∗ Group interaction.

Primary Aim: Effectiveness of the GRS Intervention

3.2.1. Perceived Effectiveness of the GRS Intervention. Overwhelmingly parents reported seeing positive changes in their children's literacy and math skills in response to their participation in the GRS intervention. Parents explained changes they saw in their children's skills and attitudes towards learning. In their own words,

> *The program introduced him to math, reading, writing... it took him to another level. This is going to help him in the future, in school.*

> *I think he learned most about math: numbers, shapes, sorting. He learned about letters too but the math was really new.*

> *I see much change in her enthusiasm. She wants to do work, she initiates it and seems to have develop a habit of wanting to read, write, draw... She asks me to read to her more often. She is always saying "please read again!"*

3.2.2. Learning about Learning. The most persistent theme in focus groups was parents' notion that GRS taught them about *how* to teach/support their children's learning. Parents frequently discussed an increased focus on valuing children's process versus outcomes, asking open-ended questions, engaging children in conversation, problem-solving activities, and learning to be patient with children and to follow their pace as they made progress. This theme may represent a potential mechanism of change underlying the improvements observed in overall school-readiness skills among the children participating in the intervention. Representative comments include the following:

> *Whenever my son made a picture, I used to always ask him "what is it?" and he usually did not say anything. Now I ask him to tell me about his*

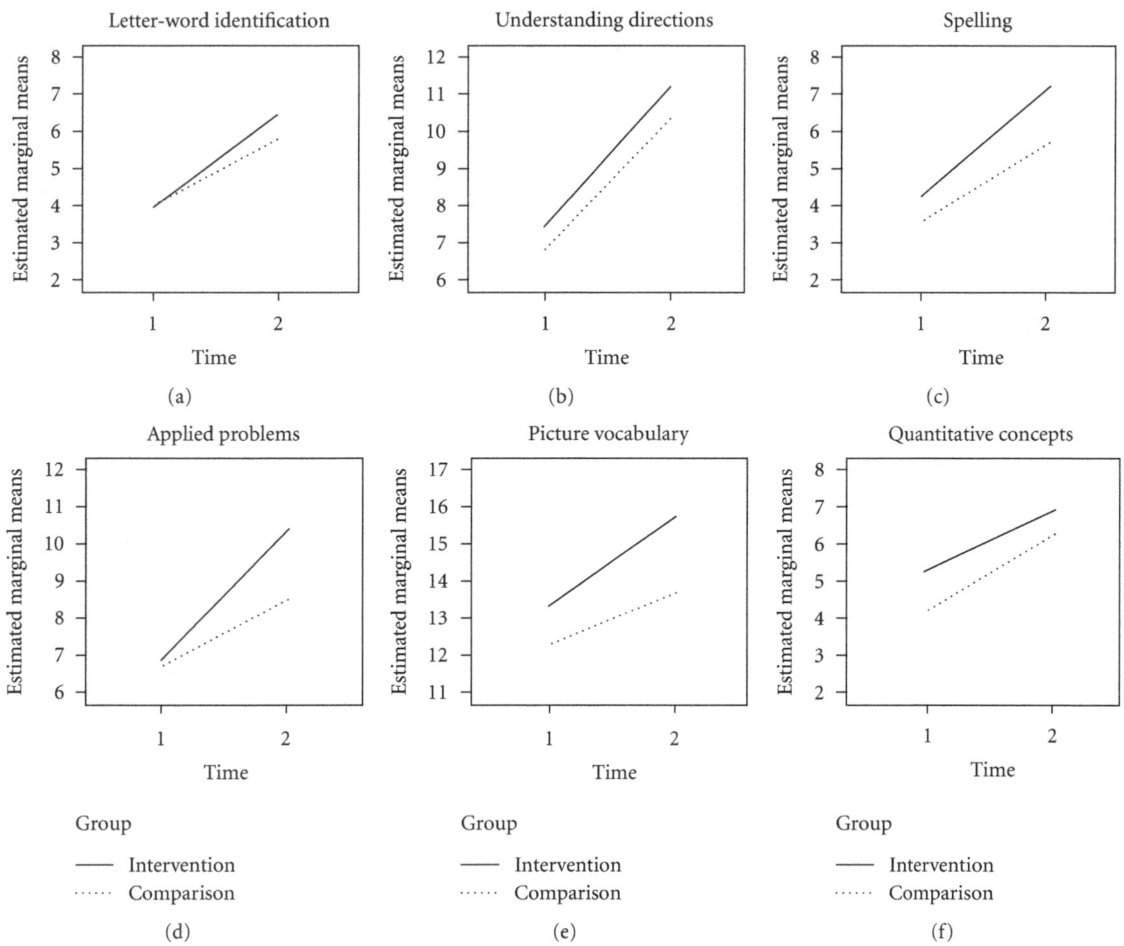

Figure 1: Language and math performance over time by group. The direction of the interaction is in the predicted direction for most subtests, with a more positive slope in the intervention group in four out of the six tests. (Note that the scale is the same for all subtests, but the intercept varies according to the range of raw scores.) This provides preliminary short-term evidence from a small sample to suggest that GRS may lead to improvement in some of children's school-readiness skills over and above a Head Start-as-usual experience.

> *picture, the colors, the shapes and we have much longer conversations.*
>
> *I really learned how to organize myself and be more patient in working with my daughter. When we are reading a story, I know what to ask her and now she asks those questions herself. I feel like reading is the base of everything. The book we got had many elements to help us read to our children, reading and understanding reading. That was excellent.*
>
> *We are our children's first teachers and these tools really helped me know how to prepare him for school.*

Secondary Aim: General response to use of the GRS intervention.

3.2.3. Need for Parent/Teacher Coordinated Efforts. Parents consistently requested that the classroom teachers should engage in similar activities in the classroom. Parents wanted playful learning for their children that focused on the same literacy and math areas targeted in the GRS curriculum. Parents reported that having a coordinated effort between them and the teachers would improve their children's outcomes and also help them provide continuity of experiences in the home. In their own words,

> *I think we should also give this book to the classroom teachers. They spend many hours with our children and... this way we would be doubly beneficial for the children and for us too, the teachers can help us keep our minds a little more open about education.*
>
> *I am a substitute teacher, as well as a parent. For me the book was very useful, not just with my daughter but in my classroom. I took many ideas from the book and it really helped me as a teacher. For example, I never really focused on mathematics, other than counting, I did not know what else to do... now I have many ideas.*

3.2.4. Making the Time. Parents were asked to work with their children on a daily basis. They talked about how challenging it was to make time when they are busy with work, other children, housework, and so forth. However, there was an overwhelming desire expressed by families to "make the time." Parents described how a little bit of time was all that was necessary and that children would frequently continue to be engaged in games or activities after parents had moved to other tasks. They also described realizing how sometimes one need not make explicit time, but rather just include the child in daily activities as these can serve as learning experiences as well.

> *There never is enough time... one has to learn what their priorities are. If your child is your priority, then you find the time.*
>
> *I did not know that my son could help me cook and that if he did, maybe I could teach him to count, measure... He loves being my helper.*

3.2.5. Involving Other Family Members. Parents described how part of making the time was also including other family members, predominantly spouses and older children. Busy lives made some parents ask other parents or older children to join in the GRS activities. Some mothers described the GRS book as a tool to explain to the child's father the kind of learning that was taking place in school.

> *I had to involve my husband. After he comes home from work and has a rest, I ask him to spend some time doing activities with our girl. This way he also joins us. When he gets home, my girl says "mami, papi...let us go do work!"*
>
> *I shared the materials with my cousin who lives in Queens. Her children do not go to any Head Start or any program so she is very interested in what I give her. I see her every weekend and pass on the materials from the class.*

3.2.6. Challenges. Families described some difficulty working with their children on the curriculum calendars. In particular, it was difficult to explain the concept of time to preschoolers. Other games, especially some of those related to math skills, were difficult to implement since parents themselves had little experience with them (e.g., Dominos). They also requested more strategies to help their children sustain attention during tasks and manage challenging behaviors that took place while engaged in the materials.

> *I also want to learn some specific ways to help him pay more attention and persist when things that he has to do are difficult. I think he has made some progress but I would like more ideas.*

3.2.7. Packaging of Materials. Families reported positive impressions of the packaging of the materials. They described their children responding positively to the pictures, the games and the backpack.

> *For Thanksgiving, we all went around the table saying what we are grateful for. When it was my son's turn, he said "I am thankful for my school backpack with games."*
>
> *I like that all the pictures are in black and white because after we played a game or talked about a picture, we would spend time coloring it. We have put some of those pictures in her room now, as decorations.*

4. Discussion

The primary objective of this study was to assess whether a parent-focused school-readiness intervention would have an effect on the early math and literacy skills of low-income children of predominantly Latino descent. In addition, we aimed to explore parents' perceptions of the effectiveness of the intervention, as well as parental responses to the day-to-day usability of the materials. The preliminary results presented previously suggest that a targeted intervention that actively involves parents has the potential to improve children's school-readiness skills over and above a Head Start-as-usual experience. Further, qualitative data obtained from focus groups highlight the overwhelmingly positive response of parents to the materials. In addition, the qualitative data point to a possible mechanism for the change observed in the quantitative study. Overwhelmingly, parents talked about learning about how their children learn and acquiring skills and tools to facilitate children's learning. Together, these results highlight the important role that parent-based, targeted interventions can have in the emergent school-readiness skills of preschool children.

Evidence-based interventions can improve the degree to which disadvantaged children are ready for school and in turn can have long-lasting ramifications for educational and life achievement. However, individual programs typically only report modest gains [22]. As parents and teachers independently influence school readiness [23], one promising approach to narrowing the gap in school readiness may be to harness the power of parents to reinforce the critical skills taught in school, thereby providing support for these two independent sources of learning. Indeed, programs targeting both parents and teachers have increased potential to affect outcomes [12, 58, 59].

This study thus provides some support to bioecological theory, which suggests that human development requires "proximal processes," or progressively complex reciprocal interactions between children and people in their immediate environment [26–28]. To the extent that parent-child interactions represent the most proximal—and thus most powerful—processes in children's lives, one would expect that interventions aimed at directly altering these processes may wield particularly strong effects on child development. Indeed, Bronfenbrenner [25] postulated that the family may be the most effective and economical system for fostering and sustaining early child development. He further stated that interventions targeted directly at parents tend to be particularly effective, as they may serve as a catalyst for sustaining and enhancing the effects of classroom intervention [25]. In the context of the preliminary results presented here, we may theorize that GRS may directly affect parenting, which in turn may amplify the effects of classroom literacy and math pedagogy.

Socioeconomically disadvantaged Latino children are at particular risk for poor school readiness [16–18] and yet remain an under-studied and underserved group. The GRS materials are available in both English and Spanish, require only a minimal parent literacy level, and in the present study were administered by a fully bilingual, bicultural team. Qualitative data obtained from focus groups suggest that parents enjoyed and felt comfortable with the materials. More detailed examination of the cross-cultural relevance of the program is warranted prior to wider dissemination of the materials.

4.1. Limitations of the Present Study. This pilot study evaluated the potential of the Getting Ready for School intervention to improve disadvantaged preschooler's early literacy and math skills. Though potentially promising, the study's small sample size renders these results preliminary. Further research must be conducted with larger groups of children and parents to fully assess the feasibility and efficacy of this intervention.

Randomization of the intervention occurred at the classroom level, rather than at the family level, to reduce contamination between the intervention and comparison groups. The lack of randomization at the family level was mitigated in part by the fact that intervention and comparison families did not differ on key demographic factors. Nonetheless, future research using a design randomized at the family level will be necessary for rigorously testing the efficacy of the program.

In addition, the data collected here have a nested structure, with families nested in classrooms. Although multilevel models would not have had sufficient power to detect treatment effects in this small pilot study, future work with a larger sample will have the power to fully consider and investigate the nested structure of the data.

The present study sample consisted nearly entirely of disadvantaged Latino preschoolers and their mothers. Further work should be conducted with a diverse population to assess the generalizability of the intervention with other socioeconomic and ethnic groups.

This study did not measure the fidelity of implementation of the GRS intervention. The results of this study would suggest that parents engaged in literacy- and math-promoting activities at home, but we are uncertain of the specific activities or processes they used. Measuring fidelity of implementation at the home level might also shed some light over the mechanisms of change for this intervention as well as allow for comparison between groups of parents who had low and high adherence to curriculum guidelines.

4.2. Future Directions. While the current implementation of GRS focuses exclusively on parents, future work will attempt to more fully integrate the GRS curriculum for use by both parents and teachers. By supporting classroom and home learning experiences in parallel, we may take advantage of these independent sources of variance, leading to an additive benefit [5, 12, 60]. This idea was often articulated by parents during focus groups who wanted their children's classroom teachers to "support the same work they were doing." Additional research on the additive effects of interventions that place equal weight on parent and classroom practices will be important in understanding the mechanisms by which interventions exert positive effects.

Additionally, the current implementation of GRS is focused on improving literacy and math readiness. While an evidence-based focus on these skills is critical, recent research highlights the complementary importance of early self-regulation skills [61–63]. Accumulating evidence suggests that both cognitive and self-regulation skills are independently important for academic success [64]. Additionally, focus groups with GRS parents noted the need for skill building to help maintain children's "attention to activities" and "reduce frustration when faced with challenges." Thus, the addition of a self-regulation component might strengthen the curriculum. In fact, several recent investigations have revealed that preschool programs focused jointly on self-regulation and other aspects of school readiness can be effective [65–69].

Finally, future research should consider additional factors and pathways that may contribute to the acquisition of literacy and math in the home, such as the availability of materials and exposure to educational programs/practices. While there is no evidence to suggest that differences in these areas were present between the intervention and the comparison classrooms in the present study, these factors may mediate or interact with school-readiness interventions in important ways.

5. Conclusions

The results of this preliminary study demonstrate that a targeted parent-focused program may be effective in supporting the development of school-readiness skills of disadvantaged preschool children. However, early childhood programs need the funding and guidance necessary to implement the kinds of interventions that will maximize parents' involvement in their children's learning. Assistance needs to be provided to Head Start programs in identifying and implementing evidence-based interventions to help build the skills of parents in supporting children's school readiness. In addition, significant professional development is needed to help staff develop the necessary skills to help parents support children's learning. Further research is necessary to understand how to best accomplish this goal. It is not just what materials we share with parents but how those materials are presented that maximizes the likelihood of feasibility, fidelity of implementation, and positive learning outcomes for children. We also must strive to understand how these programs intersect with existing cultural practices, the home learning environment, and the larger community.

Authors' Contributions

Kimberly G. Noble and Helena Duch contributed equally to this work.

Acknowledgment

The authors gratefully acknowledge the help of Maria Gonzalez, Katherine Mora, the families and children who participated, and the generous funding of the Farber Foundation. The authors thank the Open Society Foundation for their support in the initial development and implementation of the Getting Ready for School initiative.

References

[1] Task Force on Community Preventive Services, "Promoting health through the social environment: early childhood development programs," in *Guide to Community Preventive Services*, 2010.

[2] R. H. Bradley, R. F. Corwyn, H. P. McAdoo, and C. García Coll, "The home environments of children in the United States Part I: variations by age, ethnicity, and poverty status," *Child Development*, vol. 72, no. 6, pp. 1844–1867, 2001.

[3] K. G. Noble, M. F. Norman, and M. J. Farah, "Neurocognitive correlates of socioeconomic status in kindergarten children," *Developmental Science*, vol. 8, no. 1, pp. 74–87, 2005.

[4] K. G. Noble, B. D. McCandliss, and M. J. Farah, "Socioeconomic gradients predict individual differences in neurocognitive abilities," *Developmental Science*, vol. 10, no. 4, pp. 464–480, 2007.

[5] G. J. Whitehurst, "Language processes in context: language learning in children reared in poverty," in *Research on Communication and Language Disorders: Contribution to Theories of Language Development*, L. B. Adamson and M. A. Romski, Eds., pp. 233–266, Brookes Publishing, Baltimore, Md, USA, 1997.

[6] A. W. Gottfried, A. E. Gottfried, K. Bathurst, D. W. Guerin, and M. M. Parramore, "Socioeconomic status in children's development and family environment: infancy through adolescence," in *Socioeconomic Status, Parenting and Child Development*, M. H. Bornstein and R. H. Bradley, Eds., pp. 189–207, Lawrence Erlbaum Associates, Mahwah, NJ, USA, 2003.

[7] S. E. Rimm-Kaufman, R. C. Pianta, and M. J. Cox, "Teachers' judgments of problems in the transition to kindergarten," *Early Childhood Research Quarterly*, vol. 15, no. 2, pp. 147–166, 2000.

[8] C. Rouse, J. Brooks-Gunn, and S. McLanahan, "Introducing the issue. School readiness: closing racial and ethnic gaps," *Future of Children*, vol. 15, no. 1, pp. 3–14, 2005.

[9] P. C. High and Committee on Early Childhood Adoption and Dependent Care and Council on School Health, "School readiness," *Pediatrics*, vol. 121, pp. e1008–e1015, 2008.

[10] J. West, K. Denton, and E. Germino-Hausken, *America's Kindergartener's: Findings from the Early Childhood Longitudinal Study, Kindergarten Class of 1998-99*, National Center for Education Statistics, Washington, DC, USA, 2001.

[11] L. Feinstein, "Inequality in the early cognitive development of British children in the 1970 cohort," *Economica*, vol. 70, no. 277, pp. 73–97, 2003.

[12] J. Brooks-Gunn and L. B. Markman, "The contribution of parenting to ethnic and racial gaps in school readiness," *Future of Children*, vol. 15, no. 1, pp. 139–168, 2005.

[13] J. Brooks-Gunn, "Do you believe in magic? What can we expect from early childhood intervention programs?" *Social Policy Report of the Society for Research in Child Development*, vol. 17, no. 1, pp. 3–14, 2003.

[14] J. Bennett, *Investment in Population Health in Five OECD Countries*, Organization for Economic Cooperation and Development, Paris, France, 2003.

[15] N. Baydar, J. Brooks-Gunn, and F. F. Furstenberg, "Early warning signs of functional illiteracy: predictors in childhood and adolescence," *Child Development*, vol. 64, no. 3, pp. 815–829, 1993.

[16] C. Galindo and B. Fuller, "The social competence of Latino kindergartners and growth in mathematical understanding," *Developmental Psychology*, vol. 46, no. 3, pp. 579–592, 2010.

[17] M. Quirk, M. Furlong, E. Lilles, E. Felix, and J. Chin, "Preliminary development of a kindergarten school readiness assessment for Latino students," *Journal of Applied School Psychology*, vol. 27, no. 1, pp. 77–102, 2011.

[18] J. Brooks-Gunn and L. B. Markman, "The contribution of parenting to ethnic and racial gaps in school readiness," *Future of Children*, vol. 15, no. 1, pp. 139–168, 2005.

[19] M. Berends and R. V. Penaloza, "Increasing racial isolation and test score gaps in mathematics: a 30-year perspective," *Teachers College Record*, vol. 112, no. 4, pp. 978–1007, 2010.

[20] K. A. Magnuson and J. Waldfogel, "Early childhood care and education: effects on ethnic and racial gaps in school readiness," *Future of Children*, vol. 15, no. 1, pp. 169–196, 2005.

[21] L. M. Anderson, C. Shinn, M. T. Fullilove et al., "The effectiveness of early childhood development programs: a systematic review," *American Journal of Preventive Medicine*, vol. 24, supplement 3, pp. 32–46, 2003.

[22] G. D. Borman, G. M. Hewes, L. T. Overman, and S. Brown, "Comprehensive school reform and achievement: a meta-analysis," *Review of Educational Research*, vol. 73, no. 2, pp. 125–230, 2003.

[23] U. Bronfenbrenner, "Making human beings human: bioecological perspectives on human development," in *Making Human Beings Human: Bioecological Perspectives on Human Development xxix*, p. 306, Sage Publications, Thousand Oaks, Calif, USA, 2005.

[24] M. Burchinal, J. E. Roberts, S. A. Zeisel, E. A. Hennon, and S. Hooper, "Social risk and protective child, parenting, and child care factors in early elementary school years," *Parenting: Science and Practice*, vol. 6, no. 1, pp. 79–113, 2006.

[25] U. Bronfenbrenner, "Is early intervention effective?" *Early Childhood Education Journal*, vol. 2, no. 2, pp. 14–18, 1974.

[26] U. Bronfenbrenner and S. J. Ceci, "Nature-nurture reconceptualized in developmental perspective: a bioecological model," *Psychological Review*, vol. 101, no. 4, pp. 568–586, 1994.

[27] U. Bronfenbrenner and G. W. Evans, "Developmental science in the 21st century: emerging questions, theoretical models, research designs and empirical findings," *Social Development*, vol. 9, no. 1, pp. 115–125, 2000.

[28] J. R. H. Tudge, I. Mokrova, B. E. Hatfield, and R. B. Karnik, "Uses and misuses of Bronfenbrenner's bioecological theory of human development," *Journal of Family Theory & Review*, vol. 1, no. 4, pp. 198–210, 2009.

[29] M. A. Evans and D. Shaw, "Home grown for reading: parental contributions to young children's emergent literacy and word recognition," *Canadian Psychology*, vol. 49, no. 2, pp. 89–95, 2008.

[30] S. R. Hooper, J. E. Roberts, L. Nelson, S. Zeisel, and D. K. Fannin, "Preschool predictors of narrative writing skills in elementary school children," *School Psychology Quarterly*, vol. 25, no. 1, pp. 1–12, 2010.

[31] G. J. Whitehurst and C. J. Lonigan, "Child development and emergent literacy," *Child Development*, vol. 69, no. 3, pp. 848–872, 1998.

[32] G. J. Whitehurst, J. N. Epstein, A. Angell, A. C. Payne, D. Crone, and J. E. Fischel, "Outcomes of an emergent literacy intervention in head start," *Journal of Educational Psychology*, vol. 86, no. 4, pp. 542–555, 1994.

[33] G. J. Whitehurst, D. S. Arnold, J. N. Epstein, A. L. Angell, M. Smith, and J. E. Fischel, "A Picture book reading intervention in day care and home for children from low-income families," *Developmental Psychology*, vol. 30, no. 5, pp. 679–689, 1994.

[34] M. Senechal, "Testing the home literacy model: parent involvement in kindergarten is differentially related to grade 4 reading comprehension, fluency, spelling, and reading for pleasure," *Scientific Studies of Reading*, vol. 10, no. 1, pp. 59–87, 2006.

[35] M. Senechal and J. A. LeFevre, "Parental involvement in the development of children's reading skill: a five-year longitudinal study," *Child Development*, vol. 73, no. 2, pp. 445–460, 2002.

[36] B. A. Levy, Z. Gong, S. Hessels, M. A. Evans, and D. Jared, "Understanding print: early reading development and the contributions of home literacy experiences," *Journal of Experimental Child Psychology*, vol. 93, no. 1, pp. 63–93, 2006.

[37] L. M. Phillips, R. Hayden, and S. P. Norris, *Family Literacy Matters. A Longitudinal Parent-Child Literacy Intervention Study*, Temeron, Calgary, Canada, 2006.

[38] K. Denton, J. West, and J. Walston, *Reading—Young Children's Achievement and Classroom Experiences*, National Center for Education Statistics: Findings from the Condition of Education, Washington, DC, USA, 2003.

[39] D. R. Entwisle and K. L. Alexander, "Factors affecting achievement test scores and marks of black and white first graders," *The Elementary School Journal*, vol. 88, no. 5, p. 449, 1988.

[40] P. Starkey and A. Klein, "Sociocultural influences on young children's mathematical knowledge," in *Contemporary Perspectives on Mathematics in Early Childhood Education*, pp. 253–276, Information Age Publishing, 2007.

[41] H. P. Ginsburg and R. L. Russell, "Social class and racial influences on early mathematical thinking," *Monographs of the Society for Research in Child Development*, vol. 46, no. 6, pp. 1–69, 1981.

[42] N. C. Jordan, S. C. Levine, and J. Huttenlocher, "Development of calculation abilities in middle-and low-income children after formal instruction in school," *Journal of Applied Developmental Psychology*, vol. 15, no. 2, pp. 223–240, 1994.

[43] H. P. Ginsburg, A. Klein, and P. Starkey, "The development of children's mathematical thinking: connecting research with practive," in *Handbook of Child Psychology: Vol 4, Child Psychology in Practice*, pp. 401–476, John Wiley & Sons, New York, NY, USA, 5th edition, 1998.

[44] K. H. Seo and H. P. Ginsburg, "What is developmentally appropriate in early childhood mathematics education? Lessons from new research," in *Engaging Young Children in Mathematics: Standards for Early Childhood Mathematics Education*, pp. 91–105, Lawrence Erlbaum Associates, 2004.

[45] D. H. Clements, J. Sarama, and A. M. DiBiase, *Engaging Young Children in Mathematics: Standards for Early Childhood Mathematics Education*, Lawrence Erlbaum Associates, Mahwah, NJ, USA, 2004.

[46] National Association for the Education of Young Children and National Council of Teachers and Mathematics, *Early Childhood Mathematics: Promoting Good Beginnings*, Joint position statement on math, 2002.

[47] J. A. Lefevre, S. L. SKwarchuk, D. Kamawar, B. L. Smith-Chant, L. Fast, and J. Bisanz, "Home numeracy experiences and children's math performance in the early school years," *Canadian Journal of Behavioural Science*, vol. 41, no. 2, pp. 55–66, 2009.

[48] G. B. Saxe, S. R. Guberman, M. Gearhart, R. Gelman, C. M. Massey, and B. Rogoff, "Social processes in early number development," *Monographs of the Society for Research in Child Development*, vol. 52, no. 2, pp. 1–162, 1987.

[49] P. Starkey, A. Klein, I. Change, Q. Dong, L. Pang, and Y. Zhou, "Environmental supports for young children's mathematics development in China and the United States," in *Society for Research in Child Development*, Albuquerque, NM, USA, 1999.

[50] A. Klein and P. Starkey, "Preparing for the transition to school mathematics: the head start family math project," in *P. Starkey (Chair). School Readiness and Early Achievement of Impoverished Children, in Symposium Conducted at the Meeting of the Society for Research in Child Development*, Indianapolis, Ind, USA, 1995.

[51] P. Starkey and A. Klein, "Fostering parental support for children's mathematical development: an intervention with head start families," *Early Education and Development*, vol. 11, no. 5, pp. 659–680, 2000.

[52] C. Bowyer-Crane, M. J. Snowling, F. J. Duff et al., "Improving early language and literacy skills: differential effects of an oral language versus a phonology with reading intervention," *Journal of Child Psychology and Psychiatry and Allied Disciplines*, vol. 49, no. 4, pp. 422–432, 2008.

[53] C. M. Connor, F. J. Morrison, and L. Slominski, "Preschool instruction and children's emergent literacy growth," *Journal of Educational Psychology*, vol. 98, no. 4, pp. 665–689, 2006.

[54] R. W. Woodcock, K. S. McGrew, and N. Mather, *Woodcock Johnson III Nu*, Riverside Publishing, Rolling Meadows, Ill, USA, 2007.

[55] J. W. Creswell, W. E. Hanson, V. L. Clark Plano, and A. Morales, "Qualitative research designs: selection and implementation," *Counseling Psychologist*, vol. 35, no. 2, pp. 236–264, 2007.

[56] R. Whitley, "Introducing psychiatrists to qualitative research: a guide for instructors," *Academic Psychiatry*, vol. 33, no. 3, pp. 252–255, 2009.

[57] A. Strauss and J. M. Corbin, *Basics of Qualitative Research: Grounded Theory Procedures and Techniques*, Sage Publications, Thousand Oaks, Calif, USA, 1990.

[58] W. S. Barnett, "Early childhood education," in *School Reform Principles: The Research Evidence*, A. Molner, Ed., Information Age Publishing, Greenwich, Conn, USA, 2002.

[59] C. T. Ramey, S. L. Ramey, R. G. Lanzi, and J. N. Cotton, "Early educational interventions for high-risk children: how center-based treatment can augment and improve parenting effectiveness," in *Parenting and the Child's World: Influences on Academic, Intellectual, and Social-Emotional Development*, J. G. Borkowski, S. L. Ramey, and M. Bristol-Power, Eds., pp. 125–140, Erlbaum Publishers, Mahwah, NJ, USA, 2002.

[60] T. P. Beauchaine, C. Webster-Stratton, and M. J. Reid, "Mediators, moderators, and predictors of 1-year outcomes among children treated for early-onset conduct problems: a latent growth curve analysis," *Journal of Consulting and Clinical Psychology*, vol. 73, no. 3, pp. 371–388, 2005.

[61] C. Blair, "School readiness: integrating cognition and emotion in a neurobiological conceptualization of children's functioning at school entry," *American Psychologist*, vol. 57, no. 2, pp. 111–127, 2002.

[62] M. M. McClelland, C. E. Cameron, C. M. Connor, C. L. Farris, A. M. Jewkes, and F. J. Morrison, "Links between behavioral regulation and preschoolers' literacy, vocabulary, and math skills," *Developmental Psychology*, vol. 43, no. 4, pp. 947–959, 2007.

[63] F. J. Morrison, H. J. Bachman, and C. M. Connor, *Improving Literacy in America: Guidelines from Research*, Yale University Press, New Haven, Conn, USA, 2005.

[64] C. C. Raver, P. W. Garner, and R. Smith-Donald, "The roles of emotion regulation and emotion knowledge for children's academic readiness: are the links causal?" in *School Readiness and the Transition to Kindergarten in the Era of Accountability*, pp. 121–147, Paul H. Brookes Publishing, Baltimore, Md, USA, 2007.

[65] W. S. Barnett, K. Jung, D. J. Yarosz et al., "Educational effects of the Tools of the Mind curriculum: a randomized trial," *Early Childhood Research Quarterly*, vol. 23, no. 3, pp. 299–313, 2008.

[66] K. L. Bierman, C. E. Domitrovich, R. L. Nix, M. T. Greenberg, and C. Blair, "Executive functions and school readiness intervention: impact, moderation, and mediation in the Head Start REDI program," *Development and Psychopathology*, vol. 20, no. 3, pp. 821–843, 2008.

[67] C. E. Domitrovich, S. D. Gest, S. Gill, K. L. Bierman, J. A. Welsh, and D. Jones, "Fostering high-quality teaching with an enriched curriculum and professional development support: the head start REDI program," *American Educational Research Journal*, vol. 46, no. 2, pp. 567–597, 2009.

[68] A. Diamond, W. S. Barnett, J. Thomas, and S. Munro, "The early years: preschool program improves cognitive control," *Science*, vol. 318, no. 5855, pp. 1387–1388, 2007.

[69] W. S. Barnett, D. Yarosz, J. Thomas, and A. Hornbeck, *Educational Effectiveness of a Vygotskian Approach to Preschool Education: A Randomized Trial*, National Institute for Early Education Research, Rutgers University, New Brunswick, NJ, USA, 2006.

7

Moderation of Breastfeeding Effects on Adult Depression by Estrogen Receptor Gene Polymorphism

Päivi Merjonen,[1,2] Markus Jokela,[1] Johanna Salo,[1] Terho Lehtimäki,[3,4] Jorma Viikari,[5] Olli T. Raitakari,[6] Mirka Hintsanen,[1,7] and Liisa Keltikangas-Järvinen[1]

[1] *Unit of Personality, Work, and Health Psychology, IBS, University of Helsinki, P.O. Box 9, 00014 University of Helsinki, Finland*
[2] *Department of Biological Psychology, VU University Amsterdam, 1081 BT Amsterdam, The Netherlands*
[3] *Laboratory of Atherosclerosis Genetics, Department of Clinical Chemistry, Centre for Laboratory Medicine, Tampere University Hospital, P.O. Box 66, 33101 Tampere, Finland*
[4] *The School of Medicine, University of Tampere, 33014 Tampere, Finland*
[5] *Department of Medicine, University of Turku and Turku University Hospital, 20520 Turku, Finland*
[6] *Department of Clinical Physiology, Turku University Hospital and Research Centre of Applied and Preventive Cardiovascular Medicine, University of Turku, P.O. Box 52, 20521 Turku, Finland*
[7] *Helsinki Collegium for Advanced Studies, 00014 University of Helsinki, Finland*

Correspondence should be addressed to Liisa Keltikangas-Järvinen, liisa.keltikangas-jarvinen@helsinki.fi

Academic Editor: Masha Gartstein

Breastfeeding is known to benefit both the mother's and the child's health. Our aim was to test the interactive effects between estrogen receptor 1 (ESR1) rs2234693 and breastfeeding when predicting the child's later depression in adulthood. A sample of 1209 boys and girls from the Young Finns Study were followed from childhood over 27 years up to age 30–45 years. Adulthood depressive symptoms were self-reported by the participants using the Beck Depression Inventory. Breastfeeding as well as several possibly confounding factors was reported by the parents in childhood or adolescence. Breastfeeding tended to predict lower adult depression, while ESR1 rs2234693 was not associated with depression. A significant interaction between breastfeeding and ESR1 was found to predict participants' depression ($P = .004$) so that C/C genotype carriers who had not been breastfed had higher risk of depression than T-allele carriers (40.5% versus 13.0%) while there were no genotypic differences among those who had been breastfed. In sex-specific analysis, this interaction was evident only among women. We conclude that child's genes and maternal behavior may interact in the development of child's adult depression so that breastfeeding may buffer the inherited depression risk possibly associated with the C/C genotype of the ESR1 gene.

1. Introduction

Depression is a major mental health problem in western countries, affecting working-age young adults in particular [1]. The etiology of depression is complex and involves genetic, neurobiological, psychological, and social factors. Furthermore, recent research has demonstrated that adult vulnerability to depression may have its origins already in early childhood [2], which emphasizes the value of life-course studies of depression.

A large research literature has investigated the potential role of maternal behavior in the development of children's mental and behavioral problems. In particular, breastfeeding has been shown to have beneficial effects for children's physical health and cognitive development [3–5]. Emerging evidence suggests that breastfeeding might also have favorable effects on children's mental health. In a study on 5-year-olds, breastfeeding duration was associated with lower prevalence of children's mental health problems [6]. Other studies demonstrated that children who had not been breastfed in infancy had a higher risk for clinical depression in early adulthood [7] and hostility in adulthood [8].

However, genetic background may determine, in part, the sensitivity and responsiveness of individuals to environmental influences. For instance, in a study of breastfeeding and children's cognitive development, a polymorphism of the FADS2 gene (rs174575) was observed to moderate the beneficial effect of breastfeeding so that only individuals carrying the C allele of the FADS2 benefitted from breastfeeding and had higher IQ than those who had not been breastfed [9]. Genetic effects such as this may help to explain inconsistencies between different studies that have not taken genetic background into account.

In the present study, we hypothesized that a similar moderating genetic effect by estrogen-related gene might be observed in the association between breastfeeding and adult depression of offspring. We concentrated on a gene affecting estrogen functioning, estrogen receptor 1 (ESR1). Estrogen, and especially estrogen receptor functioning, has been linked to major mental health problems, for example, schizophrenia [10, 11] and depression [11, 12], and estrogen is related to breastfeeding and might therefore influence the maternal effect of breastfeeding. Estrogen receptor 1 (ESR1) gene codes for estrogen receptor α, and the ESR1 PvuII is a functional polymorphism suggestively associated with severe mental health problems [13], for example, psychosis [10] and depression [14, 15]. In a sample of individuals diagnosed with schizophrenia, the CC genotype of the ESR1 PvuII polymorphism was associated with lower expression of ESR1 mRNA in the prefrontal cortex [16], which may lead to an inability to respond normally to brain estrogen. However, breastfeeding and maternal care associated with it might buffer against this risk. High maternal care has been shown to increase levels of estrogen receptor α mRNA in female rat offspring [17, 18]. In addition, breastfeeding might increase levels of oxytocin which has been shown to increase the expression of estrogen receptor α in prairie voles [19]. Thus, it is plausible that breastfeeding increases the expression of ESR1 mRNA directly or indirectly (via oxytocin) also in human brain.

The aim of this longitudinal, prospective cohort study is to test whether there is an association between breastfeeding and adult depression of offspring and whether this association is moderated by the ESR1 genotype. We hypothesized that the coincidence of environmental and genetic risk factors is most detrimental to the child's mental health, that is, that individuals who carry the possibly vulnerable CC genotype and who lack the buffering maternal effect (i.e., breastfeeding) against it, are in especially high risk to developing depression.

2. Methods

2.1. Participants. The present study is part of a prospective longitudinal study known as the Cardiovascular Risk in Young Finns Study, which started in 1980 with 3596 participants: boys and girls from age groups of 3, 6, 9, 12, 15, and 18 years. Participants were derived from rural and urban surroundings in different parts of Finland to ensure geographical representativeness of the Finnish population. Complete details of the cohort have been published elsewhere [20, 21]. There have been seven followups of the same participants, and the present study utilizes the baseline and first (in year 1983), fourth (in year 1992), fifth (in year 1997), sixth (in year 2001), and seventh (in year 2007) followups. The study was approved by local ethics committees, and all participants gave their written informed consent.

The present sample consisted of 725 women and 484 men (1209 total participants) for whom data on the ESR1 genotype, breastfeeding in childhood, and adult depression at age 30–45 were available. Those selected for the final sample were younger (37.2 versus 37.56 years, $P = .05$), more often women (60.0% versus 46.4% $P < .001$), had higher educated mother (10.2 versus 9.9 years, $P = .001$), had more often nuclear family background (89.9% versus 83.1% $P < .001$), earlier birth order (2.0 versus 2.2 $P = .003$) and fewer siblings (2.7 versus 2.8 $P = .016$) than those who due to missing data were left out from the analyses.

2.2. Measures

2.2.1. Depressive Symptoms. Depressive symptoms were self-reported by the participants in 2007 when they were 30–45 years old using two different versions of the Beck Depression Inventory (BDI): (1) in the original 21-item BDI-II, for each item the participants choose from 4 alternative response statements the most suitable one (scored from 0 to 3), and the sum of these responses is calculated. Here, the BDI-II was scored both as a continuous and a dichotomous variable. The categorization of the latter was based on the previously established cut-off point for clinical depression (0 = 0–13, 1 = 14–63) [22]. (2) In a modified version of the BDI, which has been used in several previous studies of the present cohort [23–26], participants rated 21 items of the second mildest statements of the original BDI instrument using a 5-point Likert-type scale and the mean of these responses was calculated. The modified BDI scale was also measured in 1992, 1997, and 2001, when participants were 15–30, 20–35, and 24–39 years old. Thus, the depression outcomes included (1) continuously coded BDI-II score, (2) dichotomously coded BDI-II clinical depression, and (3) continuously coded depressive symptoms of the modified BDI instrument.

2.2.2. Breastfeeding. In 1983 parents of the participants reported (1) whether the participants had been breastfed as infants (0 = no, 1 = yes) and (2) the duration of breastfeeding in months. The questions of breastfeeding did not differentiate between partial and exclusive breastfeeding. Although the assessment of breastfeeding was retrospective, it has been shown that mothers' reports of breastfeeding history after 20 years are highly reliable and valid [27]. In Finland, practically all mothers and infants are regularly checked in antenatal clinics during pregnancy and in child health centers after birth from where parents get the child's personal record card with them. Thus, parents can check the information regarding breastfeeding from the participant's personal record cards obtained from child health centers. In a previous study with the present cohort, breastfed men were shown to have better brachial endothelial function than formula fed-men [28], supporting the validity of the breastfeeding measure.

2.2.3. ESR1 rs2234693 Genotyping. Genomic DNA was extracted from peripheral blood leukocytes using a commercially available kit and Qiagen BioRobot M48 Workstation according to the manufacturer's instructions (Qiagen Inc., Hilden, Germany). Estrogen receptor 1 (ESR1, *rs2234693*) polymorphism was genotyped by employing the 5′ nuclease assay and fluorogenic allele-specific TaqMan MGB probes [29], using the ABI Prism 7900HT Sequence Detection System (Applied Biosystems, Foster City, CA, USA) and commercially available TaqMan assay (assay ID C_3163590_10). The samples were pipetted using an automated TECAN Freedom EVO-100 instrument (Tecan Group Ltd., Männedorf, Switzerland). The PCR reactions containing genomic DNA, 1 × Universal PCR Master Mix, 900 nM of each primer, and 200 nM of each probe are performed in 384-well plates using the standard protocol in a total volume of 5 μL. End-point fluorescence is measured after PCR and genotype calling carried out by the allelic discrimination analysis module (ABI Prism SDS software, ABI, Foster City, CA, USA). Random duplicates were used as quality control.

2.2.4. Covariates. Mother's age at childbirth, her educational years, the family structure (1 = nuclear family versus 0 = single-parent household or child of only one of the parents), number of children in family, and birth order of the child (all assessed in 1980) were included as covariates because they may have affected the mother's decision to breastfeed and indicate wider family atmosphere. Child's birth weight and whether the child was born full term (1 = full term 0 = preterm) were also taken into account.

2.3. Statistical Analyses. When predicting continuously coded depression scores, the main effects of breastfeeding and ESR1, and the interaction effect between the two, were assessed with analysis of covariance, adjusted for participants' age and sex. For the dichotomous BDI-II, the corresponding analysis was carried out using logistic regression analysis. The models were then further adjusted for maternal age at childbirth, maternal educational years, family structure, number of children in family, participant's birth order, birth weight, and whether the participant was born full term. Sex differences in the ESR1-breastfeeding interaction effect were tested with three-way interactions between sex, breastfeeding, and ESR1 genotype. Given that the repeated measurements of the modified BDI were available for 4 measurement times, we also fitted a multilevel regression model in which all the measurement times were pooled together and each participant could contribute 1 to 4 person-observations to the dataset. Multilevel regression modeling takes into account the nonindependence of the observations in calculating standard errors of the estimates. All the analyses were conducted using PASW 18.0 software.

3. Results

Descriptive statistics for the sample are shown in Table 1. Age- and sex-adjusted partial correlations between the study variables are shown in Table 2. Having been breastfed at infancy was related to younger age of mother, being born full term, and having higher birth weight. Longer duration of breastfeeding was related to older mothers, later birth order, and higher number of children in the family.

Table 3 shows mean levels of depression by breastfeeding status and ESR1 genotype, which suggest no consistent main effects for these variables. There was a tendency for breastfeeding to be associated with a lower depression risk, particularly with depression assessed with the continuously coded BDI-II scores, but this association was not observed with other measures of depression.

Next we examined the interaction effects between ESR1 and breastfeeding in predicting depression. There was a significant interaction effect when predicting continuous BDI-II score ($F(2, 1201) = 5.47$, $P = .004$) and a marginally significant interaction effect in the same direction when predicting dichotomous BDI-II $P = .071$ (TC : OR (95% CI) = 0.74 (0.18–3.01) $P = .67$; CC : OR (95% CI) = 5.18 (0.92–29.14) $P = .06$; breastfed TT carriers as the reference category) and the modified BDI score ($F(2, 1201) = 2.28$, $P = .102$). The age- and sex-adjusted interaction effects are illustrated in Figure 1. Among participants who had not been breastfed, individuals carrying the C/C genotype had higher risk of BDI-II depression (40.5% versus 13.0%), higher BDI-II mean scores (12.80 versus 5.74), and higher modified-BDI mean scores (2.55 versus 2.11) when compared to combined group of carriers of T/T and T/C genotypes. The C/C genotype was not associated with increased depression risk in participants who had been breastfed. Stated the other way around, the interaction effect indicated that breastfeeding was associated with lower risk of depression in those carrying the C/C genotype but not associated with depression in carriers of T/T or T/C genotypes. These interaction effects were little affected when the models were further adjusted for childhood covariates (continuous BDI-II score ($F(2, 1194) = 5.50$, $P = .004$), BDI-II $P = .074$ (TC : OR (95%) = 0.75 (0.18–3.09) $P = .70$; CC : OR (95%) = 5.35 (0.93–30.82) $P = .06$; breastfed TT carriers as the reference category), and modified BDI score ($F(2, 1194) = 2.37$, $P = 0.094$).

Statistically significant three-way interaction effects between sex, breastfeeding status, and ESR1 were observed when predicting continuous BDI-II ($F(2, 1196) = 4.93$, $P = .007$), and modified BDI ($F(2, 1196) = 4.58$, $P = .010$). However, when predicting dichotomous BDI-II the three-way interaction was not observed ($P = 0.47$). When the above analyses were fitted separately in men and women, the interaction effect was observed only in women (Figure 2). In women who had not been breastfed in infancy, carriers of the C/C genotype had higher risk of BDI-II depression (59.8% versus 13.9%), higher BDI-II mean scores (19.46 versus 6.37), and higher modified-BDI mean scores (3.20 versus 2.12) than those carrying the T/T or T/C genotype.

In addition, when testing whether the interaction between ESR1 genotype and breastfeeding would replicate when predicting modified BDI in different years, replication was found when predicting BDI in 1992 ($F(2, 1300) = 4.86$, $P = .008$) and 2001 ($F(2, 1294) = 3.28$, $P = .038$). Although the interaction was not statistically significant when predicting modified BDI in 1997 ($F(2, 1151) = 1.322$,

TABLE 1: Characteristics of the study group ($N = 1209$).

Variable	Total sample $N = 1209$		Women $N = 725$		Men $N = 484$		P value‡
	Value†a	Range	Value†	Range	Value†	Range	
Family and childhood variables							
Maternal age at childbirth	27.30 (5.57)	16–48	27.15 (5.67)	16–48	27.52 (5.41)	18–46	.254
Maternal educational years	10.23 (3.16)	2–22	10.10 (3.05)	2–22	10.43 (3.31)	4–22	.079
Family structure§							.315
Nuclear family	1087 (89.9)		657 (90.6)		430 (88.8)		
Other	122 (10.1)		68 (9.4)		54 (11.2)		
Birth order	2.00 (1.40)	1–14	2.01 (1.42)	1–11	1.98 (1.37)	1–14	.663
Number of children in family	2.65 (1.60)	1–15	2.70 (1.68)	1–14	2.59 (1.47)	1–15	.238
Birth status§							.599
Full term	1059 (87.6)		638 (88.0)		421 (87.0)		
Premature	150 (12.4)		87 (12.0)		63 (13.0)		
Birth weight	3501 (527)	1040–5750	3463 (518)	1300–5250	3558 (535)	1040–5750	**.002**
Breastfeeding status§							.063
Breastfed	1122 (92.8)		681 (93.9)		441 (91.1)		
Not breastfed	87 (7.2)		44 (6.1)		43 (8.9)		
Duration of breastfeeding	3.82 (3.67)	0–36	3.99 (3.87)	0–36	3.57 (3.33)	0–36	**.048**
Participant's adulthood variables							
Sex§							
Male	484 (40.0)						
Female	725 (60.0)						
Age in 2007	37.21 (4.91)	30–45	37.18 (4.91)	30–45	37.26 (4.91)	30–45	.768
ESR 1 PvuII§							.052
T/T	420 (34.7)		246 (33.9)		174 (36.0)		
T/C	595 (49.2)		375 (51.7)		220 (45.5)		
C/C	194 (16.0)		104 (14.3)		90 (18.6)		
Depressive symptoms in 2007	2.06 (0.66)	1.00–4.67	2.12 (0.67)	1.00–4.67	1.97 (0.64)	1.00–4.63	**<0.001**
BDI in 2007 (continuous)	5.24 (6.41)	0–46	6.13 (6.79)	0–46	3.92 (5.58)	0–40	**<0.001**
BDI in 2007 (dichotomous)§							**.001**
Depression	127 (10.5)		93 (12.8)		34 (7.0)		
No depression	1082 (89.5)		632 (87.2)		450 (93.0)		

†Values are means (and standard deviations) unless otherwise indicated.
‡Gender differences, Pearson's chi-square for categorical variables, t-ratio for continuous variables.
§Values are numbers (and percentages) of participants.

$P = .267$), the association was in same direction. Pooling the 4 measurement times into a single multilevel model resulted in a dataset with 5017 person-observations from 1603 unique participants. In a multilevel regression, the interaction between ESR1 genotype with breastfeeding predicted modified BDI in both only age- and sex-adjusted ($F(2, 1613) = 3.59$, $P = 0.028$) and fully adjusted ($F(2, 1612) = 3.69$, $P = 0.025$) models. The three-way interaction effect between sex, breastfeeding status, and ESR1 was statistically significant ($F(2, 1621) = 4.721$, $P = 0.009$), implying that those women who had CC genotype and who had not been breastfed had higher modified-BDI mean score (2.93 versus 2.19) than T-allele carriers who had been breastfed, as suggested by the regression models for depressive symptoms in 2007 (Figure 2).

4. Discussion

The present study appears to be the first to show that an interaction between breastfeeding status and gene polymorphism may predict the development of child's depression later in life. The results suggest that whether or not the child is breastfed may modify the effect of estrogen receptor 1 (ESR1) rs2234693 on depression 30 to 45 years later in life. Those who were not breastfed and had the C/C genotype had especially high risk of developing depression compared to other groups. Gender differences were also observed, the effect being evident only among women. The interaction effect was independent of a number of childhood covariates reflecting early developmental environment.

Table 2: Age- and sex-adjusted correlations between variables.

	1	2	3	4	5	6	7	8	9	10	11	12
(1) Maternal age at childbirth												
(2) Maternal educational years	**−.06***											
(3) Nuclear family	**.07***	−.02										
(4) Birth order	**.57******	**−.21******	.04									
(5) Number of children in family	**.36******	**−.15******	**.10*****	**.80******								
(6) Full term	.04	−.04	**.08*****	**.09*****	.05							
(7) Birth weight	**.08*****	−.01	**.07***	**.11******	**.06***	**.43******						
(8) Breastfed	**−.10******	.03	.03	.01	.03	**.19******	**.18******					
(9) Duration of breastfeeding	**.15******	−.04	−.00	**.18******	**.13******	**.08*****	**.08*****	**.29******				
(10) ESR 1 PvuII	.03	.02	−.01	.02	−.02	.00	**.07***	.03	−.01			
(11) Depressive symptoms in 2007	−.02	−.02	−.03	−.00	.01	.00	−.02	−.04	.04	−.03		
(12) BDI in 2007 (continuous)	−.02	.01	−.04	−.02	−.03	−.00	−.03	**−.06***	.04	.00	**.75******	
(13) Clinical depression (BDI)	−.03	.02	−.03	−.02	−.03	−.02	−.03	−.05	.01	−.01	**.58******	**.78******

*** $P < 0.001$, ** $P < 0.01$, and * $P < 0.05$.

Table 3: Age- and sex-adjusted main effects of breastfeeding and ESR1 predicting depression.

	BDI-II dichotomous depression		BDI-II continuous depression		BDI modified depression	
	OR (95% CI)	*P*	Mean (std. error)	*P*	Mean (std. error)	*P*
Breastfeeding		.054		**.047**		.151
Yes	1.00		5.14 (0.19)		2.05 (0.02)	
No	1.82 (0.99–3.36)		6.55 (0.68)		2.16 (0.07)	
ESR1 genotype		.872		.766		.486
T/T	1.00		5.33 (0.31)		2.09 (0.03)	
T/C	0.93 (0.62–1.40)		5.11 (0.26)		2.04 (0.03)	
C/C	0.86 (0.48–1.54)		5.45 (0.46)		2.04 (0.05)	

Breastfeeding may affect child's depression through at least two different mechanisms. There may be a direct nutritional link from breast milk to child's hormone and neurotransmitter functioning. Breastfeeding is known to affect child's brain development through nutritional processes involving fatty acids [30], and this effect might be mediated via hormonal processes. On the other hand, breastfeeding may be a proxy measure of maternal behavior toward the child or of a wider family atmosphere [31]. Breastfeeding mothers may be more child-oriented, have more contact with the child, and be more sensitive and less hostile toward the child. It has been suggested that mothers have higher oxytocin release after breastfeeding, and this may intensify mother's bonding to the infant [32]. Other suggestions assume that some mothers are bonded to the infant before birth, but not all [33]. A study reported that first reaction towards their newborns among about 40 percent of first time mothers was indifference, but this was changed to affection in a week among most of the mothers [34]. Thus breastfeeding may be especially important to the maternal bonding among those whose bonding did not develop during pregnancy. Early suckling and skin-to-skin contact have been shown to predict better mother-infant interaction in one year of age as well as more self-regulated and less irritable children [35]. Thus, the idea of sensitive period shown in many other species may also be relevant in humans. Oxytocin is hypothesized to increase in both the mother's and the infant's brain when the infant starts to suckle the mother's nipple in skin-to-skin contact after birth [36, 37]. At least among rats, suckling alters brain functioning similarly as oxytocin administration as was observed in a study utilizing functional magnetic resonance imaging [38]. Skin-to-skin contact in form of massage has also shown to decrease aggression among preschool children [39], which might be related to oxytocin effects.

Oxytocin, on the other hand, alters estrogen expression, at least among prairie voles [19]. Lower expression of ESR1 mRNA may be related to many major mental health problems. C/C genotype of ESR1 rs2234693 is suggested to be "a risk genotype" related to schizophrenia and other psychoses [10, 16] and might relate to other mental health problems, like depression [14], as well. It is possible that C/C genotype carriers have inherited a vulnerability to mental health problems, which however might be neutralized by breastfeeding. Breastfeeding may increase the expression of ESR1 mRNA among C/C genotype carriers, who initially seem to have a low expression of ESR1 mRNA, and thus buffer the risk related to mental health problems among C/C genotype carriers. Finally, as estrogen is a known female sex-hormone, the observed sex difference could be expected because estrogen might be suggested to be a more important

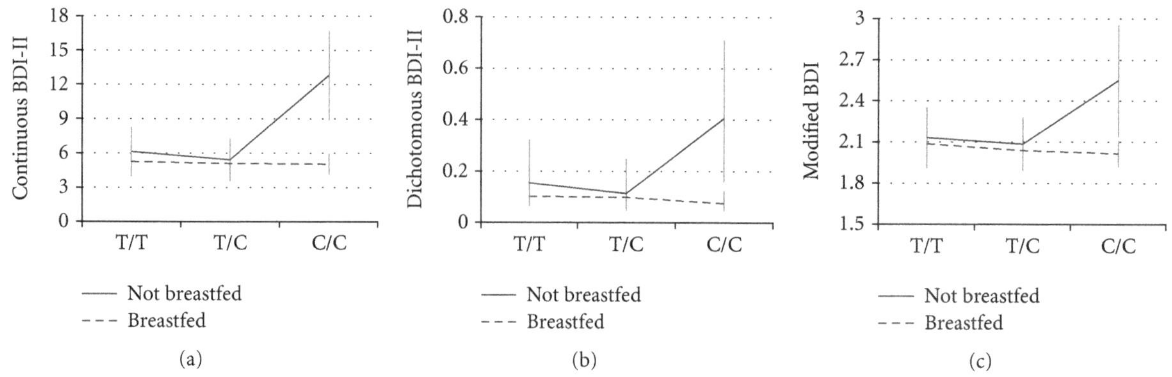

FIGURE 1: Adult depression by estrogen receptor 1 genotype (ESR1) and being breastfed at infancy. The vertical lines are 95% confidence intervals.

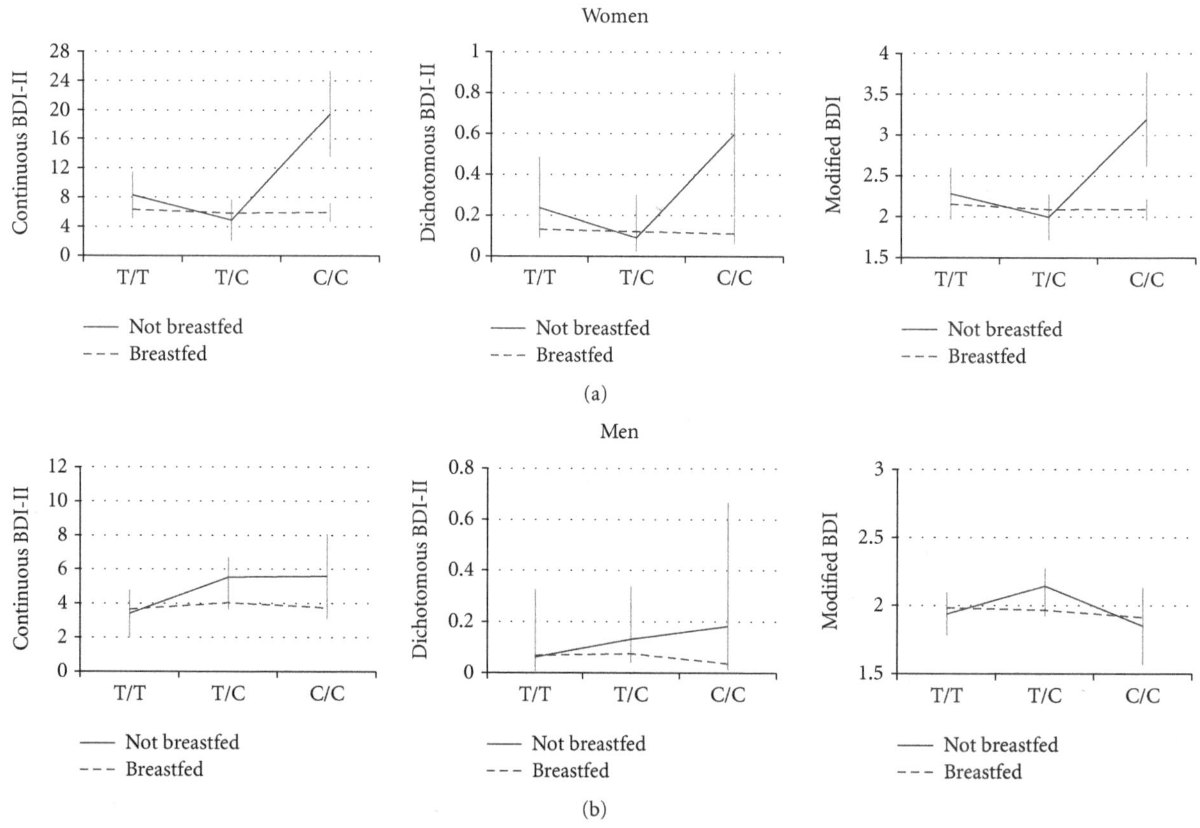

FIGURE 2: Adult depression by estrogen receptor 1 genotype (ESR1) and being breastfed at infancy separately in women and men. The vertical lines are 95% confidence intervals.

determinant of depression vulnerability in women than in men [40].

There are study limitations that need to be taken into account when interpreting the results. First, we could not control mothers' depression or their genetic background, which might introduce confounding into the results. Depressed mothers may be more reluctant to breastfeed [41, 42] and depression may pass from the mother to her child either via environmental factors or due to shared genetic background. Second, breastfeeding was assessed retrospectively when participants were 6–21 years old. However, maternal reports of duration of breastfeeding 20 years later have been shown to have high validity [27]. Third, due to selective dropout, those included in the final sample had a more advantageous family background, which may limit the generalizability of the results. In addition, the number of participants carrying the C/C genotype and who were not breastfed was relatively small ($n = 10$) which increases the risk that the present results might be due to chance. Replication of these findings is therefore essential.

Our study benefits from a large population-based sample followed over a long period of time and from the use of two different measures of depressive symptoms. Depressive symptoms were self-reported by the participants in adulthood in 30–45 years of age while breastfeeding was reported by the participants' mothers over two decades before when participants were 6–21 years old, which reduces the influence of common informant bias to the results.

In conclusion, the present study suggests that child's genes and maternal behavior interact in the development of child's adult depression. Breastfeeding—and possibly the maternal care associated with it—may confer a protective effect especially to individuals who may have inherited a possible susceptibility to mental health problems in the form of specific estrogen receptor genotype.

Abbreviations

ESR1 gene:	Estrogen receptor 1 gene
FADS2 gene:	Fatty acid desaturase 2 gene
IQ:	Intelligence quotient
mRNA:	Messenger ribonucleic acid
BDI:	Beck's Depression Inventory.

Acknowledgments

Ville Aalto and Irina Lisinen are acknowledged for skilful data management. This study was supported by the Academy of Finland Project 258578 (M. Hintsanen, and P. Merjonen) and 124399 (L. Keltikangas-Järvinen), Signe and Ane Gyllenberg Foundation (L. Keltikangas-Järvinen), Tampere University Hospital Medical Fund (T. Lehtimäki), Emil Aaltonen Foundation (T. Lehtimäki, M. Hintsanen), Ella & Georg Ehrnrooth Foundation (M. Hintsanen), Research Funds of the University of Helsinki (M. Hintsanen), Research Foundation of the University of Helsinki (J. Salo), Finnish Cultural Foundation (P. Merjonen), and Alfred Kordelin Foundation (P. Merjonen).

References

[1] C. J. L. Murray and A. D. Lopez, "Alternative projections of mortality and disability by cause 1990–2020: global Burden of Disease Study," *The Lancet*, vol. 349, no. 9064, pp. 1498–1504, 1997.

[2] R. L. Repetti, S. E. Taylor, and T. E. Seeman, "Risky families: family social environments and the mental and physical health of offspring," *Psychological Bulletin*, vol. 128, no. 2, pp. 330–366, 2002.

[3] S. Ip, M. Chung, G. Raman et al., "Breastfeeding and maternal and infant health outcomes in developed countries," *Evidence Report*, no. 153, pp. 1–186, 2007.

[4] M. S. Kramer, F. Aboud, E. Mironova et al., "Breastfeeding and child cognitive development: new evidence from a large randomized trial," *Archives of General Psychiatry*, vol. 65, no. 5, pp. 578–584, 2008.

[5] E. B. Isaacs, B. R. Fischl, B. T. Quinn, W. K. Chong, D. G. Gadian, and A. Lucas, "Impact of breast milk on intelligence quotient, brain size, and white matter development," *Pediatric Research*, vol. 67, no. 4, pp. 357–362, 2010.

[6] M. Robinson, W. H. Oddy, J. Li et al., "Pre- and postnatal influences on preschool mental health: a large-scale cohort study," *Journal of Child Psychology and Psychiatry and Allied Disciplines*, vol. 49, no. 10, pp. 1118–1128, 2008.

[7] L. Batstra, J. Neeleman, C. Elsinga, and M. Hadders-Algra, "Psychiatric morbidity is related to a chain of prenatal and perinatal adversities," *Early Human Development*, vol. 82, no. 11, pp. 721–729, 2006.

[8] P. Merjonen, M. Jokela, L. Pulkki-Råback et al., "Breastfeeding and offspring hostility in adulthood," *Psychotherapy and Psychosomatics*, vol. 80, pp. 371–373, 2011.

[9] A. Caspi, B. Williams, J. Kim-Cohen et al., "Moderation of breastfeeding effects on the IQ by genetic variation in fatty acid metabolism," *Proceedings of the National Academy of Sciences of the United States of America*, vol. 104, no. 47, pp. 18860–18865, 2007.

[10] T. Kishi, M. Ikeda, T. Kitajima et al., "A functional polymorphism in estrogen receptor alpha gene is associated with Japanese methamphetamine induced psychosis," *Progress in Neuro-Psychopharmacology and Biological Psychiatry*, vol. 33, no. 5, pp. 895–898, 2009.

[11] W. R. Perlman, E. Tomaskovic-Crook, D. M. Montague et al., "Alteration in estrogen receptor α mRNA levels in frontal cortex and hippocampus of patients with major mental illness," *Biological Psychiatry*, vol. 58, no. 10, pp. 812–824, 2005.

[12] U. Halbreich and L. S. Kahn, "Role of estrogen in the aetiology and treatment of mood disorders," *CNS Drugs*, vol. 15, no. 10, pp. 797–817, 2001.

[13] E. E. Sundermann, P. M. Maki, and J. R. Bishop, "A review of estrogen receptor α gene (ESR1) polymorphisms, mood, and cognition," *Menopause*, vol. 17, no. 4, pp. 874–886, 2010.

[14] J. Ryan, J. Scali, I. Carrière et al., "Estrogen receptor alpha gene variants and major depressive episodes," *Journal of Affective Disorders*, vol. 136, pp. 1222–1226, 2012.

[15] S. J. Tsai, Y. C. Wang, C. J. Hong, and H. J. Chiu, "Association study of oestrogen receptor α gene polymorphism and suicidal behaviours in major depressive disorder," *Psychiatric Genetics*, vol. 13, no. 1, pp. 19–22, 2003.

[16] C. S. Weickert, A. L. Miranda-Angulo, J. Wong et al., "Variants in the estrogen receptor alpha gene and its mRNA contribute to risk for schizophrenia," *Human Molecular Genetics*, vol. 17, no. 15, pp. 2293–2309, 2008.

[17] F. A. Champagne, I. C. G. Weaver, J. Diorio, S. Sharma, and M. J. Meaney, "Natural variations in maternal care are associated with estrogen receptor α expression and estrogen sensitivity in the medial preoptic area," *Endocrinology*, vol. 144, no. 11, pp. 4720–4724, 2003.

[18] F. A. Champagne, I. C. G. Weaver, J. Diorio, S. Dymov, M. Szyf, and M. J. Meaney, "Maternal care associated with methylation of the estrogen receptor-α1b promoter and estrogen receptor-α expression in the medial preoptic area of female offspring," *Endocrinology*, vol. 147, no. 6, pp. 2909–2915, 2006.

[19] K. M. Kramer, S. Yoshida, E. Papademetriou, and B. S. Cushing, "The organizational effects of oxytocin on the central expression of estrogen receptor α and oxytocin in adulthood," *BMC Neuroscience*, vol. 8, article 71, 2007.

[20] H. K. Åkerblom, M. Uhari, E. Pesonen et al., "Cardiovascular risk in young Finns," *Annals of Medicine*, vol. 23, no. 1, pp. 35–39, 1991.

[21] O. T. Raitakari, M. Juonala, T. Rönnemaa et al., "Cohort profile: the cardiovascular risk in young Finns study," *International Journal of Epidemiology*, vol. 37, no. 6, pp. 1220–1226, 2008.

[22] A. T. Beck, R. A. Steer, and G. K. Brown, *Depression Inventory*, 2nd edition, 2009, http://cps.nova.edu/~cpphelp/BDI2.html.

[23] M. Jokela, L. Keltikangas-Järvinen, M. Kivimäki et al., "Serotonin receptor 2A gene and the influence of childhood maternal nurturance on adulthood depressive symptoms," *Archives of General Psychiatry*, vol. 64, no. 3, pp. 356–360, 2007.

[24] M. Jokela, T. Lehtimäki, and L. Keltikangas-Järvinen, "The influence of urban/rural residency on depressive symptoms is moderated by the serotonin receptor 2A gene," *American Journal of Medical Genetics B*, vol. 144, no. 7, pp. 918–922, 2007.

[25] M. Elovainio, L. Keltikangas-Järvinen, M. Kivimäki et al., "Depressive symptoms and carotid artery intima-media thickness in young adults: the cardiovascular risk in Young Finns study," *Psychosomatic Medicine*, vol. 67, pp. 561–567, 2005.

[26] M. Jokela, K. Räikkönen, T. Lehtimäki, R. Rontu, and L. Keltikangas-Järvinen, "Tryptophan hydroxylase 1 gene (TPH1) moderates the influence of social support on depressive symptoms in adults," *Journal of Affective Disorders*, vol. 100, no. 1-3, pp. 191–197, 2007.

[27] J. D. Kark, G. Troya, and Y. Friedlander, "Validity of maternal reporting of breast feeding history and the association with blood lipids in 17 year olds in Jerusalem," *Journal of Epidemiology and Community Health*, vol. 38, no. 3, pp. 218–225, 1984.

[28] M. J. Järvisalo, N. Hutri-Kähönen, M. Juonala et al., "Breast feeding in infancy and arterial endothelial function later in life. The cardiovascular risk in Young Finns Study," *European Journal of Clinical Nutrition*, vol. 63, no. 5, pp. 640–645, 2009.

[29] K. J. Livak, "Allelic discrimination using fluorogenic probes and the 5' nuclease assay," *Genetic Analysis*, vol. 14, no. 5-6, pp. 143–149, 1999.

[30] J. R. Marszalek and H. F. Lodish, "Docosahexaenoic acid, fatty acid-interacting proteins, and neuronal function: breastmilk and fish are good for you," *Annual Review of Cell and Developmental Biology*, vol. 21, pp. 633–657, 2005.

[31] S. F. Virden, "The relationship between infant feeding method and maternal role adjustment," *Journal of Nurse-Midwifery*, vol. 33, no. 1, pp. 31–35, 1988.

[32] J. H. Kennell and M. H. Klaus, "Bonding: recent observations that alter perinatal care," *Pediatrics in Review*, vol. 19, no. 1, pp. 4–12, 1998.

[33] C. M. Corter and A. S. Fleming, *Psychobiology of Maternal Behavior in Human Beings*, 1995.

[34] K. M. Robson and R. Kumar, "Delayed onset of maternal affection after childbirth," *British Journal of Psychiatry*, vol. 136, no. 4, pp. 347–353, 1980.

[35] K. Bystrova, V. Ivanova, M. Edhborg et al., "Early contact versus separation: effects on mother-infant interaction one year later," *Birth*, vol. 36, no. 2, pp. 97–109, 2009.

[36] M. Klaus, "Mother and infant: early emotional ties," *Pediatrics*, vol. 102, no. 5, pp. 1244–1246, 1998.

[37] K. Uvnäs-Moberg and M. Eriksson, "Breastfeeding: physiological, endocrine and behavioural adaptations caused by oxytocin and local neurogenic activity in the nipple and mammary gland," *Acta Paediatrica*, vol. 85, no. 5, pp. 525–530, 1996.

[38] M. Febo, M. Numan, and C. F. Ferris, "Functional magnetic resonance imaging shows oxytocin activates brain regions associated with mother-pup bonding during suckling," *Journal of Neuroscience*, vol. 25, no. 50, pp. 11637–11644, 2005.

[39] A. L. Von Knorring, A. Söderberg, L. Austin, and K. Uvnäs-Moberg, "Massage decreases aggression in preschool children: a long-term study," *Acta Paediatrica*, vol. 97, no. 9, pp. 1265–1269, 2008.

[40] J. Mill, E. Kiss, I. Baji et al., "Association study of the estrogen receptor alpha gene (ESR1) and childhood-onset mood disorders," *American Journal of Medical Genetics B*, vol. 147, no. 7, pp. 1323–1326, 2008.

[41] O. G. Falceto, E. R. J. Giugliani, and C. L. C. Fernandes, "Influence of parental mental health on early termination of breast-feeding: a case-control study," *Journal of the American Board of Family Practice*, vol. 17, no. 3, pp. 173–183, 2004.

[42] T. G. Fairlie, M. W. Gillman, and J. Rich-Edwards, "High pregnancy-related anxiety and prenatal depressive symptoms as predictors of intention to breastfeed and breastfeeding initiation," *Journal of Women's Health*, vol. 18, no. 7, pp. 945–953, 2009.

8

Naturalistic Observations of Nonverbal Children with Autism: A Study of Intentional Communicative Acts in the Classroom

Samantha Drain[1] and Paul E. Engelhardt[2]

[1] *Department of Psychology, University of Chester, Parkgate Road, Chester CH1 4BJ, UK*
[2] *School of Psychology, University of East Anglia, Norwich Research Park, Elizabeth Fry Building 1.10, Norwich NR4 7TJ, UK*

Correspondence should be addressed to Paul E. Engelhardt; p.engelhardt@uea.ac.uk

Academic Editor: Cheryl Dissanayake

We examined evoked and spontaneous communicative acts in six nonverbal children with autism (10–15 years, M = 12.8, SD = 2.1). All participants attended the same special school for children with autism but were in different classes. Each was observed for 30 minutes during a typical school day. An observer coded the presence/absence of an antecedent, the form and function of the communicative act, and the teacher's response to the child. One hundred and fifty-five communicative acts were observed, 41% were spontaneous and 59% were evoked. The main antecedents to evoked communicative acts were verbal prompts, and most of the evoked communicative acts were physical in nature (i.e., motor acts and gestures). However, verbalizations and the use of the Picture Exchange Communication System (PECS) were higher for spontaneous communicative acts. The functions of spontaneous communicative acts were primarily requests. Results showed a substantial number of "nonresponses" from teachers, even following evoked communicative acts. These results suggest that teachers may not actively promote intentional communication as much as possible. Therefore, our findings provide information concerning ways in which educators could facilitate intentional communication in non-verbal children with autism.

1. Introduction

Autism is a neurodevelopmental disorder that is characterized by impairments in social, behavioral, and linguistic domains. The DSM-IV diagnostic criteria for autism are based on substantial impairments in communication and social interactions [1]. By some estimates, 25% of individuals with autism do not develop speech [2–4]. In addition, they also tend to show restrictive, repetitive, and stereotyped behaviors. However, it is important to note that most children with autism do use intentional communication even if they do not have symbolic communication abilities [5–8]. Stone et al. [9] reported that most nonverbal children with autism use less complex behaviors in their communicative acts compared to typically developing children, who use language as their primary means of communication. For example, if a child with autism wants an object, they will simply reach for it or make gesture, such as pointing, to indicate what they want. Similarly, in other cases, children with autism may use eye gaze or unusual verbalizations [10, 11], whereas a typically developing child will employ language to express their wants/desires. In general, there has been little systematic research on intentional communicative acts in nonverbal children with autism (cf. [5, 12–14]), and so, there is a need for research that examines the relationships between the antecedent of a communicative act, the form and function of the communicative act, and the response provided by a teacher to the child. In the current study, we examined both spontaneous and evoked communicative acts in nonverbal children with autism in a naturalistic (classroom) environment.

In order to improve communication, augmentative and alternative communication systems have been used to support children with autism [15–18]. There are two main types. Unaided systems refer to communication systems that do not have external devices; that is, they rely on motor actions and manual signs. Aided systems have external devices, such as communication boards or the Picture Exchange Communication System (PECS) [19–21]. The goal of both types of systems is to encourage children with autism to gain and use functional communication skills in interactive social situations. PECS has been argued to be one of the best aided systems because it tends to promote more spontaneous communicative acts, which is one of the main weaknesses in autism [22–30]. With PECS, children are encouraged and/or taught to approach a communicative partner and gain their attention by placing one of the cards in their hand. Therefore, PECS may encourage individuals with autism to communicate with other people in a more spontaneous manner [31].

Boucher and Lewis [22] argued that children with autism may not be impaired in their ability to communicate but rather that they have a deficit with regards to the spontaneity of social interactions (see also [32]). Thus, children with autism do not always display communication behaviors that they in fact have the ability to perform. Kanner [28] also noted an absence of spontaneous sentence production in children with autism who did have symbolic communication as well as those who had more limited language abilities (see also [23, 33, 34]). Spontaneous communication is important for several reasons [32, 35–37]. First, it allows a person to initiate social interactions. Second, it gives a person some control over their environment, and what they do. Third, it allows a person to convey their personal needs to others. If a person is solely reliant upon their partners' cues, then their ability to communicate will be severely restricted. Preliminary research suggests that the more children with autism respond spontaneously to natural stimuli, the more their behavior resembles that of typically developing children [35]. Spontaneity, then, appears to be a significant factor affecting children's ability to effectively communicate, and, thus, to successfully employ intentional communication.

The issue of spontaneity in communication has been operationalized in two ways (for reviews, see [25, 38]). The first way views spontaneity as a binary, which essentially is all or nothing. If there is an antecedent to the communicative act, then it is not spontaneous. In contrast, if there is no antecedent, then the communicative act is spontaneous. The second view sees spontaneity as occurring along a continuum [27, 39]. According to this conceptualization, all communicative acts have some degree of spontaneity, and the level is dependent upon the extent to which the evoking stimulus is related to the communicative act.

Carter and Hotchkins [38] devised a four-level antecedent model with regards to expressive communicative acts. The goal of their model was to provide a scheme for classifying antecedents, which then permits a closer examination of the spontaneity of a communicative act. This model has been reliable across a number of studies [24, 25, 40]. The antecedent category that is the most spontaneous is a *natural cue* (i.e., the mere presence of a desired object or communicative partner) (We refer to intentional communicative acts in response to *naturalistic cues* as spontaneous. All other antecedent types are associated with evoked communication.) The second category along the continuum is *stimulus highlighting*, which focuses on prompts that actively draw attention to an object (or a person), thereby altering the saliency of an entity in the environment. The third category is *generalized communicative cues*. These are cues that require a response but do not directly indicate what that response is (e.g., verbal prompts, such as "tell me what you want" or presenting several PECS cards). The fourth category, *direct prompts*, is deemed the least spontaneous. This type of antecedent requires a specific response (e.g., an instruction to perform an action). In the current study, we used this categorical (continuum) approach because it allowed us to investigate a range of antecedents and to more systematically study which antecedents evoked communicative acts from children with autism.

There have been four studies that investigated expressive communication by observing children with autism in a classroom setting [5, 12–14]. Stone and Caro-Martinez [14] focused on spontaneous communicative acts, which occurred on average 3-4 times per hour in their study. They found that the form of the communicative acts consisted of 52% motor acts, 26% speech acts, 16% vocalizations, and 13% gestures. (Motor acts were defined as physical communications that were nonsymbolic in nature, and gestures were symbolic.) The functions of the communicative acts were getting attention (23%), engaging in social routine (22%), requesting things (22%), commenting (15%), and rejecting things (8%). In a similar study that compared children with autism across two countries (i.e., Australia and Taiwan), Chiang and Lin [5] investigated expressive communicative acts in children with a range of verbal abilities. The purpose of the study was to examine how many children, from the sample of 32, used different forms of communication (i.e., aided communication systems, unaided communication systems, or speech), as well as the functions of their communicative acts (i.e., commenting, requesting, or rejecting). Results showed that children on average produced 44 communicative acts per hour. Unaided communicative acts were more frequent than both aided communication and speech. With regard to functions, requesting and commenting were used (significantly) more frequently compared to rejecting.

The final study was conducted by Chiang [13], and she focused primarily on the form and function of spontaneous and evoked communicative events. Results showed that spontaneous communicative acts were significantly more common than evoked communicative acts. The form of the communicative acts showed greater frequency of unaided communication and speech, and both were more frequent than aided communication. Unaided communicating was significantly higher than speech for spontaneous communicative acts, but there was no difference between the two for evoked communicative acts. The "functions" of the communicative acts showed an interaction. Requesting was higher than commenting for spontaneous and the pattern was reversed for evoked, (i.e., commenting > requesting). Partner responses were also analyzed in this particular study. The most common response to the child was to acknowledge their communication, and this held for both spontaneous and evoked communicative acts. Deny responses (i.e., verbally and/or physically refusing the child's request) and deliver responses (i.e., giving the requested object/activity to the child) were more common for spontaneous communicative acts compared to evoked communicative acts. In addition, there was a trend for more "nonresponses" with the spontaneous communicative acts.

There are a couple of limitations in these studies. First, none examined the full range of antecedents (i.e., naturalistic cues, generalized cues, stimulus highlighting, and direct prompts), and none examined the relationship between the antecedent type and spontaneous versus evoked communicative acts. To date, there has been only a single study (i.e., [13]) that examined the ratio of evoked compared to spontaneous communicative acts within the same individuals. Second, there was a great deal of variability in where the observations occurred. In Chiang's studies, some participants were observed in special schools, some in regular schools, and some in their homes. There is an additional issue in that observations within the school environment took place during quite disparate activities and/or locations (e.g. "normal" academic activities, free time, physical education, cafeteria, hallways, etc.). To our knowledge, the length of time that participants spent in the different activities was not controlled, and, thus, the mean communication rates may not truly reflect communication tendencies in the classroom. It is assumed that home observations consisted mainly of interactions with parents, which would presumably have higher communication rates compared to teacher interactions in the classroom [41, 42].

In summary, there is preliminary evidence that relationships may exist between the type of antecedent and the form and function of expressive communication that children with autism produce. We were also interested in the teacher's responses to the children and whether these differed depending on evoked or spontaneous communicative acts. As mentioned previously, there has been only a single study that has investigated spontaneous and evoked communication in children with autism [13], and, to a large extent, there has been little research on expressive communicative acts in nonverbal children with autism, despite the fact that research suggests that approximately 25% of children with autism are nonverbal [2–4]. Therefore, the primary purpose of the study was to add to the literature on intentional communicative acts in nonverbal children with autism in a classroom environment. Our specific research questions were (1) what are the most successful antecedents in evoking intentional communicative acts? (2) what are the most common forms of communicative acts used by children with autism? (3) what are the functions of those communicative acts? and (4) how do teachers respond to the intentional communicative acts made by children with autism?

2. Method

2.1. Participants. Six children with autism participated in the study, ranging in age from 10 to 15 yrs (M = 12.8, SD = 2.1). Participants were recruited through the North East Autism Society. All children had severe language impairments (i.e., fewer than five functional words) and had been diagnosed with autism by a physician or psychiatrist. Standardized assessments of language and cognitive abilities, adaptive behavior, and autism symptom severity were not available to the research team. In addition, the research team was not provided with information concerning how much the use of PECS is emphasized within classroom instruction in this particular school.

2.2. Materials. A coding sheet was used to record the spontaneous and evoked communicative acts made by the children [12, 38]. The coding sheet was divided into four main categories: the antecedent, the child's response, the function of the communicative act and the teacher's response to the child. The sheet also had a section at the bottom that allowed the observer to make notes regarding the situation, and the time the observation started and ended. The frequencies of events within each category were summed for each participant and then transformed into proportions for each child. The analyses were carried out on the proportions.

2.3. Design and Procedure. All observations were carried out in the same school, which was a special school for children with autism, located in the northeast of England. The children who were observed were permanently located in different classes from one another. However, there were three or four other children with autism or other developmental disabilities in each of the classrooms and one teacher and two teaching assistants. The observations took place over five days at various times throughout the day, and each observation took place during a structured teacher-led activity. Each child was observed in a single 30-minute session during their regular school routine. The teachers and teaching assistants were blind to the purposes of the study and were asked to maintain their normal activities. The observer was an undergraduate psychology student who was trained on the forms of communicative acts and the coding scheme used in the study. In order to assess observer reliability, we had the observer and a second trained researcher code several short videos of a nonverbal child with autism interacting with a parent or a teacher. The proportion of agreement between the two raters ranged from 1.0 for the form of the child's communicative act to .94 for the teacher/parent's response to the child. In addition, the primary observer (i.e., the first author) had extensive experience (approximately 20 hours per week over 2 years) working with children with autism in a residential care setting.

2.4. Communication Coding. A communicative act was considered expressive if there was evidence that the child was actively communicating information to a teacher (or a teachers' assistant). If the child merely complied with an instruction or request from the teacher, it was not coded as an intentional communicative act [5]. In contrast, if the child's behavior was a response to the teacher's question (e.g., "What do you want?"), then it was coded as an intentional communicative act.

Due to the limited sample size, we analyzed our data using nonparametric tests, which do not rely on the assumption of normality and are substantially more conservative than parametric tests. For analyses that compared three or more variables, we used a Friedman test, which is conceptually similar to a one-way repeated measures ANOVA. However, the test of significance is chi-square (χ^2) instead of F-ratio. For analyses that compared two variables, we used a Wilcoxon signed-rank test, which is conceptually similar to a paired samples t-test. All analyses were two tailed. Evoked communicative acts were analyzed with a Friedman test coded along a continuum with three categories: (1) stimulus highlighting (e.g., teacher comments that drew attention to an object), (2) generalized communicative cues, indicating that a nonspecific response was required (e.g., questions and the presentation of PECS cards), and (3) direct prompts, indicating that a specific response was required [38]. The category direct prompts was subdivided into four categories: verbal (e.g., questions or instructions), modeling (e.g., demonstrating a requested response), physical (e.g., giving assistance), and other. (Other responses were infrequent and excluded from the analysis.) If more than one form of prompting occurred simultaneously or in rapid succession, then all forms were coded. However, this almost never occurred during any of the observations.

A Friedman test was also used to analyze the communication forms employed by the children. Separate tests were conducted for both evoked and spontaneous communicative acts. Response types were verbal (e.g., echolalic or other verbal sound), physical (e.g., gestures and sign language), use of PECS (e.g., the child employed PECS successfully), modeling (e.g., the child copied the teachers prompting), challenging behavior (e.g., self-harm, tantrums, and physical violence), and other. (Challenging behavior and "other" turned out to be infrequent and were excluded from the analyses.)

A Friedman test was used to examine the functions of the communicative acts produced, and, again, the evoked and spontaneous communicative acts were examined separately. Functions were coded as a request (e.g., asking for an object), reject (e.g., refuse to accept an object or instruction), and other (e.g., greeting another person, commenting on an object, etc.).

Finally, a Friedman test was used to examine the responses that the teacher (or teachers' assistant) made to the child. (Participants never communicated with other children in the classroom.) For both evoked and spontaneous communicative acts, teachers' responses were coded into six categories: deny (i.e., the teacher verbally and/or physically refused the child's request), acknowledge (i.e., the teacher verbally acknowledged the child), no response (i.e., no verbal/physical reaction to the child), delivered (i.e., the referent was given to the child), removed (i.e. the referent that the child wanted or disliked was removed), and other. (The acknowledge category was used only for those instances in which the teacher acknowledged the communication but did not act on it further (i.e., deny, deliver, and remove).) (Again, "removed" and "other" responses were very infrequent and so, were excluded from the analyses.)

3. Results

Results showed that 63 of the 155 communicative events were spontaneous. The other 92 were evoked from generalized cues, stimulus highlighting, and direct prompts. A Wilcoxon test showed no difference between spontaneous and evoked communicative acts $z = -1.15$, $P = .25$.

3.1. Antecedents. The first Friedman test revealed a significant difference between direct prompts, stimulus highlighting, and generalized prompts $\chi^2(2) = 11.56$, $P = .003$ (see Figure 1(a)). (For this analysis the direct prompts were summed.) The Wilcoxon paired comparisons revealed significant differences between generalized and direct prompts $z = -2.20$, $P = .028$, stimulus highlighting and direct prompts $z = -2.20$, $P = .028$, and stimulus highlighting and generalized $z = -2.02$, $P = .043$. Table 1 shows the frequency counts for each participant separately. A second Friedman test revealed that there was a significant difference in the types of direct prompts used by the teacher to evoke intentional communicative acts $\chi^2(2) = 6.91$, $P = .032$ (see four bars on the right side of Figure 1(a)). Wilcoxon paired comparisons were conducted to examine the differences between the different categories. Results showed a significant difference between verbal and physical prompts $z = -2.20$, $P = .028$. This shows that verbal prompts were the most effective direct prompt for evoking communicative acts from children. There were no significant differences for any of the other paired comparisons (all P's > .05).

3.2. Child's Communication. A Friedman test conducted on evoked communicative acts revealed a significant effect $\chi^2(3) = 10.44$, $P = .015$. The proportions are shown on the left side of Figure 1(b). There were significant (paired) comparisons between verbal and physical responses $z = -2.20$, $P = .028$, between PECS and physical responses $z = -2.20$, $P = .028$, and between physical responses and modeling $z = -1.99$, $P = .046$. None of the other paired comparisons were significant (all P's > .05). For *spontaneous* communicative acts, the Friedman test was not significant $\chi^2(3) = 5.59$, $P = .133$. Thus, physical communication acts were the most common response for evoked communicative acts and a similar (but not significant) trend was observed for spontaneous communicative acts.

3.3. Function of Communication. A Friedman test conducted on evoked communicative acts revealed a significant effect $\chi^2(2) = 10.57$, $P = .005$ (see Figure 1(c) and Table 2 for frequency counts for each participant). Paired Wilcoxon comparisons indicated a significant difference between "other" and requests $z = -2.20$, $P = .028$ and "other" and rejects $z = -2.02$, $P = .043$. None of the other paired comparisons were significant. For spontaneous communicative acts, the Friedman test was also significant $\chi^2(2) = 10.17$, $P = .006$. There were two significant paired comparisons. Requests were more common compared to rejects $z = -2.20$, $P = .028$, and requests were more frequent than other $z = -2.20$, $P = .028$. The difference between reject and other was not significant.

3.4. Teacher's Response. A Friedman test conducted on evoked communicative acts revealed a significant effect $\chi^2(3) = 13.18$, $P = .004$ (see Figure 1(d)). Paired Wilcoxon tests revealed significant differences between acknowledge and deny responses $z = -2.20$, $P = .028$, no responses and

TABLE 1: Frequency counts for both communication prompts and the form of communicative acts for each participant.

	Part. 1	Part. 2	Part. 3	Part. 4	Part. 5	Part. 6
Prompts						
Naturalistic (spontaneous)	15	14	11	3	5	15
Evoked	27	7	17	17	8	16
Generalized	4	1	3	3	1	5
Highlighting	4	0	0	0	0	2
Verbal	11	4	14	5	6	5
Modelling	6	0	0	8	0	0
Physical	2	2	0	0	0	3
Child's communication						
Evoked	27	7	17	17	8	16
PECS	1	0	0	0	1	2
Verbal	0	0	4	0	0	0
Modeling	5	0	0	12	0	0
Physical	21	7	9	4	6	14
Spontaneous	15	14	11	3	5	15
PECS	4	0	0	0	2	4
Verbal	0	0	7	2	0	0
Modeling	0	0	0	1	0	0
Physical	11	14	4	0	3	8

Note. PECS stands for picture exchange communication system. Part.: participant.

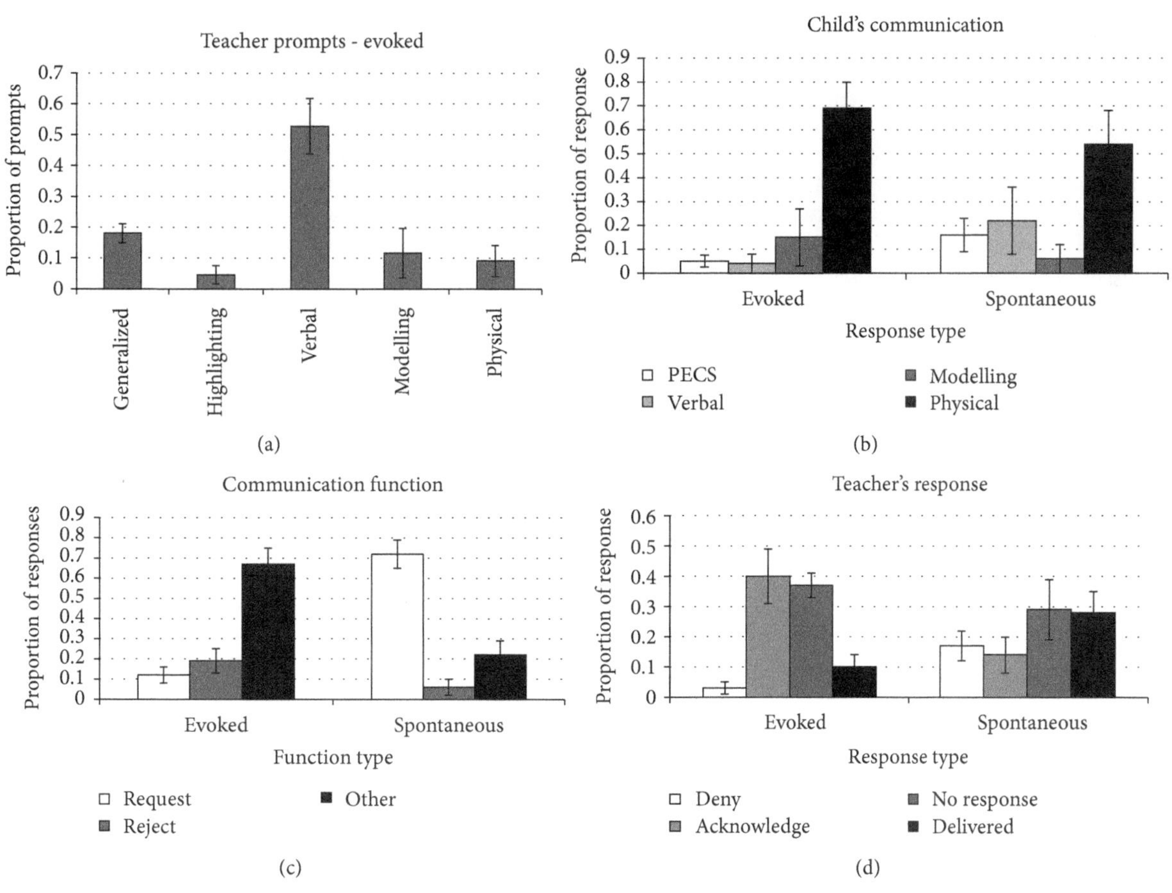

FIGURE 1: (a) shows the antecedents of evoked communicative acts. (b) shows the form of the communicative acts. (c) shows the function of the communicative acts. (d) shows the teacher's response to the child. Error bars show the standard error of the mean.

TABLE 2: Frequency counts for both communication function and the teacher response for each participant.

	Part. 1	Part. 2	Part. 3	Part. 4	Part. 5	Part. 6
Communication function						
Evoked	27	7	17	17	8	16
Request	3	0	4	1	2	1
Reject	3	0	5	2	3	4
Other	21	6	8	14	3	11
Spontaneous	15	14	11	3	5	15
Request	8	9	8	3	4	9
Reject	0	0	1	0	0	4
Other	7	5	2	0	1	2
Teacher response						
Evoked	27	7	17	17	8	16
Deny	0	0	1	0	0	2
Acknowledge	11	5	4	9	1	6
No response	8	2	9	6	3	6
Delivered	6	0	1	0	2	1
Spontaneous	15	14	11	3	5	15
Deny	3	3	2	1	0	1
Acknowledge	2	2	1	0	2	1
No response	1	5	7	0	2	4
Delivered	7	2	1	1	1	7

Notes. Part.: participant.

deny $z = -2.20$, $P = .028$, deliver and acknowledge $z = -1.99$, $P = .046$, and no responses and deliver $z = -2.20$, $P = .028$. For spontaneous communicative acts, the Friedman test was significant $\chi^2(3) = 9.75$, $P = .02$, but none of the paired comparisons achieved significance. The most common response to evoked communicative acts was acknowledgement and non-response. The most common response to spontaneous communicative acts was non-response and delivered, but these effects were not statistically significant.

4. Discussion

The primary goal of this study was to investigate the intentional communicative acts of nonverbal children with autism in a classroom environment, and we were particularly interested in the differences between spontaneous and evoked communicative acts. The results showed that every child displayed intentional communication, despite their lack of symbolic communication. We investigated four main research questions, each of which focused on a different aspect of the communicative acts. The first question looked at what are the most successful antecedents in evoking expressive communication. Results showed, similar to Chiang [12], that verbal prompts were the most common antecedents. The second and third research questions looked at the form and function of the communicative acts displayed by the children, respectively. The final research question looked at the teacher's responses to the child. Overall, the children in this study showed somewhat higher rates of intentional communication compared to earlier work (51 per hour in the current study versus 44 per hour in Chiang and Lin's study). (Stone and Caro-Martinez [14] focused on spontaneous communicative acts and they reported only 3-4 communicative acts per hour in their study.) Chiang [12] focused only on evoked communication from teacher instructions, and she reported a rate of ten per hour. As discussed in Section 1, we used a continuum approach with regard to antecedents, and we distinguished between evoked and spontaneous communicative acts.

This study found that 41% of the communicative acts were spontaneous. Chiang [13] also reported a high percentage of spontaneous communicative acts, and, in fact, spontaneous communicative acts were more common than evoked communicative acts in her study. There are two points that should be made concerning the rates of spontaneous communication that we observed. First, the spontaneous communicative acts were primarily instances in which the child wanted something (see also [13]). Thus, communication was driven by an internal desire for some object [20]. Second, the school in which the observations occurred does not adhere to highly structured teaching methods. Preliminary evidence indicates that structured teaching methods are successful in improving working skills and functional communication abilities of children with autism and other types of developmental disorders [43]. In contrast, Chiang and Carter [25] argued that structured teaching methods may stifle communicative spontaneity. Our data do not directly support this conjecture. However, given that the classroom environment in which the observations occurred was less structured, and when combined with the (relatively) high rates of spontaneous communication (i.e., 21 per hour), our data at least indirectly suggest that less-structured environments result in more spontaneous communicative acts.

If this conjecture is true, it would provide important information for educators on how to facilitate and encourage more spontaneous communication. Of course, there would likely be a tradeoff in that less structure would presumably come at the cost of less learning. That is, minimizing the structure within the classroom environment may adversely affect the development of the children's working skills and other forms of learning. Thus, it may be that an equal balance of structured and nonstructured activities needs to be integrated into daily school timetables. A further point worth considering is whether the frequency and duration of unstructured activities should be dependent upon the child's current ability to communicate spontaneously. For example, if a child with autism demonstrates limited ability to spontaneously communicate, it may be beneficial for the child to develop their spontaneous communication skills compared to other alternative working skills (e.g., drawing or painting). The National Research Council [44] stated that the development of functional spontaneous communication is the most important goal in educating children with autism. However, these issues can only be speculated on at this time and are beyond the scope of the current investigation.

With regards to the second research question, we found that physical forms of communication were the most frequent, which is in line with the results from Chiang [13]. This finding is also consistent with other studies, in that children with autism, who are nonverbal, showed a preference for less complex communication forms, for example, physical gestures and modeling [9, 11]. Often the signals that children with autism provide are idiosyncratic and subtle [45]; thus, in some instances, educators may miss communication signals displayed by the children. In addition throughout this study PECS was not frequently used by the children. However, we do not know how much or how often the teachers in this particular school actively promote the use of such devices. On the other hand, the severity of symptoms in these particular children may prevent them from using more complex forms of communication, such as PECS, and sign language, functional spoken language. We did find that the frequency of PECS was slightly higher when the child produced spontaneous communicative acts compared to evoked communicative acts. Thus, our data would suggest that children with autism are more likely to use PECS when requesting an object they want. Recall that the primary function of spontaneous communicative acts was requests for objects (i.e., > 70%). On the other hand, children with autism may have a tendency (or preference) for communicating with their teachers using physical communicative acts, such as physical gestures and/or actions. Our data does not provide a base rate for physical versus PECS, and, so, we cannot determine what causes the differences we observed. Further research is needed in order to determine whether the use of PECS increases when the child is requesting something they want or whether the rate decreases because the teacher is attempting to get the child to comply with educational instructions.

The teacher's responses followed straightforwardly from the trends in the functions of the communicative acts. The spontaneous acts were responded to more frequently by denying and delivering the requested object compared to the evoked communicative acts. In contrast, when the teacher evoked the communication, their responses were more frequently to acknowledge the communication. Acknowledging and commending communicative behavior is one way of enacting a positive change in communication abilities in autism [46–48]. There was no difference in the rates of nonresponding by the teacher depending on whether the communication was evoked or spontaneous. However, about one-third of the communicative acts displayed by the children in this study did not evoke a response from the teacher (cf. [13]).

There are several potential reasons for this finding. First, the communicative behaviors of children with autism are often subtle and may be missed. Second, in the classroom setting, teachers have plans and goals for each lesson. Thus, in many instances, the goals of the teacher and the goals of the student conflict with one another, and nonresponses by the teacher may be cases in which the child's communicative act is not relevant to what the teacher is attempting to accomplish. This explanation is more likely following spontaneous, as opposed to evoked communicative acts. Related to this point, we found that challenging behavior was relatively infrequent [49–52]. Some have argued that challenging behavior is a form of communication in which the child is deliberately seeking attention [53], as well as to escape demands and gain access to objects and/or activities [52]. In either case, challenging behavior was infrequent in our observations.

4.1. Educational Implications. It is important to note that the results obtained from this study should be considered preliminary, due to the restricted sample size and observer-reliability limitations. However, we believe that this study has several implications for educational practices for children with autism. The first is that our study supports previous research and provides clear examples that children with autism do communicate spontaneously, and they are more likely to do so when they want something [13]. Even though this study only had six participants, it provides empirical support for several teaching methods that are commonly used with nonverbal children with autism (e.g., making objects inaccessible, the Mand technique). The second point is also related to spontaneous communicative acts. We found somewhat higher rates of PECS use and more verbal communications when the children were communicating spontaneously. Thus, placing desired objects away from the child and having them communicate what they want should tend to evoke more desirable communicative behaviors [54–57]. This strategy is commonly employed in early interventions but may not be appropriate for school-aged pupils with autism. A further suggestion with regards to spontaneous communicative acts is for schools to incorporate more frequent unstructured activity sessions. The duration and frequency of such sessions could be altered depending on the ability of the pupils within the class to spontaneously communicate.

A final point concerns the rate of nonresponses by the teacher. There were a few instances of challenging behavior, and in the majority of these, the teacher did not respond.

However, the vast majority of non-responses did not follow challenging behavior. As mentioned above, there may be good reasons why the teacher did not respond to the child in certain situations. In this study, we cannot say whether teacher non-responses had a positive or negative effect on communication development. Keen et al. [46] argued that the best practice for nonverbal children with autism is to provide frequent and consistent responses, and that this is the best way to facilitate and improve communication development [58, 59]. Our data suggest that there is room for improvement in providing consistent feedback, at least for the teaching method/environment that we observed in.

4.2. Limitations and Future Directions. Several limitations need to be highlighted. First, we acknowledge that this study observed participants for a shorter period of time compared to previous studies (e.g., [5]), and of course, we recommend replication with a larger sample in order to ensure generalizability of the results. A larger sample would also obviate concerns about the statistical assumptions and permit the use of more standard parametric analyses. The second limitation was that there was no reliability check on the actual data. There were a couple of reasons why this was not possible; however, we did have two individuals independently code secondary data in order to ensure some level of reliability on the observations. We admit that this situation is less than ideal, and, again, we would encourage replication with a larger sample and reliability checks on the actual observations. The third limitation is that the activities that the child engaged in during the observation period were not always consistent. It is possible that certain classroom activities may have encouraged more communicative acts compared to others. However, all observations in this study took place in the classroom, and so, our data was collected in a more consistent environment compared to earlier work [5, 12–14]. The final limitation is that we did not have developmental assessments (e.g., language and cognitive measures, autism symptom severity, etc.) for the participants in the study. Thus, we were not able to assess differences between individuals and their communicative tendencies.

We think that one important avenue for future work is to investigate whether communicative behaviors differ in the home, as compared to the school environment. In particular, the home and school differ in the number of structured activities, and so, it would be interesting to investigate how unstructured activities affect communicative behavior across settings.

5. Conclusions

The children in this study all showed intentional communication, and we found that the most successful antecedents for evoking intentional communication were verbal prompts and naturalistic cues. The most common intentional communicative acts were physical. They accounted for approximately one-third of all communicative acts in this study. However, we also found that with spontaneous communication (i.e., those due to naturalistic cues), the use of PECS increased compared to the use of PECS in evoked communication. The spontaneous communicative acts were primarily requests for objects [13]. Finally, a substantial percentage of intentional communicative acts resulted in a nonresponse from the teacher. Future work will need to be conducted to determine whether nonresponses in certain situations (e.g., following challenging behavior) have positive or negative effects on communication development. In summary, this study largely supports previous research with respect to the form and function of spontaneous and evoked communication. However, it also extends existing literature by examining the antecedents to the intentional communicative acts.

Acknowledgments

The authors would like to thank Sean N. Veld and Kerry Shields for help with data analysis and for constructive discussions of the findings. They would also like to thank the Northeast Autism Society and Margaret Burton for arranging the observation sessions.

References

[1] American Psychiatric Association, *Diagnostic and Statistical Manual of Mental Disorders*, American Psychiatric Association, Washington, DC, USA, 4th edition, 2000.

[2] E. Fombonne, "The epidemiology of autism: a review," *Psychological Medicine*, vol. 29, no. 4, pp. 769–786, 1999.

[3] C. Lord, S. Risi, and A. Pickles, "Trajectory of language development in autistic spectrum disorders," in *Developmental Language Disorders: From Phenotypes to Etiologies*, M. L. Rice and S. F. Warren, Eds., pp. 7–29, Lawrence Erlbaum Associates, Mahwah, NJ, USA, 2004.

[4] F. R. Volkmar, C. Lord, A. Bailey, R. T. Schultz, and A. Klin, "Autism and pervasive developmental disorders," *Journal of Child Psychology and Psychiatry and Allied Disciplines*, vol. 45, no. 1, pp. 135–170, 2004.

[5] H.-M. Chiang and Y.-H. Lin, "Expressive communication of children with autism," *Journal of Autism and Developmental Disorders*, vol. 38, no. 3, pp. 538–545, 2008.

[6] A. S. Chan, J. Cheung, W. W. M. Leung, R. Cheung, and M. Cheung, "Verbal expression and comprehension deficits in young children with autism," *Focus on Autism and Other Developmental Disabilities*, vol. 20, pp. 117–124, 2005.

[7] S. Mitchell, J. Brian, L. Zwaigenbaum et al., "Early language and communication development of infants later diagnosed with autism spectrum disorder," *Journal of Developmental and Behavioral Pediatrics*, vol. 27, no. 2, pp. S69–S78, 2006.

[8] A. M. Wetherby, "Ontogeny of communicative functions in autism," *Journal of Autism and Developmental Disorders*, vol. 16, no. 3, pp. 295–316, 1986.

[9] W. L. Stone, O. Y. Ousley, P. J. Yoder, K. L. Hogan, and S. L. Hepburn, "Nonverbal communication in two- and three-year-old children with autism," *Journal of Autism and Developmental Disorders*, vol. 27, no. 6, pp. 677–696, 1997.

[10] R. Paul, "Assessing communication in autism spectrum disorders," in *Handbook of Autism and Pervasive Developmental Disorders*, F. R. Volkmar, R. Paul, A. Klin, and D. Cohen, Eds., vol. 2, pp. 799–816, John Wiley & Sons, Hoboken, NJ, USA, 2005.

[11] P. Yoder, R. B. McCathren, S. F. Warren, and A. L. Watson, "Important distinctions in measuring maternal responses

to communication in prelinguistic children with disabilities," *Communication Disorder Quarterly*, vol. 22, pp. 135–147, 2001.

[12] H.-M. Chiang, "Naturalistic observations of elicited expressive communication of children with autism: an analysis of teacher instructions," *Autism*, vol. 13, no. 2, pp. 165–178, 2009.

[13] H.-M. Chiang, "Differences between spontaneous and elicited expressive communication in children with autism," *Research in Autism Spectrum Disorders*, vol. 3, no. 1, pp. 214–222, 2009.

[14] W. L. Stone and L. M. Caro-Martinez, "Naturalistic observations of spontaneous communication in autistic children," *Journal of Autism and Developmental Disorders*, vol. 20, no. 4, pp. 437–453, 1990.

[15] D. R. Beukelman and P. Mirenda, *Augmentative and Alternative Communication. Management of Severe Communication Disorders in Children and Adults*, Paul H. Brookes Publishing, Baltimore, Md, USA, 1992.

[16] C. Lord, "Commentary: achievements and future directions for intervention research in communication and autism spectrum disorders," *Journal of Autism and Developmental Disorders*, vol. 30, no. 5, pp. 393–398, 2000.

[17] P. Mirenda, "Autism, augmentative communication, and assistive technology: what do we really know?" *Focus on Autism and Other Developmental Disabilities*, vol. 16, pp. 141–151, 2001.

[18] B. T. Ogletree and W. E. Harn, "Augmentative and alternative communication for persons with Autism: history, issues and unanswered questions," *Focus on Autism and Other Developmental Disabilities*, vol. 16, pp. 138–140, 2001.

[19] A. S. Bondy and L. A. Frost, "Mands across the water: a report of the application of the picture-exchange communication system in Peru," *The Behavior Analyst*, vol. 16, pp. 123–128, 1993.

[20] A. S. Bondy and L. A. Frost, "The picture exchange communication system," *Focus on Autistic Behavior*, vol. 9, pp. 1–19, 1994.

[21] A. S. Bondy and L. A. Frost, *Pictures Worth: PECS and Other Visual Communication Strategies in Autism*, Woodbine House, Bethesda, Md, USA, 2002.

[22] J. Boucher and V. Lewis, "Guessing or creating? A reply to Baron-Cohen," *British Journal of Developmental Psychology*, vol. 8, pp. 205–206, 1990.

[23] E. G. Carr and E. Kologinsky, "Acquisition of sign language by autistic children. II: spontaneity and generalization effects," *Journal of Applied Behavior Analysis*, vol. 16, no. 3, pp. 297–314, 1983.

[24] M. Carter, "Communicative spontaneity of children with high support needs who use augmentative and alternative communication systems I: classroom spontaneity, mode, and function," *Augmentative and Alternative Communication*, vol. 19, no. 3, pp. 141–154, 2003.

[25] M. Carter and H.-M. Chiang, "Spontaneity of communication in individuals with autism," *Journal of Autism and Developmental Disorders*, vol. 38, no. 4, pp. 693–705, 2008.

[26] M. Carter, G. D. Hotchkis, and M. C. Cassar, "Spontaneity of augmentative and alternative communication in persons with intellectual disabilities: critical review," *Augmentative and Alternative Communication*, vol. 12, no. 2, pp. 97–109, 1996.

[27] M. H. Charlop, L. Schreibman, and M. G. Thibodeau, "Increasing spontaneous verbal responding in autistic children using a time delay procedure," *Journal of Applied Behavior Analysis*, vol. 18, no. 2, pp. 155–166, 1985.

[28] L. Kanner, "Autistic disturbances of affective contact," *Nervous Child*, vol. 2, pp. 217–250, 1943.

[29] L. K. Koegel, "Interventions to facilitate communication in autism," *Journal of Autism and Developmental Disorders*, vol. 30, no. 5, pp. 383–391, 2000.

[30] J. C. Light, B. Roberts, R. Dimarco, and N. Greiner, "Augmentative and alternative communication to support receptive and expressive communication for people with autism," *Journal of Communication Disorders*, vol. 31, pp. 153–180, 1998.

[31] D. Preston and M. Carter, "A review of the efficacy of the picture exchange communication system intervention," *Journal of Autism and Developmental Disorders*, vol. 39, no. 10, pp. 1471–1486, 2009.

[32] J. Riechle and J. Sigafoos, "Establishing spontaneity and generalization," in *Implementing Augmentative and Alternative Communication: Strategies For Learners with Severe Disabilities*, J. Reichle, J. York, and J. Sigafoos, Eds., pp. 157–192, Brookes, Baltimore, Md, USA, 1991.

[33] D. Cantwell, L. Baker, and M. Rutter, "A comparative study of infantile autism and specific developmental receptive language disorder. IV. Analysis of syntax and language function," *Journal of Child Psychology and Psychiatry and Allied Disciplines*, vol. 19, no. 4, pp. 351–362, 1978.

[34] K. A. Kroeger and W. M. Nelson III, "A language programme to increase the verbal production of a child dually diagnosed with Down syndrome and autism," *Journal of Intellectual Disability Research*, vol. 50, no. 2, pp. 101–108, 2006.

[35] M. H. Charlop and L. K. Haymes, "Speech and language acquisition and intervention: behavioural approaches," in *Autism in Children and Adults: Etiology, Assessment and Intervention*, J. L. Matson, Ed., pp. 213–240, Brooks Cole, Belmont, Calif, USA, 1994.

[36] L. A. Kaczmarek, "Teaching spontaneous language to individuals with severe handicaps: a matrix model," *Journal of the Association for Persons with Severe Handicaps*, vol. 15, pp. 160–169, 1990.

[37] C. Potter and C. Whittaker, *Enabling Communication in Children With Autism*, Jessica Kingsley, London, UK, 2001.

[38] M. Carter and G. D. Hotchkis, "A conceptual analysis of communicative spontaneity," *Journal of Intellectual and Developmental Disability*, vol. 27, no. 3, pp. 168–190, 2002.

[39] J. W. Halle, "Teaching language in the natural environment: an analysis of spontaneity," *Journal of the Association for Persons with Severe Handicaps*, vol. 12, pp. 28–37, 1987.

[40] M. Carter, "Communicative spontaneity of children with high support needs who use augmentative and alternative communication systems II: antecedents and effectiveness of communication," *Augmentative and Alternative Communication*, vol. 19, no. 3, pp. 155–169, 2003.

[41] C. Kasari, M. Sigman, and N. Yirmiya, "Focused and social attention of autistic children in interactions with familiar and unfamiliar adults: a comparison of autistic, mentally retarded, and normal children," *Development and Psychopathology*, vol. 5, pp. 403–414, 1993.

[42] P. Warreyn, H. Roeyers, and I. de Groote, "Early social communicative behaviours of preschoolers with austism spectrum disorder during interaction with their mothers," *Autism*, vol. 9, no. 4, pp. 342–361, 2005.

[43] S. Panerai, L. Ferrante, V. Caputo, and C. Impellizzeri, "Use of structured teaching for treatment of children with autism and severe and profound mental retardation," *Education and Training in Mental Retardation and Developmental Disabilities*, vol. 33, no. 4, pp. 367–374, 1998.

[44] National Research Council, Committee on Educational Interventions for Children with Autism, Division of Behavioral and Social Science and Education, *Educating Children with Autism* , National Academy Press, Washington, DC, USA, 2001.

[45] J. Houghton, G. J. Bronicki, and D. Guess, "Opportunities to express preferences and make choices among students with severe disabilities in classroom settings," *Journal of the Association for Persons with Severe Handicaps*, vol. 12, pp. 18–27, 1987.

[46] D. Keen, J. Sigafoos, and G. Woodyatt, "Teacher responses to the communicative attempts of children with autism," *Journal of Developmental and Physical Disabilities*, vol. 17, no. 1, pp. 19–33, 2005.

[47] S. F. Warren, P. J. Yoder, G. E. Gazdag, K. Kim, and H. A. Jones, "Facilitating prelinguistic communication skills in young children with developmental delay," *Journal of Speech and Hearing Research*, vol. 36, no. 1, pp. 83–97, 1993.

[48] P. Yoder, S. Warren, R. McCathren, and S. Leew, "Does adult responsivity to child behavior facilitate communication development?" in *Transitions in Prelinguistic Communication*, A. Wetherby, S. Warren, and J. Reichele, Eds., vol. 7, pp. 39–58, Brookes, Baltimore, Md, USA, 1998.

[49] H.-M. Chiang, "Expressive communication of children with autism: the use of challenging behaviour," *Journal of Intellectual Disability Research*, vol. 52, no. 11, pp. 966–972, 2008.

[50] B. Holden and J. P. Gitlesen, "A total population study of challenging behaviour in the county of Hedmark, Norway: prevalence, and risk markers," *Research in Developmental Disabilities*, vol. 27, no. 4, pp. 456–465, 2006.

[51] G. H. Murphy, J. Beadle-Brown, L. Wing, J. Gould, A. Shah, and N. Holmes, "Chronicity of challenging behaviours in people with severe intellectual disabilities and/or autism: a total population sample," *Journal of Autism and Developmental Disorders*, vol. 35, no. 4, pp. 405–418, 2005.

[52] R. M. Reese, D. M. Richman, J. M. Belmont, and P. Morse, "Functional characteristics of disruptive behavior in developmentally disabled children with and without autism," *Journal of Autism and Developmental Disorders*, vol. 35, no. 4, pp. 419–428, 2005.

[53] V. M. Durand and E. G. Carr, "Functional communication training to reduce challenging behavior: maintenance and application in new settings," *Journal of Applied Behavior Analysis*, vol. 24, no. 2, pp. 251–264, 1991.

[54] C. S. Englert, "Measuring special education teacher effectiveness," *Exceptional Children*, vol. 50, pp. 247–254, 1983.

[55] C. S. Englert, "Measuring teacher effectiveness from the teacher," *Focus on Exceptional Children*, vol. 17, pp. 1–15, 1984.

[56] K. A. Quill, *Teaching Children with Autism: Strategies to Enhance Communication and Socialization*, Delmar Publishing, New York, NY, USA, 1995.

[57] J. Sigafoos, J. Reichle, S. Doss, K. Hall, and L. Pettitt, "'Spontaneous' transfer of stimulus control from tact to mand contingencies," *Research in Developmental Disabilities*, vol. 11, no. 2, pp. 165–176, 1990.

[58] H. Goldstein, "Communication intervention for children with Autism: a review of treatment efficacy," *Journal of Autism and Developmental Disorders*, vol. 32, no. 5, pp. 373–396, 2002.

[59] M. Hauck, D. Fein, L. Waterhouse, and C. Feinstein, "Social initiations by autistic children to adults and other children," *Journal of Autism and Developmental Disorders*, vol. 25, no. 6, pp. 579–595, 1995.

9

Utilizing Social Stories to Increase Prosocial Behavior and Reduce Problem Behavior in Young Children with Autism

Lisa A. Wright[1] and Rebecca B. McCathren[2]

[1] *Kaplan University, Department of Educational Studies, Davenport, IA 52807, USA*
[2] *University of Missouri, Department of Special Education, Columbia, MO 65211, USA*

Correspondence should be addressed to Lisa A. Wright, wrightla@missouri.edu

Academic Editor: Olga Capirci

The purpose of this paper was to evaluate the effects of a Social Story intervention on the behavior rates of 4 young children with autism using a multiple-baseline across participants design. The results of this paper indicate that the Social Story was modestly effective in increasing prosocial behavior rates in 3 of the 4 participants, though none of the participants reached the prosocial behavior rates of age and gender-matched peers. The problem behaviors of the participants modestly decreased with the intervention. Maintenance of skills over a 1-month period was demonstrated for all of the participants. The variable and inconsistent results of the research add to the current literature base in support of the use of Social Stories for some children with autism.

1. Introduction

Autism is a complex neurological disability that is diagnosed in increasingly large numbers of children. The Centers for Disease Control [1] estimate that 1 in 110 Americans have an autism spectrum disorder (ASD). Children with ASD often lack the ability to understand another person's perspective, which can lead to problem behavior and social deficits [2]. Problem behavior may be the single most challenging characteristic in children with autism and includes screaming, crying, aggression, and sometimes self-injurious behavior [3]. Children with ASD often exhibit social deficits including decreased eye contact, poor play skills and an inability to interact with peers and form friendships, poor appreciation of social cues, and socially inappropriate behavior [3–6]. A teaching intervention of increasing popularity used to increase prosocial behavior and decrease problem behavior in young children with autism is Social Stories [7–10].

Social Stories are individualized short stories used to assist children with ASD in understanding social situations by describing and explaining appropriate behavior and providing examples of appropriate responses. Gray and Garand [2] introduced the concept of Social Stories to decrease problem behavior in children with autism. Social Stories can be used to help children understand that other people have perspectives that may differ from their own, and that others have information that is helpful to them. These short stories outline specific steps for implementing the appropriate social skill and include short text and pictorial cues. The Social Story assists the child's accurate understanding of specific social information in a given setting or circumstance [11].

Social Stories may be a beneficial intervention for multiple reasons. First, Social Stories may help explain confusing situations and diffuse anxiety and problem behavior. Second, the Social Story uses visual learning strategies which are often a strength in children with autism [12]. Third, Social Stories do not require special training to implement and can easily be used across settings and implementers. Last, the Social Story is individually written with the child's interests and perspective in mind and can be accessed easily until the target behavior is mastered. Thus, Social Stories may be an effective intervention for children with autism. Social Stories are used extensively in the field with positive results [8, 10, 13, 14].

Social Stories are an intervention used increasingly with children with ASD and have been found by the National Autism Center to be an effective research-based intervention [7].

This discussion of the literature will only include peer-reviewed published studies that used an experimental design with sufficient experimental control (e.g., exclusion of case studies and AB designs) as recommended by leaders in the field [15, 16]. Many researchers have used Social Stories to decrease screaming and crying and aggression [17–20], or decrease inappropriate verbalizations [14, 21–23]. These studies have all shown decreases in these problem behaviors, with some variability of results.

Social Story studies have also used prosocial behavior targets including increasing peer interaction [22, 24–26], increasing appropriate play [27], increasing independent behavior [28], and increasing mouth wiping [29]. All of these studies reported increases in these prosocial behaviors with the Social Story intervention. One of the studies used typical peers as criterion measures [24], and the participants had increases in prosocial behavior that approached peer criterions.

Three studies evaluated the use of Social Stories in children not diagnosed with ASD [30–32]. In the first study of its kind, Burke and colleagues evaluated the use of Social Stories with typically developing children who were experiencing sleep disturbances. Results indicated that there was an immediate and significant decrease in problem sleep time behavior in the four children in the study. Soenksen and Alper used Social Stories to increase prosocial behavior in a 5-year-old with hyperlexia while Toplis and Hadwin reported increased prosocial behaviors in 3 of 5 boys in their study of five children with behavior difficulties.

The majority of the Social Story interventions have been implemented in the classroom setting, though Adams et al. [17] studied the home environment while Ivey et al. [28] had parents read the Social Stories prior to Speech Therapy sessions. Thiemann and Goldstein [26] trained typical peers as conversation partners for implementation of the Social Stories in the classroom.

Though the literature base for Social Stories has continued to grow and become stronger, some of the studies lack strong designs. There were vague descriptions of settings [17] and lack of demonstration of experimental control [18, 33, 34]. Adams et al. also did not adequately describe participant selection criteria. In two studies [24, 25], only two of the three participants had increases in the targeted prosocial behaviors while Toplis and Hadwin [32] increased prosocial behaviors in three of five boys in their study.

Many of the studies did not assess maintenance and/or generalization effects [21–23, 25] or reported anecdotally [17, 19]. Other researchers measured maintenance but found weak or inconsistent results [27, 29] or no maintenance of effects once the Social Story was withdrawn [20, 24, 28]. Thiemann and Goldstein [26] and Sansosti and Powell-Smith [24] found weak generalization results. Only one study [14] reported a strong maintenance effect.

The articles reviewed demonstrated positive outcomes with the use of Social Stories, though some suffered from design weaknesses [17, 18, 24, 25, 34, 35]. Eight studies [18–20, 22, 26, 27, 30, 36] used interventions in addition to the Social Stories including verbal praise, video modeling, and prompts which prevented the authors from determining which intervention was responsible for effecting change in behavior. Although many of the studies demonstrated positive results, there is a wide range of experimental rigor and future studies must use appropriately stringent design to add to the growing literature base in support of Social Stories.

The purpose of this study was to evaluate the effects of a Social Story intervention on the social behavior rates of four young children with autism. This study used a multiple-baseline across participants design to evaluate the effects of the Social Story on the prosocial and problem behaviors of each of the participants in comparison to gender and age-matched peers in the inclusive preschool classroom.

2. Method

2.1. Instruments. Each child was assessed with The Social Responsiveness Scale [37] and the Carolina Curriculum for Infants and Toddlers with Special Needs [38]. The SRS is a 65-item interview tool that utilizes a standardized scale. The SRS results are divided into 5 subscales: (1) social awareness, (2) social cognition, (3) social communication, (4) social motivation, and (5) autistic mannerisms [37]. The portion of the CCITSN used in this study assessed the ability of the children to communicate functionally. For example, the participants demonstrated the ability to (1) understand "look", (2) understand words that inhibit actions such as "wait, stop, get down, my turn", and (3) follow commands in familiar contexts.

2.2. Participants. The participants for this study were selected from a public school system in a mid-western community. All participants were selected for this study based on teacher nomination after an initial screening with the Early Childhood Special Education (ECSE) Coordinator. From the pool of possible participants nominated by the ECSE Coordinator, the four children with autism were selected based on the following criteria: (1) 3 to 7 years old, (2) regular participation in an inclusive preschool, (3) current medical diagnosis of autism, and (4) ability to communicate functionally in at least the 21–24-month developmental age as measured by the CCITSN [38]. The decision about who to include in the study was based on Gray and Garand's recommendation that Social Stories benefit children who possess basic language skills and are not severely mentally impaired [2]. Participants were free of vision, hearing, and severe motor impairments that would limit their participation in the proposed study. Written parent permission was obtained in for each child.

All four of the participants were males with previous medical diagnoses of autism who were being served by the public school district's ECSE program. All four boys had target behavior of positive peer interaction and response to peer initiation which was defined by Cooper et al. [39] as follows: (1) request for peer attention unprompted by an

Table 1: Participant characteristics.

	Age	SRS	CCITSN	Problem Behavior
Nick	4 yr, 10 m	63	30–36 months.	Instances where there is no display of any verbal, physical, or gestural initiations or responses to peers as defined by no response to peer initiation
Logan	4 yr, 1 m	74	24–30 months.	Instances of negative verbal or physical behavior, instances where there is no display of any verbal, physical, or gestural initiations or responses to peers as defined by no response to peer initiation
Trevor	4 yr, 10 m	66	30–36 months.	Instances of negative verbal or physical behavior, instances where there is no display of any verbal, physical, or gestural initiations or responses to peers as defined by no response to peer initiation
Peter	5 yr	72	21–24 months.	Instances of negative verbal or physical behavior instances where there is no display of any verbal, physical, or gestural initiations or responses to peers as defined by no response to peer initiation

adult that is directed toward a peer by using his/her name or facing him/her in close proximity (e.g., "look", "John", "do you want to play?"), (2) uses gestures or vocalizations to establish joint attention with peer (e.g., holds object to show peer, taps shoulder, "good job" directed toward peer), (3) understandable answer that is unprompted by an adult, that is directed toward a peer by using his/her name or facing him/her in close proximity, and (4) a positive behavioral response to peer initiation (e.g., scoots over for peer to sit, lending toy, cooperatively building block tower, turn taking). There are additional characteristics of the participants described in Table 1.

Nick. Nick spoke in short complete sentences and was at or above age-level in all academic readiness tasks. The teacher reported that Nick is mostly playing alone with no favorite peers, using toys in a simple way such as rolling a car back and forth and occasionally participating in pretend play such as using a farm with farm animals. He had difficulty initiating and responding to conversation and play with peers.

Logan. Logan answered *yes* and *no* questions appropriately, made verbal requests not directed to a person, and often spoke from movie scripts. He was able to compose simple sentences but had difficulty with semantics. The teacher reported that Logan mostly played alone but would occasionally hand or receive a toy from a peer in the classroom. He did not initiate or respond to peer play activity in the preschool classroom and frequently spent time wandering unengaged during free play. The use of a visual schedule was used as a cue for Logan to engage in an appropriate activity.

Trevor. His teacher reported that he was a reader and that all academic skills were at age-level or above. Trevor used age-appropriate sentence length and structure except for difficulty with pronoun usage and semantic functions. He had some difficulty initiating and sustaining conversations, though he would make requests and answer questions appropriately with adults. The teacher reported that Trevor preferred to play alone and did not seem to notice peers in the classroom. Some negative behavior was observed such as taking toys, pushing, and not responding to peer initiations. The teacher indicated that many of the peers in the classroom chose to play at a distance from Trevor due to his negative peer behavior.

Peter. Peter was able to answer *yes* and *no* questions but required prompting for simple requests and one-step commands, combined with gestural cues. He occasionally used simple sentences for requests. His teacher reported that Peter played alone and did not initiate play with peers in the classroom. He would often grab toys from peers, hit, kick, or push peers when they came near him, and he often walked away when peers came close to his play area. Peter also wandered unengaged and often escaped from activities and even the classroom during free play.

Peers. After the children with autism were identified, peers with average social skills were chosen by teacher nomination from the ECSE classrooms. Peers were chosen by teacher nomination using the following criteria: (a) average social skills as assessed by the teacher, (b) age matched to participants within 6 months [40], (c) gender matched, (d) demonstrated regular attendance, (e) parent or guardian written consent to participate in study, (f) compliant to adult instructions, and (g) willing to participate in study. A median was calculated for typical social behavior based on the social behavior of the participants.

Teachers. Three of the children shared the same teacher: Logan, Trevor and Peter. Logan was in preschool in the afternoon, while Trevor, and Peter attended preschool in the morning. The ECSE teacher who read the Social Stories each day for the three participants had Master's Degrees in Education and Communication and Science Disorders with certification in Early Childhood Special Education (ECSE), and licensure as a Speech and Language Pathologist. She had been teaching in ECSE for 5 years and worked part-time as an SLP for 4 years.

Nick's primary teacher had a Master's Degree in Education with 6 years experience teaching in the preschool setting. The Social Story was read daily by Nick's ECSE teacher who spent varying amounts of time in his classroom daily.

2.3. Settings. All baseline and intervention sessions took place during free play in the preschool classroom because this was the time and setting identified as problematic for all participants. Nick's preschool classroom consisted of 12 typically developing peers. All children were from 2 years, 6 months to 3 years, 11 months. Logan and Trevor were in the same preschool classroom. There were a total of 11 three- to five-year-old children in the class, including three typical peers. The other children had diagnoses of general language, cognitive, or motor disabilities. There were a total of 7 three-to five-year-old children in Peter's preschool classroom including one typical peer. The other children had diagnoses of language, hearing, or cognitive impairments.

2.4. Materials and Measures

Observation of Peers. Observation of two comparison peers per participant was included to determine median levels of social interactions in which typical peers engage. The peers were observed five times for 10 minutes each during free play during the baseline phase of this study.

Independent Variable. The intervention of the Social Story was the independent variable. The Social Story was read by the teacher in the preschool setting during free play for each child. The construct validity of each Social Story was assessed with the Social Story Construction Checklist by an independent professional with a Master's Degree in Special Education who had extensive experience with the use of Social Stories as an intervention with children with autism. The Social Story Construction Checklist consisted of questions concerning the correct sentence ratio and the ability of the Social Story to target the specified prosocial and problem behaviors identified for each child [24].

Copies of the Social Stories were sent home for the families to read with the child, and the Social Story was available at all times in the classroom throughout the intervention and maintenance phases. Anecdotally, the parents of all participants reported that the Social Story was frequently accessed at home. The teacher reported that only Logan and Trevor accessed the Social Stories occasionally in the classroom.

Social Story. The Social Story was type written in 16-point Times New Roman font on white 5 1/2 inch (width) × 8 inch (length) cardstock, laminated and fastened by spiral binding on the left margin. There were 5 to 11 pages in each Social Story. Photographs of the child and peers were included in each Social Story to increase the communicative intent of the story for all the books except Nick's. Photographic releases were not able to be obtained for the peers in Nick's classroom; therefore his Social Story only contained photographs of himself and his teacher. Due to the limited visuals for Nick's Social Story, picture symbols were utilized for his book from the Mayer-Johnson Writing With Symbols Windows Program [41]. Each child had two individual Social Stories written, for a total of eight Social Stories (see the Appendix).

The classroom teacher was asked to introduce the story to the preschool participant with the phrase, "I wrote this story for you" [42]. The teacher then sat to the child's side and slightly back, or the child sat in the teacher's lap while the story was read aloud by the teacher (Gray). Comprehension was assessed during each intervention by having the child answer questions about the Social Story, and/or role play [22, 43]. All children demonstrated 100% comprehension from each intervention session. The Social Story was read at least once a day, at the same designated time each day during free play, until the maintenance and fading phase of the study.

2.5. Experimental Design. A multiple baseline design across participants was utilized for this study [15]. The experiment was composed of four phases. The first phase (A1) was baseline where the observer recorded the frequency of prosocial behaviors and problem behaviors. The second phase (B1) was intervention 1, the Social Story, while the third phase was intervention 2, the modified Social Story (B2). The final phase (A2) evaluated the maintenance of the intervention. Treatment sessions commenced with the first participant once a stable baseline was reached for the dependent measure. Visual analysis was utilized to identify appropriate phase changes.

Fidelity of Treatment. The teacher recorded whether or not the Social Story was read to the child that day at the specified time during free play and whether comprehension questions were asked. For at least 25% of the intervention sessions, the researcher was present to record on a checklist the treatment integrity, while the teacher completed the checklist 100% of the time.

Interobserver Agreement. Prior to beginning the study, three observers were trained to reliably record behaviors. The two primary data collectors were the researcher and a doctoral student in special education with experience in data collection. The third observer was one of the classroom teachers. The observers read the target behavior definitions and became familiar with the data collection forms and procedures for recording observations [39]. The observers then practiced observing and recording data in the free play setting defined for each participant. All three observers established a criterion of 100% agreement for three consecutive sessions [39]. The three researchers viewed social interactions in the inclusive preschool classroom and recorded observed behaviors for each targeted skill. Interobserver agreement checks were conducted for at least 1/3 of the observation sessions to insure the integrity of data collection across each participant in each condition of the study [15].

Interobserver agreement for observations was calculated to assess the reliability of the data. Reliability checks occurred for at least 30% of baseline condition, 33% of intervention sessions, and 40% of maintenance condition for each child. Observations were considered reliable if at least 80% interrater agreement was achieved for each observation. Interrater agreement was consistently above 80% for all participants. Agreement in each condition ranged from 90% to 100% for Nick ($M = 95\%$), 82% to 100% for Logan ($M = 93\%$), from 88% to 100% for Trevor ($M = 98\%$), and 93% to 100% for Peter ($M = 97\%$).

Construct Validity. The construct validity of each Social Story was assessed with the Social Story Construction Checklist and found to comply 100% of the time with the correct sentence ratio and target for specified prosocial behavior.

Procedural Reliability. A Treatment Fidelity Checklist was used to determine the fidelity of the intervention. Procedural reliability was computed as a percentage by dividing the number of days the participant was present and available in the preschool free play setting divided by the number of days the participant was read the Social Story multiplied by 100. Treatment fidelity for all participants was 100% as recorded by the teachers. The researcher was present for 100% of interventions for Nick, Logan, and Peter and 58% of interventions for Trevor.

2.6. Experimental Procedures

Baseline. There were two variables of interest: target prosocial behavior and problem behavior. During baseline, observational data were recorded for each participant's target behavior and problem behavior for 10-minute periods at least three times a week in the free play setting until baseline data were determined to be stable with at least 5 data points [15]. Observations of the five comparison peers were also conducted in the free play setting during the baseline period. No intervention occurred during this period. If any instance of the target prosocial behavior or problem behaviors occurred during the 10 minute observation, the observer recorded the behavior on the data collection sheet.

Intervention. Once baseline data were stable, intervention 1 (I1) began, which was reading of the Social Story. Data were collected for six data points [31]. When six data points were collected during I1 and the child had not met the prosocial median criterion rate of target behavior, then the Social Story was revised as recommended by Gray [42] for Intervention 2 (I2). Revisions were made to the individual Social Stories after discussing appropriate changes with the classroom teacher. For example, Nick's initial Social Story had a sentence that said, "I can try to go up to one of my friends, stand close, look at my friend and say, "Will you play with me?" This sentence was changed to, "If a friend comes over while I'm reading a book, I can scoot over and ask my friend to read with me" with the modified Social Story in I2. Data were then taken for an additional 6 data points.

Maintenance. After intervention, the Social Story was then discontinued in the classroom and the maintenance phase began. Probes were utilized in the preschool classroom to determine if behavior changes were durable over a one-month period. Five probes took place for each participant in the free play setting over a variety of days throughout the four weeks. Data collection consisted of 10-minute event recordings in the free play setting for each child.

2.7. Data Analysis. Each participant was the component of analysis, serving as his own control [15]. All visual inspection analyses included both the changes in individual participant's data as well as comparing changes across each of the additional participants. In addition, observational data were analyzed to determine the percentage of nonoverlapping data (PND) points for each participant between baseline, intervention 1, intervention 2, and maintenance. Nonoverlapping data points were computed by comparing data points in intervention 1, intervention 2, and maintenance with baseline.

3. Results

Research Question 1. Does Social Story intervention increase socially appropriate behavior and decrease problem behavior in preschoolers with diagnoses of ASD and are these effects maintained over a one-month period?

Nick. Figure 1 indicates that with implementation of the Social Story, there was a slight increase in prosocial behaviors in I1. The modification of the Social Story for I2 indicated a somewhat variable though slightly increasing rate of instances of prosocial behavior over baseline. Maintenance data were also variable, with a general increasing trend of prosocial behaviors over baseline.

The percentage of nonoverlapping data (PND) points were calculated by counting the data points in the intervention that were higher than the highest data point in baseline, dividing this number of nonoverlapping data points in the treatment series by the total number of data points in the treatment series and multiplying this number by 100 [44, 45]. An intervention with a PND of 90% or greater is considered highly effective, 70–90% is considered moderately effective, 50–70% is considered mildly effective, and less than 50% is considered ineffective as effects can be contributed strictly to chance [45]. From baseline to I1, the PND was 67% and subsequently rose to 83% from baseline to I2, indicating a moderate effect. From baseline to maintenance, the PND was 80% which also indicates a moderate effect. These data indicate that the Social Story was mildly effective for Nick in I1 and moderately effective in I2 and maintenance.

Figure 2 indicates that there was an immediate decrease to zero problem behaviors with the implementation of I1. Though the data were variable, Nick had a decrease in problem behaviors, with no problem behaviors in maintenance.

Logan. Logan had a very stable baseline with only one instance of any target prosocial behaviors. As demonstrated in Figure 1, Logan had an immediate increase in prosocial target behaviors from baseline with a positive slope. Following introduction of I2, there was an immediate increase in target behaviors, followed by a decreasing trend in target

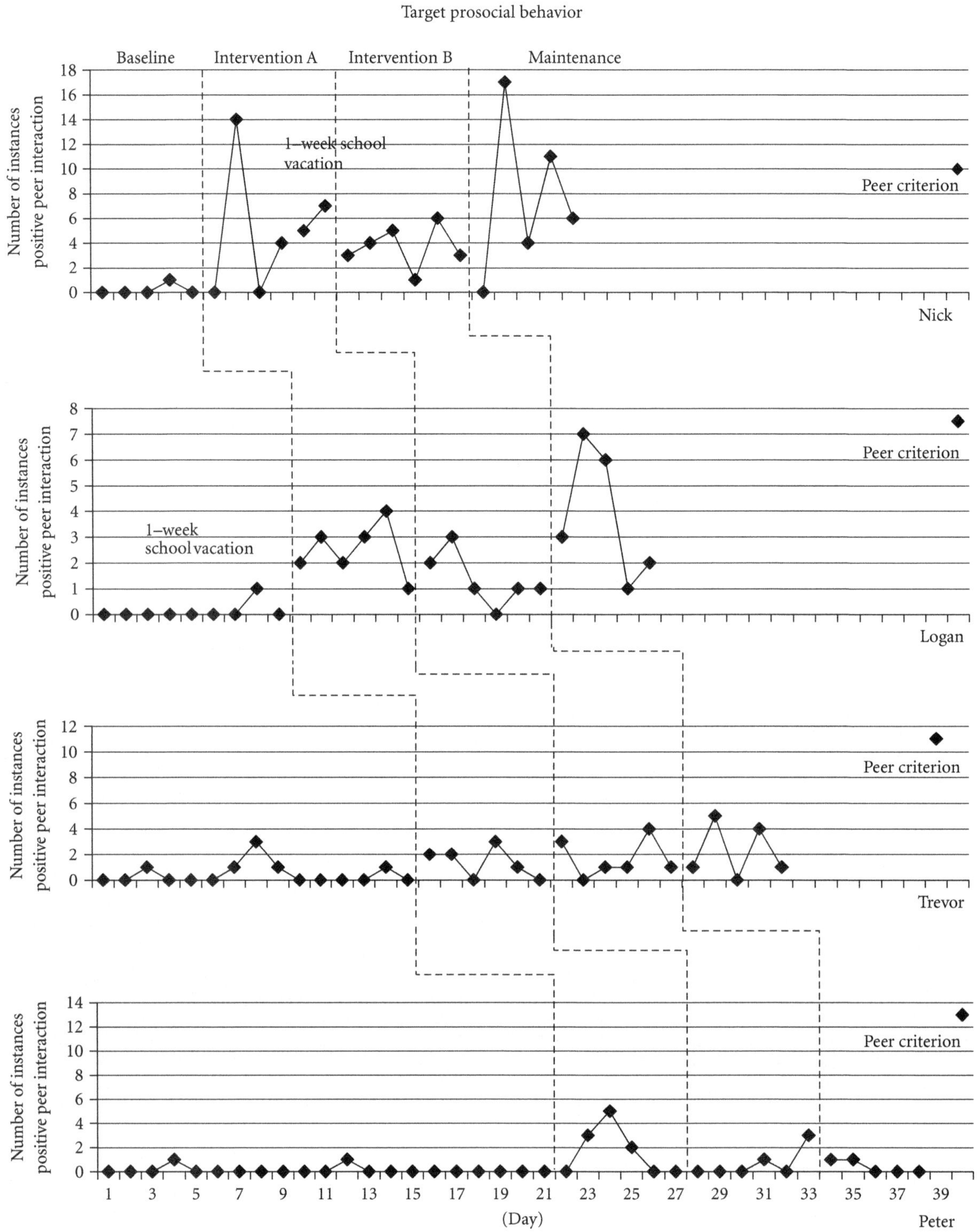

Figure 1: Target prosocial behavior.

behaviors, indicating a decreasing effectiveness of I2. Data collection in maintenance indicated an immediate increase in target prosocial behaviors.

The PND for Logan's data was 60% from baseline to I1, indicating a mild effect. From baseline to I2, the PND was only 17%, which is considered ineffective, as there were only two data points above baseline. These results indicate that the modified Social Story in I2 was not effective for increasing Logan's prosocial behaviors. The PND from baseline to maintenance was 60%, which indicates that the intervention was mildly effective in maintaining prosocial behavior after the Social Story was discontinued.

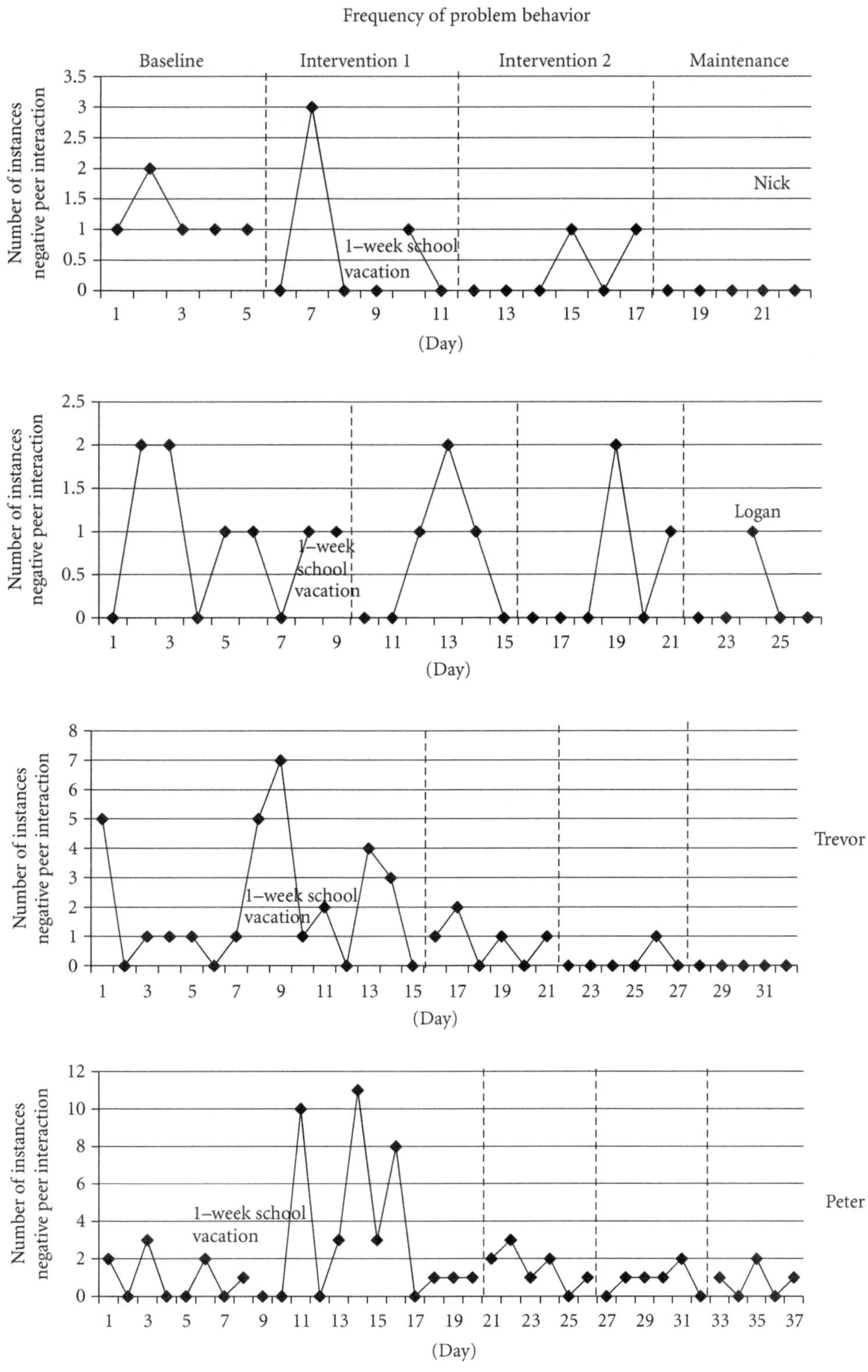

FIGURE 2: Frequency of problem behavior.

Logan's problem behavior was variable in baseline and intervention phases. It is most stable in the maintenance phase, where at 4 out of 5 days there was no problem behavior.

Trevor. In reviewing Figure 1, I1 and I2 show a slight increase in prosocial behavior from baseline, though it is inconsistent. The maintenance phase is also variable, with the highest rate of prosocial behavior of all phases, but the behavior does decrease over time.

The PND for all phases of Trevor's data was insignificant. The data points overlapped 100% from baseline to I1, while there was an 83% overlap from baseline to I2 and 60%

overlap in maintenance from baseline. The PND indicates that there was not a significant effect of I1 or I2 on Trevor's prosocial behavior.

There was a decrease in Trevor's problem behavior from baseline to I1, I2, and maintenance. Though the data were somewhat variable, with instances of no problem behavior in all of the phases of the study, visual inspection reveals a downward trend in problem behavior in I1 and I2. There were no problem behaviors in maintenance.

Peter. The data in Figure 1 indicate that upon implementation of I1, there was a slight increase in prosocial behaviors, followed by a decrease back down to zero. During I2, there were only two days of any prosocial behaviors. With discontinuation of the Social Story, there were two days of prosocial target behaviors.

The PND was only significant from baseline to I1, where it reached 50%, which is considered mildly effective. There were only 17% nonoverlapping data from baseline to I2 and 0% from baseline to maintenance. These data indicate that I1 was mildly effective, but I2 was ineffective, and there was no effect in maintenance.

Visual analysis indicates that problem behavior was variable in all phases, but there was a decrease in frequency with intervention. Peter had an increase in problem behavior following the one-week spring break vacation period, which the teacher noted occurred after a prolonged period out of the classroom.

Research Question 2. In preschoolers with diagnoses of ASD, do the social behavior rates approach those of age and gender-matched typically developing peers?

Of the four participants Nick was the closest to approaching the social behavior rate of age and gender-matched typically developing peers. On two occasions, Nick exceeded this rate though Nick's median rate of prosocial behavior fell below that of his matched peer. Logan, Trevor, and Peter did not meet or exceed the age and gender-matched peer criterion prosocial behaviors in any phase.

Research Question 3. Do teachers support the social validity of social stories?

After the intervention and maintenance sessions were completed, teacher satisfaction was assessed by a six-item questionnaire that used a 5-point scale to rate: (1) Social Story effect on the child, (2) carryover to other activities and/or settings, (3) ease of implementation, and (4) overall experience. The scale used for this tool was a Likert-type rating as follows: (1) strongly disagree, (2) disagree, (3) neutral, (4) agree, and (5) strongly agree. Both of the teachers strongly agreed with the statements that the Social Story intervention was easy to implement and that most teachers would find the intervention appropriate for a wide-range of behaviors and they would be willing to utilize the intervention again. Peter's teacher was neutral on the question of effectiveness of the intervention, though she did agree that the intervention was acceptable for the child's behavior difficulties. The other teacher either agreed or strongly agreed that the Social Story was effective. The teachers either agreed or strongly agreed that they would recommend this intervention to other teachers.

4. Discussion

The purpose of this study was to determine if using a Social Story as the sole intervention was effective in increasing prosocial interaction and decreasing problem social behavior in 4 preschoolers with autism. The results indicate that the Social Story did result in slight increases in prosocial behavior for 3 of the 4 children and some decreases in negative social interaction for all 4 of the children. The modest and inconsistent effects of the Social Story intervention are consistent with past research. The specific results are discussed hereinafter.

4.1. Increasing Prosocial Behavior. The results of this study indicate that the Social Story as a sole intervention did increase the prosocial behavior in varying though small degrees for 3 of the 4 participants. Other authors have had similar results when utilizing Social Stories without other supports [24, 25]. However, the increases in prosocial behavior were modest and none of the children approached the mean of their typically developing peers. This is not surprising given that deficits in social communication are one of the core features in autism. One of the reasons for including target levels based on the behavior of classroom peers is to ensure that our expectations for social behavior are socially valid. In this study our micronorms were based on children who were identified by teachers as being "average" in their social behavior. For children who have very low rates of prosocial behavior initially and have a disability with deficits in social communication as one of the identifying characteristics, "average" rates of social interaction may be an unrealistic criteria. Sansosti and Powell-Smith [24] had similar inconsistent results in their study of three elementary-aged children with Asperger's syndrome where only 2 of the 3 participants met or exceeded the criteria some of the time. Although having typically developing peers as the standard makes sense, it may be too rigorous a standard when used to decide whether or not an intervention has merit.

One of the benefits of using Social Stories is that they are relatively easy to make and easy to implement. As a sole intervention, particularly for young children with autism, Social Stories may be an important component, but just one piece of a more intensive systematic intervention program that includes direct teaching of the targeted behaviors. It seems likely that combining Social Stories with video [26, 36], prompting [22, 26], or response-cost systems [46] would have resulted in more robust results. We chose to not add other interventions as recommended by Ali and Frederickson [13], Nichols et al. [8], and Reynhout and Carter [9] in order to help determine the relative effectiveness of the Social Story. When multiple interventions are implemented concurrently, it is not possible to disentangle the relative contributions of each.

The inconsistent results in the published literature and in the current study make it important to identify the characteristics of children who will respond well to Social Stories. Unfortunately, our study does not help to answer this question. Since 3 of the 4 participants did have modest increases in prosocial behaviors, it is unclear which children benefit from Social Stories more than others. Scores on The CCITSN did not help predict which children would respond to the Social Story intervention. For instance, Nick and Trevor both scored in the highest range (30 to 36 months), yet Trevor did not demonstrate significant increases in prosocial behavior. It is also possible that the children who benefited from the Social Story intervention had the skills but did not use them until implementation of the intervention. The particular setting of the children in this study may have affected the results. Nick, who had the greatest prosocial behavior increase, was in a classroom with all typically developing peers. Trevor and Peter were in the same morning class and had higher gains in prosocial behavior than Logan. Perhaps the morning class had peers that positively reinforced prosocial behavior from the participants. It is also possible that the teacher gave more attention to the children in the study in addition to the Social Story, which may have affected the results of this intervention. An additional consideration is that Social Stories may be more effective in reducing inappropriate social behaviors rather than improving appropriate social behavior as discussed below.

4.2. Decreasing Problem Behavior. All four participant's problem behavior decreased modestly with the Social Story intervention. Due to the highly variable nature of behavior, it was apparent that problem behavior frequency was inconsistent for each of the participants throughout the phases of the study. It is notable that there was a possible floor effect for problem behavior instances, and this should be considered when evaluating the effectiveness of the intervention in reducing problem behaviors. Nick, Trevor, and Peter had the largest decreases in no response or negative responses to peers with the introduction of the Social Story, and these behaviors continued to decrease with intervention 2, though the behaviors were inconsistent. These results differ from the results on prosocial behavior discussed previously, where intervention 2 did not improve results. These data indicate that the modification of the Social Story was somewhat effective in decreasing problem behaviors, though the modification may not be effective in increasing prosocial behaviors. The results from this study replicate previous literature on the effectiveness of utilizing Social Stories to decrease problem behavior in children with autism [14, 19–22].

This study used Gray and Garand's [2] recommendation that the Social Story be modified if optimum results are not obtained and isolated the use of the Social Story without adding reinforcers or other confounding variables that have often been reported in the literature [25]. The results of this study indicated that it was not beneficial to modify the Social Story according to Gray and Garand's criteria, as there were not continued increases in prosocial behavior. It may be that instead of changing the Social Story, a different intervention may be necessary (e.g., prompt and praise). Problem behaviors did continue to modestly decrease with the modified Social Story, a result that is desirable in many instances.

4.3. Maintenance. After I2, the Social Story was faded for each participant while maintenance data were taken over a one month period. The maintenance data for this study were extremely encouraging. In fact, Nick, Logan, and Trevor had the highest mean prosocial behaviors in the maintenance period. Nick and Trevor had a mean of zero instances of negative behavior in maintenance. These findings are noteworthy in that prior studies utilizing Social Stories have not supported the maintenance of skills [24, 26]. Crozier and Tincani [14] reported maintenance effects in their study utilizing Social Stories with children with autism and this current study adds to the literature in support of maintenance effects of Social Story intervention. Anecdotally, the teachers indicated that the 3 children that had positive social gains with Social Stories had the targeted prosocial skills prior to implementation of the Social Story, but they did not use these skills consistently. It may be that these children had the skills but needed the Social Story to give examples of how to appropriately use the prosocial behavior in the classroom. Even once the Social Story was removed, the children still used these skills at a higher rate because they had learned how to appropriately use the social skills in the classroom.

4.4. Treatment Integrity and Social Validity. The Social Story intervention had acceptable treatment integrity and was rated as highly acceptable by the teachers. This is important as the teachers were the implementers of this intervention. These results add to the current literature base that report social validity from a teacher's perspective [47].

4.5. Limitations. Though the findings from this study are promising, there are several limitations. Both the small number of participants and the modest, inconsistent results make it difficult to generalize these findings to other children. In addition, we were unable to identify the characteristics that may help to predict which children will benefit from this intervention. Therefore, some caution must be taken in generalizing these findings to other students, types of disabilities, settings, or behaviors. The results of this study are important and help to make clear the benefits and the limitations of this particular intervention. Social Stories may have only modest effects for the types of children in this study, the study environments, and variables included. Second, the fidelity of treatment may have differed among the participants in the study. Only two teachers participated in this research. Two of the children in this study were in the same morning classroom, and a third participant also had this same teacher in the afternoon. Thus, three of the four children (Logan, Trevor, and Peter) in the study had the same teacher. It is unknown if how the teacher presents the Social Story, asks comprehension questions, and provides other extraneous variables may affect the results of a study. In addition, the teachers may have provided extra attention to the children with the addition of the Social Story intervention, and this can be a confounding variable. Also, though this study incorporated a treatment fidelity checklist, it only assessed whether the Social Story was read and if comprehension questions were asked. Future studies may need to address essential features of Social Stories through a more comprehensive treatment fidelity assessment. Though the researcher provided copies of each Social Story for home use, there was no formal assessment of how often the Social Stories were read in the home environment. Finally, we did not collect generalization data in a variety of settings as recommended by previous reviews of the literature [8, 48]. Anecdotal evidence from Nick's teacher did support the generalization of treatment gains. She stated that on two separate days she noted Nick asking peers to play during outdoor recess, which she had not observed prior to the intervention implementation.

4.6. Implications for Practice. There are several implications for practice concerning the results of this study including the call for Evidence-based practice (EBP), Social Story implementation characteristics, and the social validity of the intervention. Practitioners are utilizing Social Stories as an intervention for children with ASD yet with limited empirical support [8, 10, 48]. This study utilized rigorous experimental control which resulted in modest increases in prosocial behavior in three of the four participants and inconsistent decreases in problem behaviors in all four participants. This study raises a question about the appropriate use of peer norms for social behavior and how to determine whether an intervention is determined to be effective. Our results contribute to the body of work documenting that young children with autism need considerable instruction and support to interact appropriately with their peers. It seems likely that Social Stories may be part of a broader, more intensive set of strategies, but not enough as the sole intervention. The results also demonstrate that if the Social Story is not effective by itself, adding a different intervention rather than just changing the Social Story may yield more robust outcomes.

5. Recommendations for Future Research

It is important that future research efforts evaluate the maintenance and generalization of intervention effects. Kuttler et al. [20] found generalization of effects of Social Stories, but these results have not been replicated. There is support for the maintenance of the effects of Social Stories [14], but some reports have been anecdotal [27] or weak and inconsistent [26]. Future studies should assess maintenance after fading the Social Story and also evaluate the effectiveness of Social Stories in a variety of settings, or with a variety of behaviors.

Next, future research should evaluate the critical components required for effective Social Story implementation and how or when to use Social Stories as part of a larger intervention. This study revealed that modifying the Social Story per Gray and Garand's [2] recommendations did not result in increased prosocial behaviors. It may be that Social Stories are most effective as less intensive supports or reminders, during the generalization or maintenance phases of more intensive instructional strategies that have been successfully implemented. It is also imperative that researchers evaluate what are critical components of the Social Story intervention including number of days read, types and quality of comprehension questions, sentence ratios and types, and number and type of illustrated examples. These are many variables that have not been isolated in the current Social Story literature. The results of these types of studies can reveal the critical components for successful implementation of Social Stories [8, 10, 13].

It will be important for future researchers to continue to study peer micronorms on social behavior. Since no data could be located concerning micronorms for target prosocial behavior studied in the current research, it is imperative that researchers continue to include peer data in future studies. Only by understanding acceptable peer norms for social behavior can researchers select appropriate prosocial behavior targets for participants in studies.

Finally, since the treatment effects were variable across the four participants in this study, it is critical to determine who best benefits from Social Stories. It is essential to determine why one participant benefits from the intervention greater than another. In this study, neither the SRS nor the CCITSN scores appeared to predict increases in prosocial skills. Future research should identify the characteristics of children who respond to Social Stories. It is important for future researchers to assess the use of Social Stories with a variety of children with varying skills and diagnoses.

6. Summary

This study evaluated the effects of a Social Story intervention in four young children with ASD. The results of this study add to the current small though growing literature base in support of the use of Social Stories for some children. Though the results are promising, the current research must be replicated while addressing future research needs.

Appendix

N Plays in Preschool

Hi, my name is ___________.

I go to preschool.

Sometimes, I play alone in preschool.

Sometimes, I read with my teacher.

I can try to go up to one of my friends, stand close, look at my friend and say, "Will you play with me?"

My friends like to play with me.

When a friend calls my name, I should look at my friend and say, "Hi."

It is good to talk to my friends.

If a friend comes close to me, I can say, "Want to play?"

It is good to play with friends in preschool.

N Plays with Friends in Preschool (Modified)

Hi, my name is __________. I go to preschool.

I like to read books with my teacher at preschool.

If a friend comes over while I'm reading a book, I can scoot over and ask my friend to read with me.

My friends like to sit and read books with me.

After I read one book, I should try to go play with my friends.

My friends like to play with me.

I can try to go up to one of my friends, stand close, look at my friend and say, "Will you play with me?"

It is fun to play with friends in preschool.

When a friend calls my name, I should look at my friend and say, "Hi. Do you want to play with me?"

It is good to talk and play with my friends at preschool.

Playing with friends in preschool is fun.

L Makes a Plan, Stays, and Plays

Hi, my name is __________.

I make a plan with my teacher in preschool.

I should try to go to the area in my plan.

It is good to stay and play when I make a plan.

When a friend tries to hand me a toy, I can hold out my hand and say, "My toy."

It is good to share and talk to my friends.

Sometimes I may want a toy my friend is playing with.

I can hold out my hand and say, "My turn."

It is fun to stay, play and talk to my friends in preschool.

L Makes a Plan, Stays, and Plays (Modified)

Hi, my name is __________. I go to preschool.

I should try to join friends when I play at preschool.

My friends like to play with me in preschool.

When a friend tries to hand me a toy,

I can hold out my hand and say, "My turn."

It is good to join my friends and share and talk.

Sometimes I may want a toy my friend is playing with.

I can hold out my hand and say, "My turn."

It is fun to join my friends to play and talk in preschool.

T Shares in Preschool

Hi, my name is __________.

I go to preschool.

It's fun to play with toys in preschool. Sometimes, I may want a toy my friend is playing with.

I can hold out my hand and say to my friend, "Can I play with the toy now?"

My friends like to play with me when I share.

Usually, sharing and taking turns is a good idea.

Sometimes a friend may try to hand me a toy.

If a friend tries to hand me a toy, I can hold out my hand and say, "Thank you."

Sometimes a friend may want a toy I am playing with.

If a friend tries to take my toy, I can say, "It's my turn to play with the toy."

It is good to share with my friends in preschool.

T Shares in Preschool (Modified)

Hi, my name is __________. I like to go to preschool.

We have fun playing with toys in preschool

Sometimes, my friend is playing with a toy I want.

I can hold out my hand and say to my friend, "Can I play with the toy now?"

My friends have fun and like to play with me when I share.

Sharing and taking turns is usually a good idea.

Sometimes a friend tries to hand me a toy. If a friend tries to hand me a toy, I can hold out my hand and say, "Thank you."

Sometimes a friend may want a toy I am playing with. If a friend tries to take my toy, I can say, "It's my turn to play with the toy."

It is nice to share with my friends in preschool.

P Stays and Plays

Hi, my name is __________.

I like to play with toys.

My friends like to play too.

Sometimes a friend wants my toy.

I can say, "I want toy."

Sometimes a friend gives me a toy.

I can say, "I want toy."

It is good to stay and play with my friends at preschool.

P Stays and Plays (Modified)

Hi, my name is ___________. I go to preschool.

It is fun to play with toys.

My friends like to play with me.

Sometimes a friend wants my toy.

I can say, "I want toy."

Sometimes a friend gives me a toy.

I can say, "I want toy."

It is good to stay and play with my friends at preschool.

Disclosure

There was no funding for this research. There is no direct financial relation with the commercial identity mentioned in this paper that might lead to a conflict of interests for any of the authors.

References

[1] Centers for Disease Control and Prevention, "Autism Spectrum Disorders: Data and Statistics," 2010, http://www.cdc.gov/ncbddd/autism/data.html.

[2] C. A. Gray and J. D. Garand, "Social stories: improving responses of students with autism with accurate social information," *Focus on Autism and Other Developmental Disabilities*, vol. 8, no. 1, pp. 1–10, 1993.

[3] Centers for Disease Control and Prevention, "Autism Spectrum Disorders: Signs and Symptoms," 2010, http://www.cdc.gov/ncbddd/autism/signs.html.

[4] N. Bauminger, C. Shulman, and G. Agam, "Peer interaction and loneliness in high-functioning children with autism," *Journal of Autism and Developmental Disorders*, vol. 33, no. 5, pp. 489–507, 2003.

[5] G. Montes and J. S. Halterman, "Characteristics of school-age children with autism," *Journal of Developmental and Behavioral Pediatrics*, vol. 27, no. 5, pp. 379–385, 2006.

[6] M. Rutter, "Autistic children: infancy to adulthood," *Seminars in Psychiatry*, vol. 2, no. 4, pp. 435–450, 1970.

[7] National Autism Center, *National Standards Project: Findings and Conclusions*, National Autism Center, Randolph, Mass, USA, 2009.

[8] S. L. Nichols, S. D. Hupp, J. D. Jewell, and C. S. Zeigler, "Review of Social Story interventions for children diagnosed with autism spectrum disorders," *Journal of Evidence-Based Practices for Schools*, vol. 6, no. 1, pp. 90–120, 2005.

[9] G. Reynhout and M. Carter, "Social stories for children with disabilities," *Journal of Autism and Developmental Disorders*, vol. 36, no. 4, pp. 445–469, 2006.

[10] F. J. Sansosti, K. A. Powell-Smith, and D. A. Kincaid, "A research synthesis of social story interventions for children with autism spectrum disorders," *Focus on Autism and Other Developmental Disabilities*, vol. 19, no. 4, pp. 194–204, 2004.

[11] C. A. Gray, "Teaching children with autism to read social situations," in *Teaching Children with Autism*, K. A. Quill, Ed., pp. 219–241, Delmar, New York, NY, USA, 1995.

[12] K. A. Quill, "Instructional considerations for young children with autism: the rationale for visually cued instruction," *Journal of Autism and Developmental Disorders*, vol. 27, no. 6, pp. 697–713, 1997.

[13] S. Ali and N. Frederickson, "Investigating the effectiveness of social stories," *Educational Psychology in Practice*, vol. 22, pp. 355–377, 2006.

[14] S. Crozier and M. J. Tincani, "Using a modified Social Story to decrease disruptive behavior of a child with autism," *Focus on Autism and Other Developmental Disabilities*, vol. 20, no. 3, pp. 150–157, 2005.

[15] R. H. Horner, E. G. Carr, J. Halle, G. Mcgee, S. Odom, and M. Wolery, "The use of single-subject research to identify evidence-based practice in special education," *Exceptional Children*, vol. 71, no. 2, pp. 165–179, 2005.

[16] M. Tankersley, B. G. Cook, and L. Cook, "A preliminary examination to identify the presence of quality indicators in single-subject research," *Education and Treatment of Children*, vol. 31, no. 4, pp. 523–548, 2008.

[17] L. Adams, A. Gouvousis, M. VanLue, and C. Waldron, "Social story intervention: improving communication skills in a child with an autism spectrum disorder," *Focus on Autism and Other Developmental Disabilities*, vol. 19, no. 2, pp. 87–94, 2004.

[18] E. Agosta, J. E. Graetz, M. A. Mastropieri, and T. E. Scruggs, "Teacher-researcher partnerships to improve social behavior through social stories," *Intervention in School and Clinic*, vol. 39, no. 5, pp. 276–287, 2004.

[19] H. Kuock and P. Mirenda, "Social story interventions for young children with autism spectrum disorders," *Focus on Autism and Other Developmental Disorders*, vol. 18, no. 4, pp. 219–227, 2003.

[20] S. Kuttler, B. S. Myles, J. K. Carlson et al., "The use of social stories to reduce precursors to tantrum behavior in a student with autism," *Focus on Autism and Other Developmental Disabilities*, vol. 13, no. 3, pp. 176–182, 1998.

[21] M. D. Brownell, "Musically adapted social stories to modify behaviors in students with autism: four case studies," *Journal of Music Therapy*, vol. 39, no. 2, pp. 117–144, 2002.

[22] D. Scattone, S. M. Wilczynski, R. P. Edwards, and B. Rabian, "Decreasing disruptive behaviors of children with autism using social stories," *Journal of Autism and Developmental Disorders*, vol. 32, no. 6, pp. 535–543, 2002.

[23] K. M. Quilty, "Teaching paraprofessionals how to write and implement social stories for students with autism spectrum disorders," *Remedial and Special Education*, vol. 28, no. 3, pp. 182–189, 2007.

[24] F. J. Sansosti and K. A. Powell-Smith, "Using social stories to improve the social behavior of children with asperger syndrome," *Journal of Positive Behavior Interventions*, vol. 8, no. 1, pp. 43–57, 2006.

[25] D. Scattone, D. H. Tingstrom, and S. M. Wilczynski, "Increasing appropriate social interactions of children with autism spectrum disorders using social stories," *Focus on Autism and Other Developmental Disabilities*, vol. 21, no. 4, pp. 211–222, 2006.

[26] K. S. Thiemann and H. Goldstein, "Social stories, written text cues, and video feedback: effects on social communication of children with autism," *Journal of Applied Behavior Analysis*, vol. 34, no. 4, pp. 425–446, 2001.

[27] L. M. Barry and S. B. Burlew, "Using social stories to teach choice and play skills to children with autism," *Focus on Autism and Other Developmental Disabilities*, vol. 19, no. 1, pp. 45–51, 2004.

[28] M. L. Ivey, J. Heflin, P. Alberto et al., "The use of social stories to promote independent behaviors in novel events for children

with PDD-NOS," *Focus on Autism and Other Developmental Disabilities*, vol. 19, no. 3, pp. 164–176, 2004.

[29] R. Bledsoe, B. S. Myles, and R. L. Simpson, "Use of a social story intervention to improve mealtime skills of an adolescent with Asperger syndrome," *Autism*, vol. 7, no. 3, pp. 289–295, 2003.

[30] R. V. Burke, B. R. Kuhn, and J. L. Peterson, "Brief report: a "storybook" ending to children's bedtime problems—The use of a rewarding social story to reduce bedtime resistance and frequent night waking," *Journal of Pediatric Psychology*, vol. 29, no. 5, pp. 389–396, 2004.

[31] D. Soenksen and S. Alper, "Teaching a young child to appropriately gain attention of peers using a social story intervention," *Focus on Autism and Other Developmental Disabilities*, vol. 21, no. 1, pp. 36–44, 2006.

[32] R. Toplis and J. A. Hadwin, "Using social stories to change problematic lunchtime behaviour in school," *Educational Psychology in Practice*, vol. 22, no. 1, pp. 53–67, 2006.

[33] K. Hanley-Hochdorfer, M. A. Bray, T. J. Kehle, and M. J. Elinoff, "Social stories to increase verbal initiation in children with autism and asperger's disorder," *School Psychology Review*, vol. 39, no. 3, pp. 484–492, 2010.

[34] T. Hagiwara and B. S. Myles, "A multimedia social story intervention: teaching skills to children with autism," *Focus on Autism and Other Developmental Disabilities*, vol. 14, no. 2, pp. 82–95, 1999.

[35] K. M. Quilty, "Teaching paraprofessionals how to write and implement social stories for students with autism spectrum disorders," *Remedial and Special Education*, vol. 28, no. 3, pp. 182–189, 2007.

[36] S. Bernad-Ripoll, "Using a self-as-model video combined with social stories to help a child with Asperger syndrome understand emotion," *Focus on Autism and Other Developmental Disabilities*, vol. 22, no. 2, pp. 100–106, 2007.

[37] J. N. Constantino and C. P. Gruber, *The Social Responsiveness Scale (SRS) Manual*, Western Psych, Los Angeles, Calif, USA, 2005.

[38] N. M Johnson-Martin, S. M. Attermeier, and B. Hacker, *The Carolina Curriculum for Infants and Toddlers with Special Needs*, Brookes, Baltimore, Md, USA, 3rd edition, 2004.

[39] J. O. Cooper, T. E. Heron, and W. L. Heward, *Applied Behavior Analysis*, Pearson Education, Upper Saddle River, NJ, USA, 2nd edition, 2007.

[40] S. H. Bell and D. W. Barnett, "Peer micronorms in the assessment of young children: methodological review and examples," *Topics in Early Childhood Special Education*, vol. 19, no. 2, pp. 112–122, 1999.

[41] Mayer-Johnson, *Writing with Symbols*, Mayer-Johnson, Solana Beach, Calif, USA, 2000.

[42] C. A. Gray, *The New Social Story Book*, Future Horizons, Arlington, Tex, USA, 2000.

[43] C. Norris and J. Dattilo, "Evaluating effects of a social story intervention on a young girl with autism," *Focus on Autism and Other Developmental Disabilities*, vol. 14, no. 3, pp. 180–186, 1999.

[44] A. E. Kazdin, *Single-Case Experimental Designs: Methods for Clinical and Applied Settings*, Oxford University Press, New York, NY, USA, 1982.

[45] T. E. Scruggs and M. A. Mastropieri, "Summarizing single-subject research. Issues and applications," *Behavior Modification*, vol. 22, no. 3, pp. 221–242, 1998.

[46] B. L. Swaggart, E. Gagnon, S. J. Bock, C. Quinn, B. S. Myles, and R. L. Simpson, "Using social stories to teach social and behavioral skills to children with autism," *Focus on Autism and Other Developmental Disabilities*, vol. 10, no. 1, pp. 1–16, 1995.

[47] M. Zimbelman, A. Paschal, S. R. Hawley, C. A. Molgaard, and T. S. Romain, "Addressing physical inactivity among developmentally disabled students through visual schedules and social stories," *Research in Developmental Disabilities*, vol. 28, no. 4, pp. 386–396, 2007.

[48] J. Rust and A. Smith, "How should the effectiveness of social stories to modify the behaviour of children on the autistic spectrum be tested? Lessons from the literature," *Autism*, vol. 10, no. 2, pp. 125–138, 2006.

Relationships between 9-Year-Olds' Math and Literacy Worries and Academic Abilities

Laura Punaro and Robert Reeve

Melbourne School of Psychological Sciences, University of Melbourne, VIC 3010, Australia

Correspondence should be addressed to Robert Reeve, r.reeve@unimelb.edu.au

Academic Editor: Helga Krinzinger

We investigated whether 9-year-olds experience math and/or literacy worries and, if they do, whether it is related to problem-solving abilities. Fifty-eight children judged the correctness of math, literacy, and mental rotation problems that differed in difficulty and rated their worry level about the correctness of judgments. Nonverbal IQ, general math, and literacy abilities were also assessed. Results showed children's worry ratings varied as a function of task and problem difficulty. Latent class analyses of math and literacy worry ratings revealed high-, moderate- and low-worry subgroups in both domains. The high-worry math subgroup exhibited poorer math performance than the other math subgroups, demonstrating a link between math worry and math performance. No relationship was found between worry literacy subgroups and literacy performance. Moreover, no relationship was found between teachers' rating of children's academic and general worry and children's own worry ratings. The relevance of the findings for understanding math and literacy worry is discussed.

1. Introduction

Insofar as preadolescent children experience academic-related anxieties/worries, it is unclear whether these effects are specific to an academic domain (e.g., math) exists in other domains (e.g., literacy), or, if they exist, affect abilities similarly across domains. Although it is assumed that the trepidation associated with math is greater than other academic domains [1, 2], research into anxiety problem-solving abilities associations in areas other than math is limited, even in older students [1]. Moreover, even though academic anxieties may exist in preadolescent children, it is unclear whether children would be able to accurately describe these experiences because of immature metacognitive abilities. The research reported herein investigates 9-year-olds' academic anxiety/worry-ability relationships in math, reading, and mental rotation (a nonacademic area), where children rate anxiety level immediately after solving a problem (We use the term "worry" rather than anxiety because pilot work suggested that children could readily provide examples of their worry experiences, but had more difficulty providing examples of anxiety experiences. Moreover, the term "worry" has occasionally been used as a way of describing "anxiety" to children (see [2, 42]). Nevertheless, we also use the generic terms "math anxiety" and "literacy anxiety" because they are used in the literature). The aim is to better understand the nature of academic anxiety/worry-ability associations in preadolescent children.

Although most academic anxiety research focuses on math anxiety (MA), literacy anxiety may also exist. In one of the few studies on language anxiety, Carroll et al. [3] found that, compared to their literate peers, 5- to 15-year-olds with poor literacy tended to be more anxious about their language abilities. This is an important issue because MA might be an aspect of academic anxiety more generally. However, the reasons for literacy anxiety are not well understood, and the research considered herein mainly focuses on math anxiety/worry performance relationships.

MA is thought to emerge in the preadolescent years, peak around Grades 9 to 10, and not change thereafter [4, 5]. It is associated with poor math achievement, as well as socioemotional and behavioral difficulties in high school students [1, 5–7]. Surprisingly little is known about the impact of math anxiety/worries on preadolescent children's math abilities [8,

9]. Dowker [1] suggests that MA affects math performance only after Grade 4 (10 years old)—a claim supported by Ma [9] in his meta-analysis of research on the association between MA and math performance (note, however, Ma [9] only included three studies of children younger than 11 years old in his meta-analysis). Moreover, Krinzinger et al. [10] found no association between MA and arithmetic ability in 6- to 9-year-olds and suggested that the way young children are questioned about math-related anxieties may affect their responses. These findings suggest that young children are either not affected by math anxiety/worries, do not understand anxiety-related questions, or are unable to report their anxieties [1, 11, 12].

It is often assumed that children are able to report anxiety states—a claim that overlooks limitations in children's metacognitive capabilities, which may affect their ability to answer questions about their own cognitive or socioemotional states [13]. In questionnaires typically used to assess MA, children are asked to reflect on general events (e.g., imagine being in a math lesson) and rate their anxiety, yet this may be beyond their cognitive capabilities [9, 14, 15].

Some researchers have used simplified MA tasks to probe young children's anxiety states. Thomas and Dowker [16], for example, used a pictorial MA task in which 6- to 9-year-olds pointed to facial expressions to convey their emotional response to math events. The questions focused on children's perceived math ability, how much they enjoyed math tasks, and how worried they felt when they encountered difficult problems. Thomas and Dowker [16] found that their participants did not express anxiety or unhappiness at perceived math difficulties and concluded that MA was unrelated to poor math performance in young children. Gierl and Bisanz [12] also used a pictorial judgment paradigm to assess MA in 9- to 12-year-olds. They found that 9-year-olds reported low levels of anxiety, while 12-year-olds reported higher anxiety levels. They concluded that MA increases as students mature and become more concerned about the consequences of success and/or failure. However, both groups of researchers asked probe questions about general retrospective events (e.g., experiences with mental calculation), rather than a specific problem solving event as they occurred. It is possible that the 9-year-olds in both studies lacked the abilities to reflect on general events [13].

The question of whether MA is a manifestation of general anxiety or is specific to math has been often debated. In a meta-analysis of MA research conducted on high school and college students, Hembree [5] reported moderate correlations (0.35 and 0.40) between MA, general anxiety, trait anxiety, and state anxiety, and a stronger correlation (0.52) between MA and test anxiety. However, stronger correlations (0.5 to 0.8) have been found between MA measures (e.g., Math Anxiety Rating Scale and the Abbreviated Math Anxiety Scale), which suggests that MA is a specific anxiety—a claim supported by findings which show that general anxiety measures account for little of the variance in MA scores [6, 11]. However, these analyses do not address whether MA is unique or a part of academic anxiety more generally. Findings from a study by Faust [17] suggest that MA is unique in older students, at least. He found that high MA students did not show anxiety on a verbal anagram task. A question of some interest is whether preadolescent children exhibit similar across-domain anxieties/worries. Indeed, Gierl and Bisanz [12] found that preadolescent children's MA ratings did not differ from their general school anxiety ratings, which could be interpreted as suggesting that children exhibit anxiety across academic domains.

A key aim of studying MA is to understand its impact on math abilities. Higher levels of MA are often linked to lower levels of math achievement [2, 7, 18]. However, the relationship between MA and math ability is complex. For instance, MA is often associated with avoidance behaviors, less time spent studying, and lower class engagement [10, 19], factors that can impact the acquisition of math skills. Poor performance by high MA students may also reflect the intrusion of worrisome thoughts while solving math problems. A reduced processing efficiencymodel was proposed by Eysenck and Calvo [20] who suggest that worries limit working memory capacity because they take up problem-solving resources [4, 10, 11, 21]. Consistent with this claim, Ashcraft and Faust [22] found that MA had minimal impact on simple arithmetic problems, but had substantial impact on more difficult multiplication problems. However, not all researchers support the cognitive resources hypothesis. For arousal theorist, worry may motivate some students to increase efforts, while extreme worry may impede effort [2, 9]. Also, Wigfield and Meece [2] and Ho et al. [7] suggested that it is the affective-emotional component (i.e., tension, unpleasant physiological reactions) rather than the cognitive component that affects (correlates negatively) with math performance.

In the present study we investigate 9-year-olds' academic worry-performance associations, by probing their "worry" reactions using a "faces worry scale" immediately following problem solving (i.e., deciding whether two problems presented side by side represent the same solution to a problem). We are interested in whether worry judgments vary as a function of to-be-judged problem difficulty and problem correctness for math, literacy and, a nonacademic domain (mental rotation). If they do, it would confirm that children experience worry, whether or not they are able to report it. Of interest is whether math and language tasks elicit distinct patterns of worry judgments compared to the nonacademic task. If academic worries are unique, math and language worry judgments would be expected to differ from nonacademic worry judgments. Insofar as children's patterns of worry judgments differ, of interest is whether judgments are related to ability. On the basis of research with adolescents, it is expected that children's academic worry ratings would be associated with ability.

2. Method

2.1. Participants. Fifty-eight Grade 4 children (32 boys and 26 girls: M = 117.55 months, SD = 6.91) from an urban primary school in a large Australian city participated. Common to Australian urban schools, the sample comprised children from diverse multicultural and socioeconomic backgrounds. All children had normal or correct-to-normal vision; and, according to school personnel, none had known learning difficulties. The research was, approved by, and conducted in accordance with, the authors' university human ethics committee requirements.

2.2. Materials and Procedures. To determine whether worry level differed as a function of math, literacy, or nonacademic (mental rotation) problems, children were presented two problems side by side from the three domains and (1) judged whether the solution to the pair of problems was the same or not and (2) rated their worry about the confidence they had in their decision using a face worry scale (described above) (see Table 1 for examples of pairs of to-be-judged problems for each of the three domains). Children judged 48 separate problems in each of the three domains ($n = 144$ problems across the three domains) comprising pairs of to-be-judged problems that were easy or difficult to judge and for which the solutions were either equivalent or not ($n = 12$ for each difficulty/equivalence combination within each domain: see Table 1 e.g., of these combination for each domain).

Children completed the Ravens Colored Progressive Matrices nonverbal IQ measures two weeks before judgment tasks [23]. They also completed a general numeracy and literacy worry test one week before completing judgment tasks. This task was used to (1) introduce children to the face worry judgment procedure, described above (see Figure 1), and (2) assess children's general retrospective worries. The term worry rather than anxiety was used in discussing faces with children because pilot work revealed it was more meaningful to them. Children were able to point to faces corresponding to "not worried at all," "a little bit worried" and "very worried" without hesitation and grasped the purpose of these procedures without difficulty.

Teachers rated children's general school-related anxiety prior to the judgment tasks. They also rated children's literacy and numeracy competency. Teachers were encouraged to consult children's formal test scores in making competency judgments—Australian children complete national numeracy and literacy tests throughout the primary (elementary) school years.

To avoid fatigue, the three domain judgment tasks were completed in three 15-minute sessions on consecutive days. Task procedures were explained before each session using four practice problems. Children were reintroduced to the faces worry scale (introduced one week earlier for use in the general numeracy and literacy worry judgment task) and encouraged to use the range of anxiety/worry faces to judge worry level if they felt it was appropriate to do so. Task order presentation was randomized across the three days; however within-task problems were presented in a fixed order.

The three domain judgment task problems were presented on a 15″ laptop screen, and children judged whether to-be-judged problem pairs were equivalent by pressing the left-shift key (for equivalent/similar) or the right-shift key (for not equivalent/not similar). Task problems remained on the screen for a fixed time (math problems = 16 seconds; language problems = 11 seconds; mental rotation problems = 5 seconds). Presentation times were based on pilot data from a separate group of 10-year-olds and reflected the average time taken to complete easy and difficult problems. It was expected that children would have sufficient time to complete easy, but not hard problems, before problems disappeared from the screen. The perception of insufficient time to complete tasks is known to increase worry in children [24]. Although children could make a judgment before problems disappeared, few did so, and thus it was not possible to assess the function of response time.

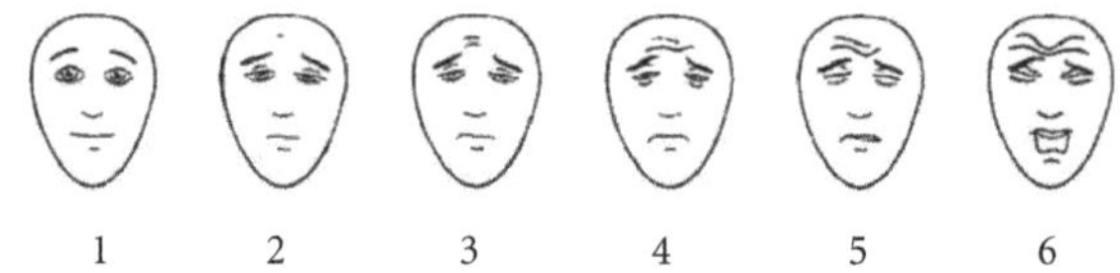

Figure 1: The faces worry scale.

As soon as children made a judgment, the faces worry scale appeared on the screen (see Figure 1 and description below). Children judged how worried they felt about the "correctness" of their equivalence judgment by pressing the numeric computer key corresponding to their worry face choice. Of interest were (1) judgment correctness and (2) worry ratings.

2.3. Judgment Tasks. For the math judgment task children judged whether two addition equations were equivalent. The problems were instances of associativity problems (e.g., $4 + 3 = 3 + 2 + 2$) [25]. Difficulty was determined by the number of terms in the equation. Easy problems comprised equations of the form of "$a + b = b + c + d$" and difficult problems comprised equations of the form of $a + b + c = c + d + e + f$. Research shows that 8-year-olds are able to solve the *easy* associativity problems, and 10-year-olds are able to solve difficult problems [25]. Equations, terms comprised single-digit numbers between 2 and 9 (excluding doubles: e.g., $6 + 6$) and summed to 20 or less. Children's task was to judge whether both sides of the equal sign were equal or unequal. The task comprised 12 easy/same (correct), easy/different (incorrect), difficult/same, and difficult/different problems (see Table 1, e.g., of each).

The language judgment task comprised a synonym judgment test [26], designed to assess literacy (verbal reasoning, reading ability, vocabulary knowledge, and comprehension). Children were presented with two sentences, which differed in a single word and were asked to decide whether the two sentences were equivalent in meaning (e.g., "Elephants are larger than mice/Elephants are bigger than mice" and asked: "Do these sentences mean the same thing?"). Level of difficulty was determined by selecting synonym pairs that were appropriate for Grade 2 (easy) and Grade 4/5 (difficult). Example stimuli are presented in Table 1.

Quaiser-Pohl's [27] mental rotation test was used as the *nonacademic* task—we regarded it as a nonacademic measure because it requires skill not taught in school. It comprised a spatial ability measure designed for primary school aged children. Stimuli comprised colored pictures of two animals or humans, one of which was rotated around a central axis. Children judged whether the rotated figure was the same as

TABLE 1: Example stimuli used in the math, literacy, and mental rotation tasks.

	Task		
	Math	Literacy	Mental rotation
Easy/Same	4 + 2 + 3 = 6 + 3 3 + 7 = 2 + 3 + 5	Peter RAISED/LIFTED the trophy after winning the Grand Final. Mark is STRONG/POWERFUL enough to lift a truck.	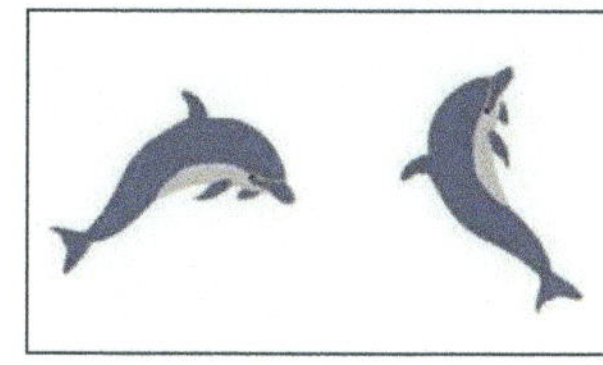
Easy/Different	3 + 4 + 1 = 2 + 5 4 + 1 + 6 = 8 + 6	Mum's dinner was a major FAILURE/SUCCESS. Kate's pet turtle was very LIGHT/HEAVY.	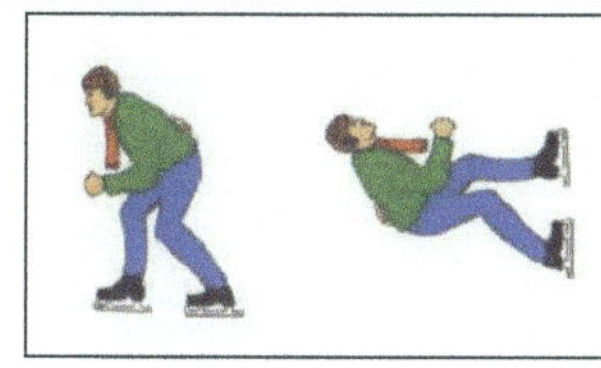
Difficult/Same	4 + 3 + 6 = 2 + 7 + 3 + 1 2 + 4 + 9 = 3 + 7 + 4 + 1	The policeman PURSUED/CHASED the thief through the alley. Frank's CONDUCT/BEHAVIOUR in the playground was atrocious.	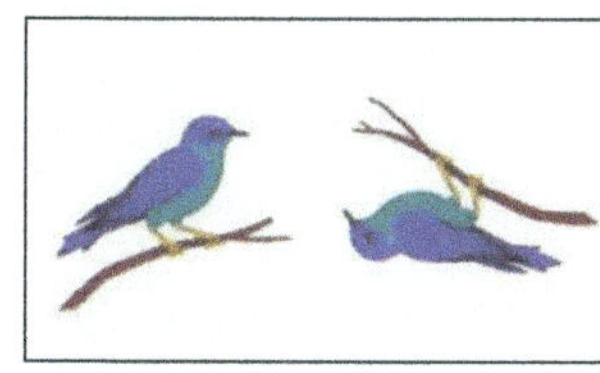
Difficult/Different	4 + 8 + 5 + 3 = 3 + 9 + 5 3 + 5 + 9 = 6 + 2 + 3 + 4	Steven waited PATIENTLY/RESTLESSLY for his mother. Roger was HOPEFUL/PESSIMISTIC about getting the job.	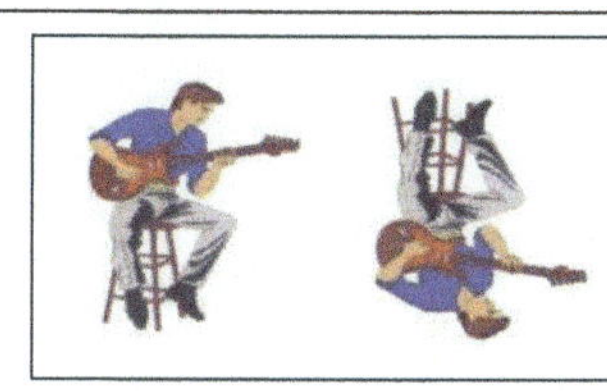

the target figure. Difficulty was determined by the rotation angle between the comparison pictures; *easy* problems were rotated less than 90 degrees (45 or 90 degrees), and difficult items were rotated more than 90 degrees (135 or 180 degrees).

Children's worry ratings for the math, literacy, and mental rotation tasks were computed for the problem difficulty and equivalence conditions (i.e., mean ratings were computed for the four within-task conditions for each of the tasks).

2.3.1. Worry Judgments. Worry judgment was assessed using the Faces Pain Anxiety Scale [28] (see Figure 2). The "faces scales" have been used in medical contexts to measure anxiety/worry [28–30]. The faces depict six different facial expressions in a graded sequence from nonanxious "1" to very anxious "6". The faces are claimed to represent approximately equal intervals in anxiety representations [28]. The Faces Anxiety Scale has a test-retest reliability of 0.79 [28] over a two-week period and correlates with similar scales $r = 0.8$ on average [31]. The scale has been used with 3-year-olds to older adults.

2.3.2. General Math and Literacy Worry. To assess children's general math and literacy worry, they were asked to rate their level of worry for math and literacy. Children rated "How worried do you usually feel when you are doing x"? (x = working on computers, sport, playing music, addition, subtraction, multiplication, reading, and writing stories). These questions were developed by the authors and served to (1) introduce children to the "faces worry scale" and (2) assess possible differences in children's general retrospective math and literacy worries. Children were introduced to the faces worry scales by judging their worry about working on computers, sports, and playing music. The purpose of using these neutral questions was to familiarize children with the worry judgment procedure and to answer questions if they arose. Following the so-called neutral questions, children made worry judgments about the addition, subtraction, multiplication, reading, writing stories questions. Children's math worry ratings were averaged across the three math items and literacy ratings were averaged across the two literacy ratings.

2.3.3. Teacher Judgment of Children's General Anxiety. Teachers completed the modified version of the *School Anxiety Scale Teacher Report* [32], which examines children's general and social anxiety in the school environments. This test has good test-retest reliability ($r = 0.93$) over an eight-week period), and is correlated ($r = 0.83$) with the Strengths and

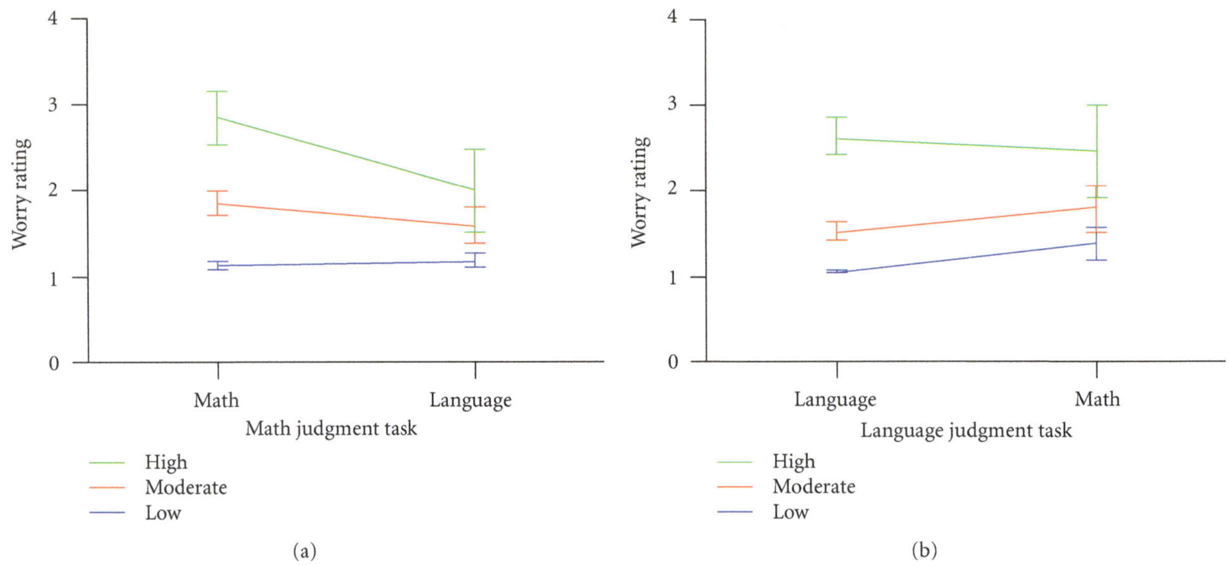

FIGURE 2: The relationships between math and literacy subgroup membership and literacy (a) and math (b) worry ratings, respectively.

Difficulties Questionnaire Internalizing Symptoms Scale, a widely used measure of teacher-rated anxiety. Seven general anxiety items were administered (e.g., "This child is afraid of making mistakes"; "This child worries about things"; "This child worries that (s)he will do badly at school"). Teachers rated anxiety on a four-point scale (0: never, 1: sometimes, 2: usually, 3: always). Teachers' ratings were averaged across the seven items.

2.3.4. Teacher Judgment of Children's Competency. Teachers rated children's ability in three areas—math, literacy (reading and writing), and general problem solving—on a five-point scale (1: poor, 2: not good, 3: average, 4: very good, and 5: superior). As noted earlier, teachers were encouraged to consult children's formal test results in rating their competencies.

2.4. Analytic Approach. Because we were not confident that the measurement scale properties of the math, literacy, and mental-rotation judgments tasks were sufficiently similar to combine them in analyses, we used separate ANOVAs to identify judgment correctness and worry rating for each task separately. Because we were also interested in identifying different patterns of worry as a function of within-task manipulations, we used latent class methods to isolate possible subgroup patterns of performances. Latent class (LC) methods [33] are a specific form of finite mixture modeling [34] approaches, which aim to uncover two or more subgroups of individuals characterized by distinct patterns of responding. A fundamental aspect of such models is the assumption of a categorical latent variable. The latent (unobserved) categories represent qualitatively different states of the underlying latent variable. Models are estimated with successively more latent classes, with the final model best capturing the structural representation of covariance between the indicator (observed) variables. Information criteria indices (e.g., AICc [35], CAIC [36]) were used to determine the best fitting model to the data, penalising increasingly complex specifications.

Unlike proximity-based cluster approaches (such as K-means), LC approaches offer a formal, model-based approach to the classification of individuals to unique clusters [37, 38]. An important outcome of using this approach is probabilistic estimates of every individual's likelihood of belonging to each class of the latent variable, in this case, levels of worry.

Latent profile analysis (LPA) is a particular type of LC modelling [39]. What separates LPA from other LC models is that the profiles are formed based on continuous indicator variables; in this case, online worry judgments. Models were successively estimated from a two- to four-class specification. The relatively small sample size resulted in idiosyncratic classes beyond this range.

3. Results

Preliminary analyses showed no relationship between gender, Ravens measures, and any of the other measures of interest and so they were not included in analyses reported herein.

Three separate ANOVAs examined judgment accuracy of the to-be-judged problem pairs for the three tasks (math, literacy, and nonacademic tasks) as a function of the difficulty (easy or difficulty) and the similarity (same or different) of the two problems (see Table 2 for the means and standard deviations associated with these analyses). For math judgment accuracy, main effects of problem difficulty ($F(1,57) = 80.83$, $P < 0.001$, $\eta^2 = 0.59$) and problem similarity ($F(1,57) = 23.38$, $P < 0.001$, $\eta^2 = 0.29$) were found. In addition, the interaction between them was also significant ($F(1,57) = 8.30$, $P < 0.01$, $\eta^2 = 0.13$). For literacy judgment accuracy, main effects of problem difficulty ($F(1,57) = 349.00$, $P < 0.001$, $\eta^2 = 0.86$) and problem

TABLE 2: Mean worry ratings and problem correctness (and standard deviations) for the math, literacy, and mental rotation tasks as a function of the difficulty and similarity of the to-be-judged problem pairs.

Easy		Difficult	
Same	Different	Same	Different
Math problems			
1.48 (0.56)	1.55 (0.67)	1.83 (0.79)	1.93 (0.83)
89.22 (11.47)	92.96 (10.79)	70.69 (22.03)	83.19 (13.92)
Literacy problems			
1.21 (0.40)	1.34 (0.44)	1.73 (0.80)	1.61 (0.70)
95.98 (8.58)	93.97 (6.58)	60.78 (18.67)	73.85 (15.88)
Mental rotation problems			
1.22 (0.35)	1.35 (0.51)	1.35 (0.46)	1.38 (0.46)
88.51 (23.04)	86.06 (13.00)	79.60 (28.02)	81.18 (17.49)

similarity ($F(1,57) = 7.93$, $P < 0.001$, $\eta^2 = 0.12$) were found. In addition, the interaction between them was also significant ($F(1,57) = 23.21$, $P < 0.01$, $\eta^2 = 0.29$). For mental rotation nonacademic accuracy, only a main effect of difficulty was found ($F(1,57) = 22.69$, $P < 0.001$, $\eta^2 = 0.29$).

Three separate ANOVAs also examined judgment worry ratings for the three tasks as a function of the problem difficulty (easy or difficulty) and the similarity (same or different) of the to-be-judged problem pairs. For math judgment worry ratings, main effects of difficulty ($F(1,57) = 50.72$, $P < 0.01$, $\eta^2 = 0.47$) and problem similarity ($F(1,57) = 8.10$, $P < 0.01$, $\eta^2 = 0.12$) were found. For literacy judgment worry ratings, only a main effect of difficulty was found ($F(1,57) = 42.72$, $P < 0.01$), $\eta^2 = 0.43$). In addition, the interaction between them was also significant ($F(1,57) = 18.38$, $P < 0.001$, $\eta^2 = 0.24$). For mental rotation-nonacademic worry ratings, main effects of difficulty ($F(1,57) = 7.92$, $P < 0.01$, $\eta^2 = 0.12$) and problem similarity ($F(1,57) = 11.94$, $P < 0.01$, $\eta^2 = 0.17$) were found. In addition, the interaction between them was also significant ($F(1,57) = 4.19$, $P < 0.05$, $\eta^2 = 0.07$).

These findings show that manipulating the difficulty and similarity of the to-be-judged problem pairs affected judgment accuracy and worry ratings for the math and literacy tasks; however, only task difficulty affected accuracy judgments in the nonacademic task.

The next set of analyses investigated the relationship between the math and literacy worry ratings and accuracy measures. Because of the relatively large math and literacy worry SD's, two separate latent profile analysis [39] were employed to identify possible worry subgroups in the two domains. Specifically, mean worry ratings for problem similarity and problem difficulty were used to identify cluster membership. Different criteria were used to identify the best fitting model (see Table 3). The AICc and CAIC values indicated a three-cluster solution for both the patterns of math and literacy worry judgments (see Table 3). In particular, the solutions revealed low-, moderate- and high-worry subgroups for both domains. Classification errors, defining the degree of uncertainty between probabilistic cluster proportions and cluster membership using maximum class assignment, were acceptably small, indicating that the subgroups were valid.

TABLE 3: Latent class analysis of the math and literacy worry ratings.

Cluster	LL	AICc	CAIC	BIC	CE (%)
Math worry clusters					
2-cluster	−104.83	224.95	295.68	278.68	0.62
3-cluster	**−68.75**	**182.78**	**269.07**	**243.07**	**2.14**
4-cluster	−49.98	214.50	277.07	242.07	1.99
Literacy worry clusters					
2-cluster	−38.02	91.34	162.07	145.07	0.36
3-cluster	**25.40**	**−5.51**	**80.78**	**54.78**	**0.76**
4-cluster	45.81	22.92	85.50	50.50	1.87

TABLE 4: Worry subgroups membership cross-classification across the math and literacy domains.

Literacy worry subgroup	Math worry subgroup		
	Low	Moderate	High
Low			
Count	18	8	1
Expected count	12.6	9.8	4.7
Adjusted residual	2.9*	−1	−2.5*
Moderate			
Count	9	9	5
Expected count	10.7	8.3	4
Adjusted residual	−0.9	0.4	0.7
High			
Count	0	4	4
Expected count	3.7	2.9	1.4
Adjusted residual	−2.8*	0.9	2.6*

* $P < 0.05$.

The relationship between low, moderate, and high subgroups across the math and language domains was significant ($\chi^2(4, N = 58) = 15.26$, $P < 0.001$), with a significant ordinal-by-ordinal association ($\gamma = 0.67$, $P < 0.001$: see Table 4 for the cross-classification of the math and literacy subgroups). Table 4 reports differences between expected and observed cell frequencies, and the associated adjusted standardized residuals for significant differences among cells. The information in Table 4 could be interpreted as suggesting that there is a tendency to belong to similar worry groups in both the math and literacy domains; however, the information in Table 4 does not provide information about the within-domain differences on across-domain measures.

Figure 2 shows the mean worry ratings for math and literacy, respectively, as a function of the math and literacy subgroups. Figure 2 suggests a differential impact of subgroup membership on across-domain measures, which was confirmed by analyses of the across-domain worry ratings. Specifically, for the math worry subgroups, a significant interaction between math subgroup and literacy worry rating was found ($F(2,55) = 12.47$, $P < 0.001$, $\eta^2 = 0.31$). However, for the literacy worry subgroups, no significant interaction between literacy subgroup and math worry ratings was found ($F(2,55) = 2.26$, $P > 0.05$, $\eta^2 = 0.08$). (Note, only interactions are important here). These results suggest that literacy subgroup worry ratings might reflect general worry ratings, whereas the math worry subgroup ratings reflect unique within-domain differences in worry ratings.

The analyses reported thus far do not address directly the question of whether worry subgroup memberships predict judgment accuracy. These relationships are reported in Table 5, which appears to show that judgment accuracy is indeed associated with worry. In the next set of analyses we report findings from regression analyses in which within-domain worry subgroup membership respectively predicted within-domain judgment accuracy over and above the effect of teachers competence ratings and children's own general worry ratings. The latter two factors are included in the analyses to determine whether teachers' assessment of children's competence and children's general retrospective worry judgments moderate the relationship between worry subgroup membership and judgment accuracy.

Two separate multiple regression analyses were conducted predicting math and literacy correctness judgments, respectively, subgroup membership was entered as a dummy variable (the low-worry subgroup was used as the reference category in both analyses). (Note: we only used the accuracy for difficult judgments because of ceiling effects associated with easy accuracy judgments—see Table 5).

VIF scores were low, suggesting that multicollinearity was not an issue in the analyses. The overall model for math problem judgments was significant ($F(4,53) = 5.50$, $P < 0.01$, $R^2 = 0.29$) (see Table 6 for the regression parameters). Two significant predictors emerged: teacher rating of math competency and worry subgroup membership. Specifically, teacher math competency ratings predicted math task judgment performance ($\beta = 0.46$, $P < 0.01$) and membership of the high worry subgroup predicted poorer math task judgment performance, relative to belonging to the low-worry subgroup ($\beta = -0.33$, $P < 0.05$). Retrospective worry ratings did not predict difficult math judgment performance. The overall model for literacy problem judgments was significant ($F(4,53) = 2.97$, $P < 0.05$, $R^2 = 0.18$) (see Table 7 for the regression parameters). Only children's own retrospective literacy worry rating predicted literacy problem judgment correctness ($\beta = 0.46$, $P < 0.01$). It is evident that different factors predict math and literacy correctness judgments.

4. Discussion

The aim of the research was twofold. The first was to determine whether 9-year-olds report differences in math, literacy, and nonacademic worry immediately after solving a problem using the "faces worry scale." The second was to see whether differences in worry ratings were related to problem solving. Three findings are of note. First, worry ratings were higher for more difficult math, language, and mental rotation problems, indicating that children were sensitive to task demands. Second, overall, worry levels were higher for the math problems, compared to language and nonacademic (mental rotation) problems. Three meaningful worry subgroups were identified from worry ratings for both the math and the language tasks (but not for the nonacademic mental rotation task). Importantly, children with high math worry were less successful in making correct math judgments compared to children with low math worry. As noted earlier, neither gender nor general ability effects were observed.

The faces worry scale was used (1) immediately after children made judgment about the equivalence of pairs of math, literacy, and mental rotation problems and (2) to assess children's general math and literacy worries. Children's worry ratings increased as math and literacy judgment task difficulty increased, which shows that children were sensitive to task difficulty (however, worry ratings did not increase as the difficulty of the mental rotation problems increased). This particular finding stands in contrast to Thomas and Dowker's [16] and Gierl and Bisanz's [12] findings that most 6- and 9-year-olds' did not exhibit math performance-related anxiety. Our finding adds weight to claims that math anxiety symptoms may be displayed in primary-aged children [9, 10, 40] and is inconsistent with claims that math anxiety symptoms only appear in late primary/elementary school students [1, 11]. It is possible of course that the latter studies may have underestimated young children's academic anxieties because of difficulties associated with assessing affective states retrospectively [13]. In the present study, this difficulty was minimized by asking children about their worry immediately after solving a problem. Nevertheless, it is also evident that children in the current study were able to use the "faces worry scale" to rate general math and literacy worries.

MA is considered a unique anxiety linked specifically to math [5]. Math is thought to elicit greater worry than other academic domains [1, 17]. Wigfield and Meece [2] suggest that math is particularly anxiety provoking because of its emphasis on precision, logic, and problem solving. While our findings support this claim (worry ratings were higher for math than language), it is evident that 9-year-olds also experienced language worries. This finding suggests that both math and language elicit worry reactions. Interestingly, a similar differential in worry ratings was found in the general academic worry ratings: math problems were rated as more worrisome than literacy problems.

It is noteworthy that associations were found between the math and language subgroups and other tasks. It is evident that (1) children in the low math anxiety/worry subgroup showed equally low levels of worry on all three judgment tasks; (2) children in the high math anxiety/worry subgroup found the math task more worrisome than the language task; (3) some children only showed high levels of worry on the math task, but not on other tasks. The latter finding is important because it provides support for the specificity of math anxiety.

The fact that some children reported high levels of worry in the literacy judgment task suggests literacy per se may evoke anxiety. Indeed, the link between reading difficulties and anxiety symptoms has been noted by researchers [41]. It is assumed that anxiety arises in response to experiences

Table 5: Worry ratings and problems corrects as a function of math and literacy worry groups.

	Math worry group					
	Low (n = 27)		Moderate (n = 21)		High (n = 10)	
	Mean	SD	Mean	SD	Mean	SD
Mean worry rating						
Math easy	1.08	0.09	1.57	0.28	2.60	0.49
Math difficult	1.22	0.20	2.15	0.39	3.10	0.57
Percent correct						
Math easy	90.43	11.25	92.46	8.80	90.00	7.91
Math difficult	80.56	15.33	76.79	13.34	67.50	13.15
	Literacy worry group					
	Low (n = 27)		Moderate (n = 23)		High (n = 8)	
Worry rating						
Literacy easy	1.03	0.04	1.27	0.18	2.12	0.33
Literacy difficult	1.10	0.11	1.82	0.39	3.14	0.41
Percent correct						
Literacy easy	95.99	4.40	95.11	5.43	91.15	9.03
Literacy difficult	68.98	12.73	66.67	10.59	63.54	13.50

Table 6: Predicting math judgment correctness: multiple regression parameters.

	B	Std. Error	β	t	Sig.
(Constant)	57.09	8.89		6.42	0.000
Moderate worry subgroup[1]	−0.09	4.20	−0.00	−0.02	0.983
High worry subgroup[1]	−12.71	5.13	−0.33	−2.48	0.016
Teacher rating math competency	6.73	1.86	0.46	3.61	0.001
Children's retrospective math worry	0.11	2.79	0.01	0.04	0.968

[1]Reference category is low subgroup.

Table 7: Predicting literacy judgment correctness: multiple regression parameters.

	B	Std. Error	β	t	Sig.
(Constant)	45.65	8.91		5.13	0.000
Moderate worry subgroup[1]	−2.14	3.18	−0.09	−0.67	0.505
High worry subgroup[1]	−2.86	4.62	−0.08	−0.62	0.539
Teacher rating literacy competency	1.61	2.73	0.08	0.59	0.559
Child retrospective reading worry	6.01	1.89	0.42	3.19	0.002

[1]Reference category is low subgroup.

of failure rather than literacy anxiety per se. Our results suggest that literacy anxiety is not necessarily a reflection of poor ability, but can arise in children with age-appropriate reading skills. Indeed, our results showed that children in the high language worry subgroup also found the math task worrisome (see Figure 2). However, it should be noted that children in the high math worry subgroup did find the language task worrisome. The difference in the direction of these relationships suggests that language worry might reflect general academic-related worries, whereas math worry is unique to math.

Interestingly, teachers' ratings of children's general anxiety (as assessed on the School Anxiety Scale) were unrelated to children's immediate or general worry ratings. This finding is consistent with previous research with adolescent and adult samples [4, 5, 11].

Some researchers have identified math anxiety in young children that was unrelated to math performance [10, 40]. The failure to find a relationship has led some researchers to question the existence of a math anxiety performance link in children [1, 9]. However, Krinzinger et al. [10] suggest that the failure to find a math anxiety-performance link might be due to methodological issues rather than an absence of math anxiety. In the present study, we found meaningful relationships between worry ratings and problem solving judgments. Similar to Krinzinger et al. [10, 42] we assessed "worry" using a faces rating scale. However, there are two key differences between our scale and the scale used by Krinzinger et al. [10, 42]. First, children rated worry immediately after making problem solving judgments. Second, our worry scale was unipolar in nature (neutral face to worried face); in contrast, Krinzinger et al.'s [10, 42] scale was bipolar in nature (from happy to neutral to worried). Tomlinson et al. [43] suggest that showing a range of emotions on the same scale that require anxiety judgment maybe difficult for children to understand. Nevertheless, it is evident that the children in our study were also able to use our faces worry scale to rate their worry about general math and literacy abilities.

It has been claimed that worry interferes with cognition because it focuses attention on intrusive thoughts rather than the task at hand [10, 11, 21]. Further, MA is claimed to reduce working memory capacity, which in turn affects math performance. Two findings from the present study are relevant here. First, a relationship between worry subgroup and performance emerged in comparing performance among the three math worry subgroups. Children in the high-worry group made fewer correct judgments than children in the low-worry group judging difficult problems. In the literacy task, overall worry groups differed in judgment accuracy, although no specific subgroup differences were identified. However, recent research suggests that the relationship between numerical cognition and MA is complex. For example, individuals with high MA also possess poor (1) spatial processing ability [42, 44], (2) dot enumeration [45], and (3) symbolic number comparison abilities [46]. These findings suggest that much more work needs to be undertaken to unpack the relationships between MA, numerical cognitive abilities, and math performance.

The present research findings have implications for educational practitioners. In particular, our findings show that it is possible to identify "at risk worry"-children earlier than previously thought. Moreover, it might be valuable to inform teachers of the consequences of academic-related worry on performance so that they can help at risk children minimize worry. Future research should focus on the impact on children's academic performance of reducing worry (see [47], e.g., on reducing, alleviating, and managing anxiety in students).

Although the current research findings provide evidence for a relationship between academic-related worry and the associated academic competencies, it is limited in at least three respects. First, the sample size ($n = 58$) was relatively small and limited possible analyses. In particular, with a larger sample we would have been able to investigate the direction of causal effects more explicitly. Second, it is evident the future research should examine the relationships between general cognitive factors (e.g., different measures of working memory), specific aspects of numerical cognition (e.g., dot enumeration, number comparison), problem solving, and worry. Third, in the present study, we were unable to examine the sequelae associated with response times. Studies have shown that time pressure affects anxiety ratings, and manipulating time requirements might shed more information about the relationships between worry, problem solving, and cognition.

Interestingly, similar to other researchers who have examined MA in preadolescent children, we found no sex differences in worry judgments [2, 12, 40]. The absence of a gender effect stands in contrast to research with adolescent samples [9, 48] in which gender differences have been found in MA. The developmental context in which MA gender effects emerge requires research.

The present study investigated 9-year-olds' worries using a sensitive measure in two academic domains—math and language—and the relationship between worry and problem solving ability. Results showed that children's worry varied with problem difficulty, and that math and literacy worry differed from nonacademic worry. Moreover, math worry predicted math ability, and a negative association was observed between high math worry and math performance. It is evident that the faces worry scale is a sensitive worry measure for assessing both immediate problem solving and more general academic worries. Nevertheless, more research is needed to investigate worry ratings across a broader range of academic-related problems that differ in difficulty, as well as to investigate how worry ratings change over time.

Acknowledgments

The authors would like to thank our colleagues Jacob Paul and Kelly Trezise for their willingness to discuss the research described herein: the paper benefitted greatly from their input. They would also like to thank Dr. Krinzinger and three anonymous reviewers for the helpful comments made on an earlier draft of the paper.

References

[1] A. Dowker, *Individual Differences in Arithmetic: Implications For Psychology, Neuroscience and Education*, Psychology Press, Hove, UK, 2005.

[2] A. Wigfield and J. L. Meece, "Math anxiety in elementary and secondary school students," *Journal of Educational Psychology*, vol. 80, no. 2, pp. 210–216, 1988.

[3] J. M. Carroll, B. Maughan, R. Goodman, and H. Meltzer, "Literacy difficulties and psychiatric disorders: evidence for comorbidity," *Journal of Child Psychology and Psychiatry and Allied Disciplines*, vol. 46, no. 5, pp. 524–532, 2005.

[4] M. H. Ashcraft and A. M. Moore, "Mathematics anxiety and the affective drop in performance," *Journal of Psychoeducational Assessment*, vol. 27, no. 3, pp. 197–205, 2009.

[5] R. Hembree, "The Nature, effects, and relief of Mathematics Anxiety," *Journal For Research in Mathematics Education*, vol. 21, pp. 33–46, 1990.

[6] M. H. Ashcraft and K. S. Ridley, "Math anxiety and its cognitive consequences," in *Handbook of Mathematical Cognition*, J. I. D. Campbell, Ed., pp. 315–327, Psychology Press, New York, NY, USA, 2005.

[7] H. Z. Ho, D. Senturk, A. G. Lam et al., "The affective and cognitive dimensions of math anxiety: a cross-national study," *Journal for Research in Mathematics Education*, vol. 31, no. 3, pp. 362–379, 2000.

[8] W. S. Bush, "Factors related to changes in elementary students' mathematics anxiety," *Focus on Learning Problems in Mathematics*, vol. 13, pp. 33–43, 1991.

[9] X. Ma, "A meta-analysis of the relationship between anxiety toward mathematics and achievement in mathematics," *Journal for Research in Mathematics Education*, vol. 30, no. 5, pp. 520–540, 1999.

[10] H. Krinzinger, L. Kaufmann, and K. Willmes, "Math anxiety and math ability in early primary school years," *Journal of Psychoeducational Assessment*, vol. 27, no. 3, pp. 206–225, 2009.

[11] M. H. Ashcraft, J. A. Krause, and D. R. Hopko, "Is math anxiety a mathematical learning disability?" in *Why is Math So Hard For Some Children? the Nature and Origins of Mathematical Learning Difficulties and disabilities*, D. B. Berch and M. M. Mazzocco, Eds., pp. 329–348, Paul H. Brookes Publishing, Baltimore, Md, USA, 2007.

[12] M. J. Gierl and J. Bisanz, "Anxieties and attitudes related to mathematics in Grades 3 and 6," *Journal of Experimental Education*, vol. 63, pp. 139–158, 1995.

[13] M. A. Campbell and R. M. Rapee, "Current issues in the assessment of anxiety in children and adolescents: a developmental perspective," *Behaviour Change*, vol. 13, no. 3, pp. 185–193, 1996.

[14] C. R. Brewin, B. Andrews, and I. H. Gotlib, "Psychopathology and early experience: a reappraisal of retrospective reports," *Psychological Bulletin*, vol. 113, no. 1, pp. 82–98, 1993.

[15] P. Harris, *Children and Emotion: The Development of Psychological Understanding*, Basil Blackwell, Oxford, UK, 1989.

[16] G. Thomas and A. Dowker, "Mathematics anxiety and related factors in young children," in *Proceedings of the British Psychological Society Developmental Section Conference*, Bristol, UK, September 2000.

[17] M. W. Faust, *Analysis of physiological reactivity in mathematics anxiety [doctoral dissertation]*, Bowling Green State University, Columbus, Ohio, USA, 1992.

[18] E. Satake and P. P. Amato, "Mathematics anxiety and achievement among Japanese elementary school students," *Educational and Psychological Measurement*, vol. 55, pp. 1000–1008, 1995.

[19] F. Yϋksel-Şahin, "Mathematics anxiety among 4thand 5th Grade Turkish elementary school students," *International Electronic Journal of Mathematics Education*, vol. 3, pp. 179–192, 2008.

[20] M. W. Eysenck and M. G. Calvo, "Anxiety and performance: the processing efficiency theory," *Cognition and Emotion*, vol. 6, pp. 409–434, 1992.

[21] X. Ma and J. Xu, "The causal ordering of mathematics anxiety and mathematics achievement: a longitudinal panel analysis," *Journal of Adolescence*, vol. 27, no. 2, pp. 165–179, 2004.

[22] M. H. Ashcraft and M. W. Faust, "Mathematics anxiety and mental arithmetic performance: an exploratory investigation," *Cognition and Emotion*, vol. 8, no. 2, pp. 97–125, 1994.

[23] J. C. Raven, J. H. Court, and J. Raven, *Manual For Raven's Progressive Matrices and Vocabulary scales*, Lewis, London, UK, 1986.

[24] R. F. Salame, "Test anxiety: its determinants, manifestations, and consequences," in *Advances in Test Anxiety Research*, H. M. van der Ploeg, R. Schwarzer, and C. D. Spielberger, Eds., pp. 83–119, Lawrence Erlbaum Associates, Hillside, NJ, USA, 1984.

[25] K. H. Canobi, R. A. Reeve, and P. E. Pattison, "Young children's understanding of addition concepts," *Educational Psychology*, vol. 22, no. 5, pp. 513–532, 2002.

[26] W. A. Garnham, J. Brooks, A. Garnham, and A. M. Ostenfeld, "From synonyms to homonyms: exploring the role of metarepresentation in language understanding," *Developmental Science*, vol. 3, no. 4, pp. 428–441, 2000.

[27] C. Quaiser-Pohl, "The mental cutting test "schnitte" and the mental rotation rotation test—two new measures to assess spatial ability," *International Journal of Testing*, vol. 3, pp. 219–231, 2003.

[28] D. Bieri, R. A. Reeve, G. D. Champion, L. Addicoat, and J. B. Ziegler, "The faces pain scale for the self-assessment of the severity of pain experienced by children: development, initial validation, and preliminary investigation for ratio scale properties," *Pain*, vol. 41, no. 2, pp. 139–150, 1990.

[29] H. R. Chapman and N. Kirby-Turner, "Visual/verbal analogue scales: examples of brief assessment methods to aid management of child and adult patients in clinical practice," *British Dental Journal*, vol. 193, no. 8, pp. 447–450, 2002.

[30] K. E. Howard and R. Freeman, "Reliability and validity of a faces version of the modified child dental anxiety scale," *International Journal of Paediatric Dentistry*, vol. 17, no. 4, pp. 281–288, 2007.

[31] J. N. Stinson, T. Kavanagh, J. Yamada, N. Gill, and B. Stevens, "Systematic review of the psychometric properties, interpretability and feasibility of self-report pain intensity measures for use in clinical trials in children and adolescents," *Pain*, vol. 125, no. 1-2, pp. 143–157, 2006.

[32] H. J. Lyneham, A. K. Street, M. J. Abbott, and R. M. Rapee, "Psychometric properties of the school anxiety scale—teacher report (SAS-TR)," *Journal of Anxiety Disorders*, vol. 22, no. 2, pp. 292–300, 2008.

[33] L. A. Goodman, "Latent class analysis: the empirical study of latent types, latent variables, and latent structures," in *Applied Latent Class Analysis*, J. A. Hagenaars and A. L. McCutcheon, Eds., pp. 3–53, Cambridge University Press, Cambridge, UK, 2002.

[34] G. J. McLachlan and D. Peel, *Finite Mixture Models*, John Wiley & Sons, New York, NY, USA, 2000.

[35] C. M. Hurvich and C. L. Tsai, "Regression and time series model selection in small samples," *Biometrika*, vol. 76, no. 2, pp. 297–307, 1989.

[36] H. Bozdogan, "Model selection and Akaike's Information Criterion (AIC): the general theory and its analytical extensions," *Psychometrika*, vol. 52, no. 3, pp. 345–370, 1987.

[37] J. Magidson and J. K. Vermunt, "Latent class clustering as a probabilistic extension of K-Means," *Quirk's Marketing Research Review*, vol. 20, pp. 77–80, 2002.

[38] J. Magidson and J. K. Vermunt, "Latent class models for clustering: a comparison with K-means," *Canadian Journal of Marketing Research*, vol. 20, pp. 36–43, 2002.

[39] L. M. Collins and S. T. Lanza, *Latent Class and Latent Transition Analysis For the Social, Behavioral, and Health Sciences*, John Wiley & Sons, New York, NY, USA, 2010.

[40] C. B. Young, S. S. Wu, and V. Menon, "The neurodevelopmental basis of math anxiety," *Psychological Science*, vol. 23, pp. 492–501, 2012.

[41] J. M. Carroll and J. E. Iles, "An assessment of anxiety levels in dyslexic students in higher education," *British Journal of Educational Psychology*, vol. 76, no. 3, pp. 651–662, 2006.

[42] H. Krinzinger, G. Wood, and K. Willmes, "What accounts for individual and gender differences in the multi-digit number processing of primary school children?" *Zeitschrift für Psychologie*, vol. 220, pp. 78–79, 2012.

[43] D. Tomlinson, C. L. von Baeyer, J. N. Stinson, and L. Sung, "A systematic review of faces scales for the self-report of pain intensity in children," *Pediatrics*, vol. 126, no. 5, pp. e1168–e1198, 2010.

[44] E. A. Maloney, S. Waechter, E. F. Risko, and J. A. Fugelsang, "Reducing the sex difference in math anxiety: the role of spatial processing ability," *Learning and Individual Differences*, vol. 22, no. 3, pp. 380–384, 2012.

[45] E. A. Maloney, E. F. Risko, D. Ansari, and J. Fugelsang, "Mathematics anxiety affects counting but not subitizing during visual enumeration," *Cognition*, vol. 114, no. 2, pp. 293–297, 2010.

[46] E. A. Maloney, D. Ansari, and J. A. Fugelsang, "The effect of mathematics anxiety on the processing of numerical magnitude," *Quarterly Journal of Experimental Psychology*, vol. 64, no. 1, pp. 10–16, 2011.

[47] E. A. Maloney and S. L. Beilock, "Math anxiety: Who has it, why it develops, and how to guard against it," *Trends in Cognitive Sciences*, vol. 16, no. 8, pp. 404–406, 2012.

[48] X. Ma and F. Cartwright, "A longitudinal analysis of gender differences in affective outcomes in mathematics during middle and high school," *School Effectiveness and School Improvement*, vol. 14, no. 4, pp. 413–439, 2003.

11

A New Tool to Explore Children's Social Competencies: The Preschool Competition Questionnaire

Daniel Paquette,[1] Marie-Noëlle Gagnon,[2] Luc Bouchard,[2] Marc Bigras,[3] and Barry H. Schneider[4]

[1] *École de Psychoéducation, Université de Montréal, Case postale 6128, Succursale Centre-Ville, Montréal, QC, Canada H3C 3J7*
[2] *Département de psychologie, Université de Montréal, Case postale 6128, Succursale Centre-Ville, Montréal, QC, Canada H3C 3J7*
[3] *Département de psychologie, Université du Québec à Montréal, Case postale 8888, Succursale Centre-Ville, Montréal, QC, Canada H3C 3P8*
[4] *School of psychology, University of Ottawa, Ottawa, Canada K1N 6N5*

Correspondence should be addressed to Daniel Paquette; daniel.paquette@umontreal.ca

Academic Editor: Annie Vinter

This paper presents the validation of *Preschool Competition Questionnaire* (PCQ). The PCQ was completed by the childcare teachers of 780 French-speaking children between the ages of 36 and 71 months. The results of exploratory factor analysis suggest three dimensions involving neither physical nor relational aggression: other-referenced competition, task-oriented competition, and maintenance of dominance hierarchy. The three dimensions are positively correlated with dominance ratings and are linked to social adjustment. Girls are just as competitive as boys in the dimensions of other-referenced competition and dominance hierarchy maintenance. Task-oriented competition is relatively more important in older children and girls. Classification analysis reveals that the children who obtain the highest dominance ratings are the ones who employ a variety of competition strategies.

1. Introduction

In highly industrialized societies, interindividual competition is omnipresent, for example, at work, in sports, and at school. Several researchers have adopted a multidimensional approach to the study of competition among university students. The Griffin-Pierson [1] questionnaire on competition explores two dimensions, interpersonal competitiveness and goal competitiveness, with respect to performance in both academics and games. Interpersonal competitiveness is defined as the desire to do better than others and to win in interpersonal situations and the enjoyment of interpersonal competition. Goal competitiveness is defined as the desire to excel, achieve a goal, and do one's best. The two competition perspectives are not mutually exclusive: "They are ways of construing achievement situations, and thus are viewed as general dispositional tendencies to perceive achievement situations in a certain manner" [1]. Ryckman and his collaborators [2–4] have also highlighted two dimensions of competition in sports: the hypercompetitive attitude scale and the personal development competitive attitude scale. Hypercompetitiveness refers to the indiscriminate need to compete and win (and to avoid losing) at all costs as a means of maintaining or enhancing feelings of self-worth, with attendant orientations of manipulation, aggressiveness, exploitation, and derogation of others across a myriad of situations [4]. Personal development competitiveness refers to an attitude in which the primary focus in competition is not upon winning, but rather upon using the competitive experience to foster personal growth. The emphasis is on self-discovery and self-improvement, and not on comparison with others [4]. Two distinct dimensions have also been observed in eight- and nine-year-olds with respect to both academics and athletics [5]. Whereas other-referenced competition is fuelled by the desire to prove oneself superior to others, task-oriented competition is undertaken with the aim of measuring one's own performance against that of others in order to improve oneself [6].

Until now, there has been no instrument to evaluate competition in preschool children. Some researchers have studied conflicts and aggression in toddlers and preschoolers. Conflicts with peers occur over access to resources (food, toys, adult attention, social partners, etc.), especially when resources are limited [7, 8]. Physical aggression is one means used by young children in competition for access to environmental resources and for dominance rank, the latter determining priority of access to resources and reducing the need for further aggression [9–11]. However, most conflicts do not entail the use of physical aggression [8, 12]: in a study by Hay et al. [8], half of the children between the ages of 18 and 30 months did not use physical aggression with peers, but 80% took objects away from peers at least once.

From both an ethological and an evolutionist perspective, aggression is an adaptive behavior, a competitive conflict-resolution strategy to ensure survival and reproduction [13, 14]. Aggression and intimidation also permit ascension to a high level of dominance, providing priority of access to varied resources during childhood and greater access to sexual partners later on [15]. Physical aggression appears early in young children, around 8 to 9 months [16], reaches a peak between 15 and 24 months in the vast majority of children [17, 18], and is used more by boys as of the age of three years [12]. So, contrary to common belief, physical aggression does not increase with age, but rather decreases in most cases between the ages of 2 and 5 [17–19]. This decrease, however, does not mean a reduction of competition as well. On the contrary, children learn other means of obtaining what they desire by, for example, trading, sharing, and collaborating, or through the use of less peaceful forms such as intimidation and verbal aggression [12, 20]. With the development of language, prosocial conflict resolution is increasingly possible. But language is also positively correlated with another competitive strategy [21] that is relatively stable over time [22] and can be observed in children beginning at age three, especially girls [23]: relational aggression. Relational aggression is a form of aggressive behavior that intentionally damages, or threatens to damage, a relationship with a peer [24]. It includes both direct relational aggression (e.g., telling a peer that you will not invite him to your party) and indirect relational aggression (e.g., ignoring the peer and spreading rumors, malicious lies, and gossip [25]). This form of aggression permits a child to isolate a peer with the ultimate aim of increasing the initiator's own network of influence given that relationally aggressive preschool children have more mutual friends [26].

Our objective was to develop an instrument for assessing styles of competition for resources in preschoolers, other than the specific behaviors of physical aggression and relational aggression. So, the main objective of this paper is to validate a questionnaire, completed by childcare teachers, for the assessment of several dimensions of competition in preschool-aged children, dimensions involving neither physical nor relational aggression, but including observable behaviors during daily childcare centre activities.

Our second objective was to verify whether children who use a variety of competition strategies are more dominant and therefore get more resources. A person-centered typological approach will then be used with respect to the different dimensions to verify if children who obtained high scores for several dimensions of competition displayed greater social adjustment and obtained more resources. The use of this approach by other researchers has revealed clearer and more complex patterns than the variable-centered approach [27, 28]. Charlesworth's [29] study of children aged from 4 to 8 years from four different cultures demonstrated that cooperation is an effective strategy in competition for access to play materials. According to LaFrenière and Charlesworth [30], preschool-aged children who are equally skilled in the use of both cooperative and assertive behaviors are more successful at obtaining resources in problem-solving situations. The works of Vaughn et al. [31] in preschool children and those of Hawley [27] on school children showed that bistrategic children (prosociality and coercion) control more resources. Game theory specialists from different disciplines have shown cooperation to be the strategy (decision rule) that obtains the most resources in the long term [32], while coercion obtains the most resources in the short term. Ethological studies suggest that in social species the survival of individuals depends on the balance between competition and cooperation [33]. The increased complexity of social life over the course of primate evolution has necessitated equilibrium in the use of coercive and cooperative strategies to ensure optimal access to local resources. Individuals who always employ aggression/assertion may wind up socially isolated, which would prevent them from enjoying the benefits of social life. On the other hand, individuals who only develop cooperation skills may not know how to defend or assert themselves in the many competitive situations that may arise.

2. Method

2.1. Sample and Data Collection Procedure. Our sample included 780 French-speaking children between the ages of 36 and 71 months ($M = 49.23$ months, $SD = 7.20$). Forty-nine percent (48.7%) were girls, and 51.3% were boys. We recruited participants through the intermediary of 20 publicly funded childcare centres in the Montréal region. The project was first presented to childcare directors and teachers. The 106 consenting childcare teachers then completed a separate questionnaire for each child between the ages of 3 and 5 in their groups (each child was rated by a single childcare teacher). In childcare centers, parents were required to sign a consent form for their children to be evaluated. Two months later, 32 of the childcare teachers completed the *Questionnaire sur la compétition au préscolaire* (Preschool Competition Questionnaire) a second time to verify test-retest reliability.

2.2. Instruments. For practical, time-related considerations, it was decided to use self-report questionnaires completed by the children's childcare teachers rather than direct observation. The childcare teachers were considered to be in the best position to report valid information regarding children's interactions with other children of the same age.

The childcare teachers completed two questionnaires: the *Questionnaire sur la compétition au préscolaire* (Preschool Competition Questionnaire (PCQ)) and the *Social Competence and Behaviour Evaluation* (SCBE [34]). They also rated the children in their groups in terms of dominance.

2.2.1. PCQ. To begin with, thirty-six (36) items were formulated describing behaviors observable in preschool-aged children during daily childcare centre activities (e.g., "Is angry when does not win at a game," "Perseveres when confronted with a difficult task," and "Objects when another child takes toy away or usurps place"); the number of items in the PCQ was subsequently reduced to 17 during validation. Childcare teachers assessed each child using the same six-point scale employed in the SCBE (1 = never, 2 = rarely, 3 = occasionally, 4 = regularly, 5 = often, 6 = always, and 0 = unable to assess). Psychometric information for the PCQ will be provided later in Section 3.

2.2.2. SCBE. Child socioaffective adjustment was measured using the short version of the *Social Competence and Behaviour Evaluation* (SCBE [35]), which consists of 30 items, each describing a developmental or emotional indicator related to the expression of affectivity, interaction with peers, or interaction with adults (e.g., "Easily frustrated," "Helps with everyday tasks," and "Sad, unhappy or depressed"). The short version of the SCBE generates three scores: an anxiety/withdrawal score (sample items: "Worries" and "Goes unnoticed in a group"), an anger-aggression score ("Irritable, gets mad easily," and "Hits, bites or kicks other children"), and a social competence score ("Accepts compromises when reasons are given," and "Works easily in groups"). Internal consistency for the French version is .92 for the anger-aggression scale, .87 for the anxiety/withdrawal scale, and .85 for the social competence scale. The test-retest measure of temporal stability after an interval of three months is .93 for the anger-aggression scale, .74 for the anxiety/withdrawal scale, and .86 for the social competence scale.

2.2.3. Dominance Hierarchy. Childcare teachers were asked to rank the children in their groups from the most dominant to the most subordinate based on the following definitions [36]: children who most frequently won conflicts with peers or who most frequently obtained what they wanted (toys, space, access to the teacher, etc.) by imposing their will were considered dominant; and children who most frequently lost conflicts or avoided them by exhibiting a submissive attitude and who had less access to resources (toys, space, teacher, etc.) were considered subordinate. The dominance hierarchy provided a dominance rating for each child, based on the following formula:

DOMINANCE RATING

$$= 1 - \left[\frac{(\text{child's hierarchical ranking} - 1)}{(\text{number of children in the hierarchy} - 1)}\right]. \quad (1)$$

Thus, the most dominant child in each group would obtain a dominance rating of 1, while the most submissive child would obtain a rating of 0. If only a small proportion of a childcare teacher's class participated in the study, we asked the teacher to replaced nonparticipating children with an "X" on the hierarchy, thus permitting us to know where participating children were situated relative to others, regardless of whether the others took part in the study or not. The mean dominance rating for the sample (n = 590, as some childcare teachers did not complete the hierarchy) was 0.521 (SD = .331), and the range was 1.0.

3. Results

3.1. Factorial Structure of the PCQ. Before factor analysis of the data was conducted, 13 items were removed from the database for one or more of the following reasons: test-retest correlations for four items were nonsignificant ($P \geq .05$); six items received a very high number of "0—Unable to assess" ratings from childcare teachers, mainly because these items did not apply to children between 3 and 5 or to a childcare centre context; finally, other items were removed because variance in the childcare teachers' answers was too small to provide informative data about the children.

Principal components factor analysis with varimax rotation was performed on the 23 remaining items. The three-factor solution appeared the most appropriate, both on a conceptual level and in terms of eigenvalues. However, it was necessary to eliminate a few items as their loadings were either inferior to .32 [37, 38] or high (≥.32) for more than one component. Five new successive factor analyses were performed to eliminate these items and produce the clearest factorial structure possible. The final factorial structure included 17 items, which are presented in Table 1, grouped according to the factor for which they received the highest loading. It should be noted that even the lowest loading obtained (.513) was excellent.

3.2. Descriptive PCQ Statistics. Table 2 indicates that internal consistency scores (Cronbach's alpha) varied between .74 and .89, which represents satisfactory levels of homogeneity. Moreover kurtosis and skewness coefficients were within ±1.96, and the average was close to the median, indicating that questionnaire scales satisfied normality criteria. Temporal stability of the *PCQ* was also satisfactory for all scales, as test-retest correlations varied between .69 and .92 ($P < .001$). Intercorrelation analysis revealed that the *Hierarchy Maintenance* scale was positively linked to the two other scales ($r = .45$, $P < .001$ for *other-referenced competition* and $r = .26$, $P < .001$ for *task-oriented competition*), while no relation was found between the *task-oriented competition* and *other-referenced competition* scales themselves ($r = -.02$, $P > .05$).

3.3. Construct Validity of PCQ. Table 3 presents correlations among children's scores on the three PCQ scales and the three SCBE scales, as well as dominance ratings. These correlations support the validity of the PCQ. Thus, the

TABLE 1: Factors including item loadings, averages, and standard deviations ($N = 597^1$).

	Factor loading	Mean	SD
Factor 1: Other-referenced competition			
Is angry when does not win at a game (poor loser)	.795	2.46	1.15
Contests when another child wins	.793	2.32	1.04
Is envious when the good performance of another child is praised	.791	2.17	1.06
Likes to compare own performance and achievements to those of others	.756	2.50	1.17
Is motivated to win or to come first at games	.707	3.09	1.30
Is angry when another child gets something he/she desires first	.702	2.79	1.27
Is disappointed when does not succeed in achieving own goals	.688	2.96	1.07
Tends to abandon games when not winning	.577	2.63	1.05
Factor 2: Task-oriented competition			
Perseveres when confronted with difficult tasks	.785	3.82	1.13
Actively seeks to improve own performance and abilities	.740	3.60	1.13
Is enthusiastic about challenges posed by adult	.641	3.85	1.18
Prefers difficult games	.637	2.72	1.05
Plays according to rules of the game	.631	4.25	1.04
Tolerates compromise as a solution to conflict	.513	3.74	1.14
Factor 3: Maintenance of dominance hierarchy			
Objects when another child takes toy away or usurps place	.770	4.34	1.21
Does not let other children grab toys away or usurp place	.768	3.99	1.36
Defends self when attacked by another child	.763	4.31	1.30

Notes: the factors, respectively, explain 28.53%, 18.58%, and 12.87% for a total of 59.98% of the variance.
[1] The final analysis was conducted using a sample of 597 children.

TABLE 2: Descriptive statistics for the PCQ scales.

Scales	Alpha	Average	Standard deviation	Skewness	Kurtosis index	Test-retest correlation[1]	Intercorrelation 1	2	3
(1) Other-referenced competition (8 items)	.89	2.61	0.86	.468	.113	$.92^{***}$	—	−.02	$.45^{***}$
(2) Task-oriented competition (6 items)	.75	3.65	0.75	−.071	−.385	$.80^{***}$		—	$.26^{***}$
(3) Dominance maintenance hierarchy (3 items)	.74	4.22	1.06	−.255	−.434	$.69^{***}$			—

Notes. [1] The test-retest correlation was calculated for a sample of 27 children.
$^{***}P < .001$.

greater the tendency of children to display other-referenced competition behaviors, the greater their tendency to occupy higher ranks in the dominance hierarchy, the more they were perceived as anger-aggressive by their childcare teachers, and the less they were perceived as socially competent. The more children engaged in task-oriented competition, the greater their tendency to occupy higher ranks in the dominance hierarchy, the more they were perceived as socially competent, and the less they were perceived as anxious/withdrawn or anger-aggressive. Finally, the more children displayed behaviors aimed at maintaining or improving their ranks in the hierarchy, the more they were perceived as dominant, socially competent and anger-aggressive, and the less they were seen as anxious/withdrawn.

Correlations between the PCQ, the SCBE, and dominance ratings were the same for girls and boys, and test-retest correlation was significant for girls and boys on the three PCQ scales ($P < .05$).

3.4. Differences by Child Age and Sex. Given that sex differences in the social development of preschool-aged children are commonly observed, it was important to verify the existence of such differences for the different dimensions of competition. A MANOVA conducted on the three competition

TABLE 3: Competition scale correlation with SCBE scores (n = 774) and dominance rating (n = 586).

	Other-referenced competition	Task-oriented competition	Maintenance of dominance hierarchy
SCBE: social competence	$-.16^{***}$	$.69^{***}$	$.12^{***}$
SCBE: anxiety/withdrawal	$-.01$	$-.40^{***}$	$-.39^{***}$
SCBE: anger-aggression	$.67^{***}$	$-.26^{***}$	$.41^{***}$
Dominance rating	$.36^{***}$	$.17^{***}$	$.42^{***}$

$^{***}P < .001$.

TABLE 4: Comparison of average scores for boys (n = 398) and girls (n = 375)[1] on PCQ and SCBE scales.

	Boys M (SD)	Girls M (SD)	t	P
PCQ				
Other-referenced competition	2.60 (0.86)	2.54 (0.84)	1.04	.297
Task-oriented competition	3.57 (0.77)	3.74 (0.71)	−3.32	.001
Maintenance of dominance hierarchy	4.23 (1.10)	4.16 (1.07)	0.99	.325
SCBE				
Social competence	3.95 (0.75)	4.24 (0.76)	−5.37	.000
Anxiety/withdrawal	2.17 (0.75)	2.16 (0.76)	0.24	.813
Aggressiveness/irritability	2.49 (0.93)	2.32 (0.81)	2.69	.007

[1]For subjects with missing values, scores were weighted according to the number of missing items.

scales showed a main effect for age on competition ($F = 1.25$, $P = .05$) and a main effect for sex on competition ($F = 3.89$, $P < .01$). Tests for between-subject effects showed an effect for age ($F = 1.51$, df = 32, $P < .05$) and for sex ($F = 6.00$, df = 1, $P < .05$) on task-oriented competition, but not on the other two dimensions ($P > .05$). Thus, task-oriented competition behaviors increased with age and were used by girls more than by boys on average. Table 4 presents the effects of sex differences on PCQ and SCBE dimensions. It shows that girls, on average, engaged in significantly more task-oriented competition behaviors than boys. Also, the girls had a higher average social competence score than the boys, in keeping with what is generally reported in the literature. On the other hand, the boys had a higher average aggressiveness/irritability score than the girls, again as reported in the literature. It should be noted that the size of the differences is very small ($d = 0.229$, $r = 0.114$ for task-oriented competition; $d = 0.384$, $r = 0.189$ for social competence; $d = 0.195$, $r = 0.097$ for aggressiveness/irritability).

In order to assess the relative importance of the three dimensions of competition with respect to one another, we transformed the data into z-scores. Figure 1 compares the scores for the three- to five-year-olds in the sample. It shows that the average other-referenced competition score for four-year-olds was higher than their average scores for the other two dimensions, while, at the age of five, children had a higher average score for task-oriented competition than for the other two dimensions.

3.5. Child Typology: Prevalences and Relation to Social Adjustment. Classification analysis (hierarchical cluster analysis using Ward's method, with square Euclidian distances as measures of dissimilarity) was performed on z-scores for the three competition scales, revealing the existence of four groups of children.

One-way ANOVAs among the four groups of children showed significant differences in group means for the three dimensions of competition (Table 5). Children in group 1 (10.3%) had high scores for all three dimensions of competition; we therefore named this the "high competitive" group. Children in Group 2 (39.5%) had task-oriented competition scores every bit as high as the "high competitive" children but had fairly low scores for other-referenced competition and average scores for hierarchy maintenance. We named this the "assertive/task-oriented" group. Children in Group 3 (22.1%) had relatively high other-referenced competition scores, very low task-oriented competition scores, and average hierarchy maintenance scores. These were the "assertive/other-referenced" children. Finally, Group 4 (28.0%) had average task-oriented competition scores and very low scores for the other two dimensions. These were the "low competitive" children.

Children in the "assertive/task-oriented" group and the "high competitive" group had higher social competence scores and lower anxiety scores (see Table 6). However, the "high competitive" children were more aggressive and had higher dominance ratings than the "assertive/task-oriented" children. "Low competitive" children had the highest anxiety scores and the lowest aggressiveness and dominance scores (Table 6). "Assertive/other-referenced" children had anxiety and aggressiveness scores comparable to those of the "high competitive" children, but had social competence scores similar to those of the "low competitive" children and dominance scores analogous to those of "assertive/task-oriented" children (Table 6). Several conclusions may be drawn from these results. First, it was the "high competitive" children who obtained the highest dominance ranks (and possibly more of

Table 5: Comparison of means (standard deviation) for dimensions of competition for the four groups of children.

	Group 4 ($n = 217$) low competitive	Group 3 ($n = 171$) assertive/other-referenced	Group 2 ($n = 306$) assertive/task-oriented	Group 1 ($n = 80$) high competitive	Oneway ANOVA F (3, 770)
Other-referenced	1.90^{b} (0.54)	3.04^{a} (0.86)	2.43^{c} (0.50)	3.87^{d} (0.55)	246.06^{3}
Task-oriented	3.20^{b} (0.63)	3.02^{a} (0.45)	4.19^{c} (0.48)	4.20^{c} (0.39)	286.57^{3}
Maintenance of dominance hierarchy	2.99^{b} (0.71)	4.72^{a} (0.85)	4.53^{a} (0.74)	5.07^{c} (0.82)	258.74^{3}

$^{3}P \leq .001$.
^{a,b,c,d}Different letters mean significant differences in two by two comparisons (Scheffé: $P < .05$).

Table 6: Comparison of means (standard deviation) for different variables for the four groups of children.

	Low competitive	Assertive/other-referenced	Assertive/task-oriented	High competitive	Oneway ANOVA F (3, 765)^{A}
Social competence	3.82^{a} (.80)	3.64^{a} (.66)	4.49^{b} (.63)	4.26^{b} (.64)	70.54^{3}
Anxiety/withdrawal	2.56^{b} (.97)	2.27^{a} (.62)	1.86^{ac} (.52)	2.03^{a} (.58)	44.62^{3}
Aggressiveness/irritability	1.92^{b} (.61)	3.05^{a} (.91)	2.18^{c} (.59)	3.21^{a} (.95)	120.20^{3}
Dominance rating	0.31^{b} (.29)	0.60^{a} (.32)	0.58^{a} (.30)	0.75^{c} (.30)	39.27^{3}

^{A}F (3, 535) for dominance rating.
$^{3}P \leq .001$.
^{a,b,c,d}Different letters mean significant differences in two by two comparisons (Scheffé: $P < .05$).

the resources in their environment). These children displayed just as much aggressive behavior as social competence in their daily lives. Other-referenced competition was a good strategy for obtaining resources for children who also made ample use of the other two strategies (task-oriented competition and dominance). Secondly, it was the "low competitive" children who obtained the lowest dominance ranks (and possibly the fewest resources). These children were primarily characterized by their greater anxiety/social withdrawal. Thirdly, the comparison between the "assertive/other-referenced" group and the "assertive/task-oriented" group showed dominance ranks to be equivalent in three- to five-year-old children characterized by social competence or aggression.

4. Discussion

There is an apparent continuity in the dimensions of competition present from preschool age to adulthood. Our study confirms the existence in preschoolers of two dimensions of competition previously observed in eight- and nine-year-olds [6] and in university students [1, 4]. The two dimensions, which correspond roughly to other-referenced competition and task-oriented competition, are independent of one another in preschoolers, as they are in adults [1, 3], although Tassi and Schneider [5] have obtained significant positive correlation between the two dimensions (in physical as much as in cognitive domains) for eight- and nine-year-olds. Moreover, our questionnaire assesses "dominance hierarchy maintenance," a third dimension of competition in preschoolers that relates to child social status. Dominance hierarchy is a mechanism that determines priority of access to resources by minimizing interpersonal conflict and thus the risk of injury [39]. Theoretically, this dimension could also be assessed in school-aged children and adolescents [40].

Like Tassi and Schneider's findings [5] involving school-aged children, our research revealed a positive relation between task-oriented competition and prosocial behaviors, as well as a positive relation between other-referenced competition and aggressiveness in preschool-aged children. Whereas Tassi and Schneider assessed the two dimensions by means of peer nominations, we have assessed them through the intermediary of the childcare teachers. Among adults, hypercompetitiveness (which corresponds most closely to other-referenced competition) has been linked to aggression and dominance. Personal development competitiveness (closest to task-oriented competition) has been linked to self-esteem and psychological health [3]. Our results reveal a negative relation in preschoolers between anxiety/withdrawal, and task-oriented competition and hierarchy maintenance.

By identifying four different groups of children, the person-centered typological approach allowed the independence of the PCQ scales to be confirmed. Classification analysis reveals that children who employ a variety of competition strategies—including other-referenced competition, highly correlated with aggressiveness in children—receive the highest dominance ratings. Hawley [27] has shown that bistrategic controllers (nearly 18% of fifth- through tenth-graders), who employ coercive strategies as frequently as prosocial strategies, report themselves to be those most effective at resource control. The quest for and maintenance of a high dominance rank appears likely to be a major consideration at preschool age. In addition to having access to more physical resources, dominant preschoolers are socially central in that they are watched, imitated, and liked more than

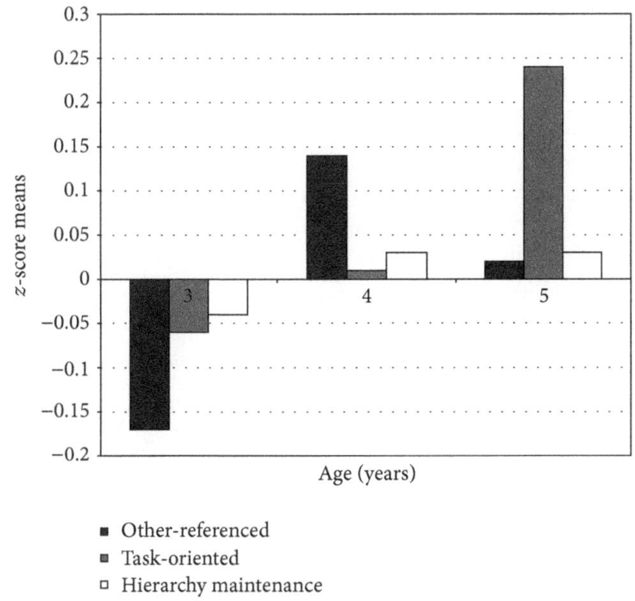

FIGURE 1: Relative importance of the three dimensions of competition.

subordinate children [41]. However, as Hawley [27] has stated with regards to prosociality and coercion, we do not know how the different dimensions of competition are employed by the best controllers of resources. Thus, it is important that we gain a better understanding of the balance between competition and cooperation required for optimal adaptation to the social environment. Vaughn et al. [31] have shown socially competent preschoolers to be relatively more coercive and dominant than their peers.

According to some researchers [41–43], social dominance in human beings is the differential ability to acquire or control resources independent of the means used, that is, that children use prosociality (i.e., persuasion, negotiation, helping, sharing, or cooperation) as much as coercion (i.e., aggression, intimidation) to obtain a high dominance rank. According to us, social dominance in humans is only one of many types of power relationship for acquiring environmental resources, one that is established and maintained by agonistic and coercive behaviors, just as it is among many animals. This misapprehension is probably based on the data of Savin-Williams [44], who showed that socially dominant boys at school have high rates of prosocial behaviors with peers during their kindergarten year. Cooperation also permits access to resources but do not lead to a high dominance rank. In other words, the individual who obtains the most resources is not necessarily the most dominant. One may well suppose that cooperation leads to another type of power relationship that has assumed special importance over the course of human evolution: leadership. According to a review of the literature by Van Vugt [45], there is no association between dominance and leadership, which are two different forms of power [46], the first resulting from coercion and the second from influence. The most constant element in the various proposed definitions of leadership involves an influence process between the leader and those who follow the leader towards the accomplish of a common goal [47]. Leadership is the result of an individual's prosocial skill in convincing others, in order to be "elected" by the group, that he or she, rather than someone else, can serve the group most usefully by helping it to attain its objectives [48, 49]. One could say that leadership is a form of cooperation between a group and an individual that provides the group with a structured approach to accomplishing a common goal. It goes without saying that the two phenomena of social dominance and leadership may in reality be combined, which makes it easy to think that one is a component of the other.

Boys are generally considered to be more competitive than girls [1]. Tassi and Schneider's [5] study has shown that eight- and nine-year-old boys engage in more other-referenced competition (both physical and cognitive) and more task-oriented competition (physical only) than girls. Moreover, longitudinal studies have shown that, between the ages of 4 and 11, boys are more likely than girls to use physical aggression, while girls are more likely than boys to engage in relational aggression [50]. The sexual dimorphism favoring males (with males being bigger, stronger, and more physically aggressive than females) found in many nonhuman primate species as well as in the human species would appear to indicate that, in earlier stages of human phylogenetic history, males had to compete for access to sexual partners and that females chose the more dominant males in order to transmit to their children traits that would facilitate the offspring's survival and reproduction [15, 51, 52]. With respect to other-referenced competition, our study shows preschool-aged girls to be just as competitive for local resources as boys, even if they are significantly less physically aggressive (see Table 4). Furthermore, girls are shown to engage in more task-oriented competition than boys, which is probably related to their greater social competence (see Table 4). According to Hawley [27], boys are overrepresented among coercive controllers and girls are overrepresented among prosocial controllers but there is no difference between boys and girls in the bistrategic group. *A posteriori* analysis of our data confirms the presence of as many girls as boys in the group of children with high scores for all three dimensions of competition (high competitive group), as well as in the assertive/task-oriented group and the low competitive group. However, there is a trend towards boys in the assertive/other-referenced group ($P = .07$). In order to comprehend these results fully, a deeper understanding of the most important physical, cognitive, and social resources based on child sex and age is needed. Competition among women for men has been documented cross-culturally [53]: several authors have documented the use of physical aggression or the spreading of malicious rumors about rivals by women in competition for men with access to subsistence products. In the context of the human species' recent evolution towards monogamy [54], one might expect to find an interfemale competition for exclusive access to the best male provider (of food resources and care for the young).

The PCQ will allow researchers to explore the development of different types of competition in preschool children in relation to the human ontogenesis of dominance and leadership, in relation to individualist/collectivist values and in relation to parental types of power (i.e., authoritative, authoritarian [55–57]). One might, for example, expect to observe the transmission by parents to children of types of power relationships either directly through the parent-child relationship, or indirectly through the child's witnessing of the parents' conjugal relationship [58]. This instrument will be particularly useful in verifying the existence of a relation between father-child rough-and-tumble play and competition in preschoolers [59]. According to the activation relationship theory [54], fathers play a primary role in the development of competition skills (including aggression) in children. In this context, children theoretically have more chances of developing varied repertories of competitive strategies if they enjoy positive affective relationships with at least one paternal figure. Finally, the PCQ may also be used as a supplement to the SCBE to provide a more complete assessment of social adjustment in preschool-aged children.

Our study's main weakness is its use of single respondents (the childcare teachers) for all assessments. It would therefore be useful to carry out a confirmatory factor analysis with another sample, using different respondents to assess social adjustment and using observation to assess social dominance, as submissive responses to attacks and threats have been shown to be the best means for assessing dominance relationships in both nonhuman primates and human children [11, 60–62]. Moreover, longitudinal studies should be conducted to confirm the competition pathways established in our transversal study, that is, the transition between 3 and 5 years of age from other-referenced competition to task-oriented competition.

References

[1] S. Griffin-Pierson, "The competitiveness questionnaire: a measure of two components of competitiveness," *Measurement and Evaluation in Counseling and Development*, vol. 23, pp. 108–115, 1990.

[2] R. M. Ryckman, M. Hammer, L. M. Kaczor, and J. A. Gold, "Construction of a hypercompetitive attitude scale," *Journal of Personality Assessment*, vol. 55, pp. 3630–4639, 1990.

[3] R. M. Ryckman, M. Hammer, L. M. Kaczor, and J. A. Gold, "Construction of a personal development competitive attitude scale," *Journal of Personality Assessment*, vol. 66, no. 2, pp. 374–385, 1996.

[4] R. M. Ryckman, C. R. Libby, B. Van den Borne, J. A. Gold, and M. A. Lindner, "Values of hypercompetitive and personal development competitive individuals," *Journal of Personality Assessment*, vol. 69, no. 2, pp. 271–283, 1997.

[5] F. Tassi and B. H. Schneider, "Task-oriented versus other-referenced competition: differential implications for children's peer relations," *Journal of Applied Social Psychology*, vol. 27, no. 17, pp. 1557–1580, 1997.

[6] F. Tassi, B. H. Schneider, and J. F. Richard, "Competitive behavior at school in relation to social competence and incompetence in middle childhood," *Revue Internationale de Psychologie Sociale*, vol. 14, no. 2, pp. 165–184, 2001.

[7] M. Caplan, J. Vespo, J. Pedersen, and D. F. Hay, "Conflict and its resolution in small groups of one- and two-year-olds," *Child Development*, vol. 62, no. 6, pp. 1513–1524, 1991.

[8] D. F. Hay, J. Castle, and L. Davies, "Toddlers' use of force against familiar peers: a precursor of serious aggression?" *Child Development*, vol. 71, no. 2, pp. 457–467, 2000.

[9] R. Gauthier and M. Jacques, "La dominance et l'affiliation chez les enfants d'âge pré-scolaire: analyse transversale," in *ÉthoLogie et DéveLoppement de L'Enfant*, R. E. Tremblay, M. A. Provost, and F. F. Strayer, Eds., pp. 309-327, Stock/Laurence Pernoud, Paris, France, 1985.

[10] P. H. Hawley and T. D. Little, "On winning some and losing some: a social relations approach to social dominance in toddlers," *Merrill-Palmer Quarterly*, vol. 45, no. 2, pp. 185–214, 1999.

[11] F. F. Strayer and M. Trudel, "Developmental changes in the nature and function of social dominance among young children," *Ethology and Sociobiology*, vol. 5, no. 4, pp. 279–295, 1984.

[12] J. D. Coie and K. A. Dodge, "1998Aggression and antisocial behavior," in *Handbook of Child Psychology: Social, Emotional and Personality Development*, W. Damon and N. Eisenberg, Eds., vol. 3, pp. 779–862, Wiley & Sons, New York, NY, USA.

[13] J. Archer, *The Behavioural Biology of Aggression*, Cambridge University Press, Cambridge, UK, 1988.

[14] I. Eibl-Eibesfeldt, *Human Ethology*, Aldine de Gruyter, New York, NY, USA, 1989.

[15] L. M. Fedigan, *Primate Paradigms. Sex Roles and Social Bonds*, Eden Press, Montreal, Canada, 1982.

[16] D. F. Hay, A. Nash, and J. Pedersen, "Interaction between Six-month-old peers," *Child development*, vol. 54, no. 3, pp. 557–562, 1983.

[17] A. Restoin, H. Montagner, D. Rodriguez et al., "Chronologie des comportements de communication et profils de comportement chez le jeune enfant," in *ÉthoLogie Et DéveLoppement de L'Enfant*, R. E. Tremblay, M. A. Provost, and F. F. Strayer, Eds., pp. 93–130, Stock/Laurence Pernoud, Paris, France, 1985.

[18] R. E. Tremblay, C. Japel, D. Pérusse et al., "The search for the age of 'onset' of physical aggression: Rousseau and Bandura revisited," *Criminal Behaviour and Mental Health*, vol. 9, no. 1, pp. 8–23, 1999.

[19] E. M. Cummings, R. J. Iannotti, and C. Zahn-Waxler, "Aggression between peers in early childhood: individual continuity and developmental change," *Child development*, vol. 60, no. 4, pp. 887–895, 1989.

[20] F. L. Goodenough, *Anger in Young Children*, University of Minnesota Press, Minneapolis, Minn, USA, 1931.

[21] C. Bonica, D. H. Arnold, P. H. Fisher, A. Zeljo, and K. Yershova, "Relational aggression, relational victimization, and language development in preschoolers," *Social Development*, vol. 12, no. 4, pp. 551–562, 2003.

[22] N. R. Crick, "The role of overt aggression, relational aggression, and prosocial behavior in the prediction of children's future social adjustment," *Child Development*, vol. 67, no. 5, pp. 2317–2327, 1996.

[23] N. R. Crick, J. F. Casas, and M. Mosher, "Relational and overt aggression in preschool," *Developmental psychology*, vol. 33, no. 4, pp. 579–588, 1997.

[24] N. R. Crick and J. K. Grotpeter, "Relational aggression, gender, and social-psychological adjustment," *Child development*, vol. 66, no. 3, pp. 710–722, 1995.

[25] A. D. Pellegrini and C. J. Roseth, "Relational aggression and relationships in preschoolers: a discussion of methods, gender differences, and function," *Journal of Applied Developmental Psychology*, vol. 27, no. 3, pp. 269–276, 2006.

[26] J. E. Burr, J. M. Ostrov, E. A. Jansen, C. Cullerton-Sen, and N. R. Crick, "Relational aggression and friendship during early childhood: 'I won't be your friend!'," *Early Education and Development*, vol. 16, no. 2, pp. 161–183, 2005.

[27] P. H. Hawley, "Prosocial and coercive configurations of resource control in early adolescence: a case for the well-adapted Machiavellian," *Merrill-Palmer Quarterly*, vol. 49, no. 3, pp. 279–309, 2003.

[28] T. D. Little, J. Brauner, S. M. Jones, M. K. Nock, and P. H. Hawley, "Rethinking aggression: a typological examination of the functions of aggression," *Merrill-Palmer Quarterly*, vol. 49, no. 3, pp. 343–369, 2003.

[29] W. R. Charlesworth, "Co-operation and competition: contributions to an evolutionary and developmental model," *International Journal of Behavioral Development*, vol. 19, no. 1, pp. 25–38, 1996.

[30] P. J. LaFrenière and W. R. Charlesworth, "Effects of friendship and dominance status on preschooler's resource utilization in a cooperative competitive paradigm," *International Journal of Behavioral Development*, vol. 10, pp. 345–358, 1987.

[31] B. E. Vaughn, M. Vollenweider, K. K. Bost, M. R. Azria-Evans, and J. B. Snider, "Negative interactions and social competence for preschool children in two samples: reconsidering the interpretation of aggressive behavior for young children," *Merrill-Palmer Quarterly*, vol. 49, no. 3, pp. 245–278, 2003.

[32] R. Axelrod, *The Evolution of Cooperation*, Basic Books, New York, Ny, USA, 1984.

[33] J. Flanders, K. N. Herman, and D. Paquette, "Rough-and-tumble play and the cooperation-competition dilemma: Evolutionary and developmental perspectives on the development of social competence," in *Evolution, Early Experience and Human Development: from Research to Practice and Policy*, D. Narvaez, J. Panksepp, A. Schore, and T. Gleason, Eds., Oxford University Press, New York, NY, USA, 2013.

[34] P. J. LaFrenière, J. E. Dumas, F. Capuano, and D. Dubeau D, "The development and validation of the Preschool socioaffective profile," in *Journal of Consulting and Clinical Psychology*, vol. 4, no. 4, pp. 442–450, 1992.

[35] M. Venet, M. Bigras, and S. Normandeau, "Les qualités psychométriques du PSA-A," *Revue Canadienne des Sciences du Comportement*, vol. 34, no. 3, pp. 163–167, 2002.

[36] M. A. Provost, "Description de catégories de compétence sociale chez des enfants d'âge préscolaire," in *Les Relations SociaLes Entre les Enfants*, R. Tessier, G. Tarabulsy, and M. A. Provost, Eds., Monographies de psychologie, pp. 19–43, Presses de l'Université du Québec, 1996.

[37] A. L. Comrey and H. B. Lee, *A First Course in Factor Analysis*, Hillsdale, NJ, USA, Lawrence Erlbaum Associates, 2nd edition, 1992.

[38] B. G. Tabachnick and L. S. Fidell, *Using Multivariate Statistics*, Allyn & Bacon, Needham Heights, Mass, USA, 4th edition, 2001.

[39] D. Paquette, "Fighting and playfighting in captive adolescent chimpanzees," *Aggressive Behavior*, vol. 20, pp. 49–65, 1994.

[40] R. C. Savin-Williams, "Dominance hierarchies in groups of early adolescents," *Child Development*, vol. 50, pp. 923–935, 1979.

[41] P. H. Hawley, "The ontogenesis of social dominance: a strategy-based evolutionary perspective," *Developmental Review*, vol. 19, no. 1, pp. 97–132, 1999.

[42] P. H. Hawley, "Social dominance and prosocial and coercive strategies of resource control in preschoolers," *International Journal of Behavioral Development*, vol. 26, no. 2, pp. 167–176, 2002.

[43] A. D. Pellegrini, C. J. Roseth, S. Mliner et al., "Social dominance in preschool classrooms," *Journal of Comparative Psychology*, vol. 121, no. 1, pp. 54–64, 2007.

[44] R. C. Savin-Williams, *Adolescence: An Ethological Perspective*, Spinger, New York, NY, USA, 1987.

[45] M. Van Vugt, "Evolutionary origins of leadership and followership," *Personality and Social Psychology Review*, vol. 10, no. 4, pp. 354–371, 2006.

[46] D. C. Jones, "Power structures and perceptions of power holders in same-sex group of young children," in *Biopolitics and Gender*, M. W. Watts, Ed., pp. 147–164, Haworth Press, New Yorkm, USA, 1984.

[47] E. P. Hollander, "Leadership and power," in *Handbook of Social Psychology*, G. Lindzey and E. Aronson, Eds., pp. 485–537, Random House, New York, NY, USA, 3rd edition, 1985.

[48] B. M. Bass and R. M. Stogdill, *Handbook of Leadership: Theory, Research and Managerial Applications*, The Free Press, New York, NY, USA, 3rd edition, 1990.

[49] W. W. Hartup, "Peer relations," in *Handbook of Child Psychology, Socialization, Personality and Social Development*, E. M. Hetherington, Ed., vol. 4, pp. 103–196, Wiley, New York, NY, USA, 1983.

[50] N. R. Crick, J. M. Ostrov, J. E. Burr, C. Cullerton-Sen, E. Jansen-Yeh, and P. Ralston, "A longitudinal study of relational and physical aggression in preschool," *Journal of Applied Developmental Psychology*, vol. 27, no. 3, pp. 254–268, 2006.

[51] D. P. Barash, *Sociobiology and Behavior*, Elsevier, Amsterdam, The Netherlands, 2nd edition, 1982.

[52] D. C. Geary, "Evolution and proximate expression of human paternal investment," *Psychological Bulletin*, vol. 126, no. 1, pp. 55–77, 2000.

[53] A. Campbell, *A Mind of Her Own: The Evolutionary Psychology of Women*, Oxford University Press, Oxford, UK, 2002.

[54] D. Paquette, "Theorizing the father-child relationship: mechanisms and developmental outcomes," *Human Development*, vol. 47, no. 4, pp. 193–219, 2004.

[55] D. Baumrind, "Child care practices anteceding three patterns of preschool behavior," *Genetic Psychology Monographs*, vol. 75, no. 1, pp. 43–88, 1967.

[56] D. Baumrind, "Current patterns of parental authority," *Developmental Psychology*, vol. 4, no. 1, pp. 1–103, 1971.

[57] D. B. Bugental, J. Krantz, J. E. Lyon, and V. Cortez, "Who's the boss? Differential accessibility of dominance ideation in parent-child relationships," *Journal of Personality and Social Psychology*, vol. 72, no. 6, pp. 1297–1309, 1997.

[58] D. Paquette, M. Bigras, and M. A. Crepaldi, "La violence: un jugement de valeur sur les rapports de pouvoir," *Revue de Psychoéducation*, vol. 39, no. 2, pp. 245–274, 2010.

[59] D. Paquette, R. Carbonneau, D. Dubeau, M. Bigras, and R. E. Tremblay, "Prevalence of father-child rough-and-tumble play and physical aggression in preschool children," *European Journal of Psychology of Education*, vol. 18, no. 2, pp. 171–189, 2003.

[60] I. S. Bernstein, "Dominance: a theoretical perspective for ethologists," in *Dominance Relations: An Ethological View of Human Conflict and Social Interaction*, D. R. Omark, F. F. Strayer, and D. G. Freedman, Eds., pp. 71–84, Garlend STPM Press, New York, NY, USA, 1980.

[61] T. E. Rowell, "Hierarchy in the organization of a captive baboon group," *Animal Behaviour*, vol. 14, no. 4, pp. 430–443, 1966.

[62] J. Strayer and F. F. Strayer, "Social aggression and power relations among preschool children," *Aggressive Behavior*, vol. 4, no. 2, pp. 173–182, 1978.

12

Parent-Initiated Motivational Climate, Self-Esteem, and Autonomous Motivation in Young Athletes: Testing Propositions from Achievement Goal and Self-Determination Theories

Daniel J. O'Rourke,[1] Ronald E. Smith,[1] Frank L. Smoll,[1] and Sean P. Cumming[2]

[1] *Department of Psychology, University of Washington, Seattle, WA 98195-1525, USA*
[2] *School of Health, University of Bath, Bath BA2 7AY, UK*

Correspondence should be addressed to Daniel J. O'Rourke, djo13@uw.edu

Academic Editor: Cheryl Dissanayake

Interactions with parents are known to have a significant impact on children's self-esteem. In this study, designed to test propositions derived from Achievement Goal Theory and Self-Determination Theory, we assessed the influence of perceived parent-initiated mastery and ego motivational climates on self-esteem and self-esteem change in competitive youth swimmers over the course of a 32-week sport season. At each of three measurement points (early, mid, and late season), mastery climate scores on the Parent-Initiated Motivational Climate Questionnaire-2 scale were positively related to global self-esteem scores and to a measure of relative motivational autonomy that reflects the intrinsic-extrinsic motivation continuum, whereas ego climate scores were negatively related to self-esteem and autonomy. Longitudinal analyses revealed that early-season mastery climate predicted positive changes in self-esteem over the course of the season, whereas ego climate predicted decreased self-esteem. Consistent with predictions derived from Self-Determination Theory, a meditational analysis revealed that these self-esteem changes were mediated by changes in autonomous motivation.

1. Introduction

The centrality of the self-concept has been emphasized by many theorists as an object of self-awareness and a determinant of behavior [1–6]. The evaluative aspect of the self-system is commonly referred to as self-esteem. Historically, few personality constructs have received greater theoretical and empirical attention than self-esteem. Although self-evaluations may relate to specific areas of experience, such as social, academic, and athletic domains, most theorists also posit a superordinate construct that refers to a generalized sense of self-worth [3, 7]. Global self-esteem is an important indicator of psychological well-being [2, 4, 8, 9].

Developmental factors that influence self-esteem have attracted the attention of both theorists and researchers. Within a variety of settings, interactions with significant others provide important feedback in the form of reflected appraisals, and social comparison processes evoke self-evaluative inferences about one's traits and competencies [10, 11]. One such domain in which specific personal and reflected evaluations of self-worth can be generated is sport [12–14]. In part, this is because the environmental conditions created by significant others, such as coaches or parents, reinforce specific behaviors in youth athletes that contribute toward attaining psychological well-being [5, 13–16]. In addition, sport exposes athletes to environmental influences that affect motivational processes thought to contribute to well-being and self-esteem [5, 17].

The relation between motivation and self-esteem is the focus of the present research. Motivational factors are thought to be critical to the development and maintenance of self-esteem [14, 18]. Researchers have also suggested that the social environment is a main contributor to the quality of motivation and therefore to self-esteem [4, 5, 13]. In this paper, we link self-esteem, and changes in self-esteem, to theoretical concepts drawn from two prominent motivational theories, namely, Achievement Goal Theory and Self-Determination Theory [4, 5, 16, 19].

Achievement Goal Theory (AGT) focuses on how the social environment influences achievement goals and competence evaluations. Although the theory continues to evolve, the key principle in AGT is that individuals vary in their conceptions of what constitutes success. In a task, or mastery conception, success evaluations are self referenced rather than other-referenced, and people view themselves as successful when they give maximal effort, increase their skill level, demonstrate personal mastery, and learn from mistakes. The focus is on personal improvement "become the best you can be" and on enjoyment of the process involved in gaining competencies. In an ego conception, success perceptions are based on social comparison processes, and success perceptions are contingent on "winning" by outperforming others using equal or less effort, often in the service of attaining recognition and status [19–22].

In an achievement situation such as sport, individuals adopt specific conceptions of success and attempt to achieve the success criterion and/or to avoid a failure criterion. Whether an individual is focused on mastery or ego goals in a particular moment is influenced by interacting dispositional and environmental factors. The most important dispositional factor is a general orientation toward mastery or ego-oriented goals (i.e., a mastery orientation or an ego orientation). The environmental factor of importance is the motivational climate, comprised of the communicated values and reinforcement contingencies created by significant others. Corresponding to mastery and ego achievement goal orientations are mastery and ego motivational climates [18, 19]. A mastery climate reinforces self-referenced improvement, learning from mistakes, effort, and enjoyment, whereas an ego climate rewards outperforming others using the minimal required effort, while punishing mistakes [19, 21, 22]. Research demonstrates that the motivational climate strengthens its corresponding goal orientation and that modifying the motivational climate can result in shifts in the nature and/or strength of young athletes' goal orientations [23–25].

In general, a mastery climate has more salutary effects than does an ego climate in both academic and athletic settings. These benefits include lower performance anxiety [23, 26], higher feelings of competence, greater enjoyment of the activity, and higher intrinsic motivation and effort [20, 27]. A mastery orientation (particularly in combination with a low ego orientation) is also related to a variety of adaptive achievement behaviors, such as exerting consistent effort, persistence in the face of setbacks, and sustained and improved performance [19, 20, 28]. Researchers have also found that a mastery climate created by teachers and athletic coaches is linked to higher self-esteem, while an ego climate predicts lower self-esteem [14, 18, 28, 29]. Moreover, coach training interventions that promoted a mastery climate have demonstrated a self-esteem enhancing effect on young athletes [30, 31].

Mechanisms whereby a mastery climate influences self-esteem have also been the focus of research. One line of research, inspired by Self Determination Theory [4, 5], has focused on externally controlled versus autonomous aspects of motivation. SDT posits that there are three basic human needs necessary for psychological well-being. These needs include competence (perceived mastery over behavior), relatedness (perceived sense of belonging), and autonomy (perceived sense of self-determination over behavior). According to SDT, behavioral regulation varies from being highly controlled to highly autonomous, and the degree to which motivation is autonomous determines need satisfaction. In particular, the need for autonomy is satisfied to the extent that the locus of motivation is internally rather than externally based [5]. This proposition has received strong empirical support from findings that when behavior is perceived as more self-determined, general well-being is enhanced [27, 29, 32–34]. Of particular significance is the finding that environments that produce greater intrinsic motivation are associated with higher levels of self-esteem [13, 14, 17, 18, 35]. One such environment, derived from AGT, is a mastery climate [14, 18]. However, López-Walle and colleagues [18] and Standage and Gillison [14] found that although a coach-initiated mastery climate predicts higher self-esteem in athletes, this effect appears to be mediated by of the athlete's level of intrinsic motivation for the activity. The researchers concluded that the encouragement of more intrinsic forms of motivation is one mechanism through which a mastery climate helps to foster high self-worth. This makes conceptual sense given that autonomous motivation should help engender a sense of self-worth compared to conditions in which behavior is dictated by external and more controlled outcomes.

Combining concepts from AGT and SDT provides a theoretical and empirically supported framework in which to study self-esteem in young athletes. SDT predicts that an autonomy-supportive environment fosters self-esteem through increasing levels of internally-motivated behavior. From an AGT perspective, previous research [14, 18] suggests that one way in which a mastery climate is conducive to higher self-esteem is by promoting autonomous forms of motivation that enhance well-being, including self-esteem.

The present study builds upon previous results in three major ways. First, all previous research has focused on the motivational climate initiated within the athletic setting by the coach. However, parents also create a parallel motivational climate to which their children are exposed. To this point, the role of parent-initiated motivational climate has received far less attention, even though parents are acknowledged as an essential contributor to well-being and motivational development in children [36–39]. In addition, youth athletes typically experience extensive parental exposure to achievement-related values and across a broad range of settings. In this study, we therefore focus on the athlete-perceived parent-initiated motivational climate and its influence on both self-esteem and autonomy.

A second focus of this study is on potential *changes* in self-esteem as a function of the motivational climate. To this point, research linking motivational climate and self-esteem has been cross-sectional in nature. In this study, we examine the role of perceived parent-initiated motivational climate upon youth athletes' self-esteem longitudinally over the course of a 32-week sport season. Drawing upon previous findings derived from AGT and SDT, we also examined the possible meditational role of climate-linked autonomy change to changes in self-esteem within this longitudinal framework. Specifically, we tested the mediational model shown in Figure 1. Previous research [14, 18] has focused on the role of intrinsic motivation. We build upon this by considering the relative strength of autonomous (intrinsically and extrinsically regulated) motivation, thereby addressing the dimensional approach of SDT and building on its theoretical and empirical foundations. Finally, the sample we studied is younger than most previous samples that have examined parent-initiated motivational climate, falling within a late childhood-early adolescence age range in which, according to theorists, self-esteem is more malleable and strongly influenced by relevant experiences and self-evaluations [3, 6, 8].

This study tests three hypotheses involving constructs derived from AGT and SDT. First, we hypothesize that athlete-perceived behaviors that define a parent-initiated mastery climate will be positively related to athletes' self-esteem in cross-sectional analyses conducted over the course of a sport season, whereas an ego climate will exhibit a negative relation with self-esteem. Second, we believe that if the motivational climate is influential over this period of time, we would expect a mastery climate to promote positive changes in self-esteem and that an ego climate will not enhance and may even decrease self-esteem. Finally, based on previous findings that autonomous motivation enhances well-being, including self-esteem, by enhancing one's sense of personal control and self-determination [4], we hypothesize that changes in autonomous motivation for participation will contribute to (i.e., at least partially mediate) the relation between perceived motivational climate and athletes' self-esteem change.

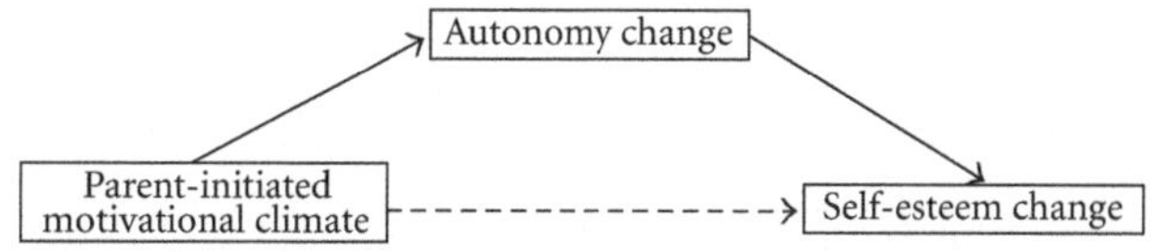

Figure 1: The proposed mediational model of the current study. Parent-initiated motivational climate is hypothesized to predict self-esteem change from early to late season. This relation is thought to be mediated by autonomy change from early to late season.

2. Method

2.1. Participants. Participants were 304 athletes (123 boys and 181 girls, M age = 11.88, SD = 1.34, age range = 9–14 years) from three elite swim clubs in a regional swimming program associated with USA Swimming. The ethnic membership was 71.0% Caucasian, 13.2% Asian, and 15.8% representing other ancestries. On average, athletes were club members for 3.30 (SD = 2.03) years and had engaged in competitive swimming since age 7 (M = 7.27, SD = 2.22). Competitive swimming occurred on a year-round basis, comprising daily weekday practices with competitive meets on many weekends. The competitive season was most intense from August to May, and athletes were coached by professionals employed by the clubs. The attrition rate was 0.03% from Time 1 to Time 2, and 22.74% from Time 2 to Time 3 because of lowered attendance at practices by season end. Athletes who failed to provide data at Time 3 did not differ significantly at Times 1 or 2 from those who did.

2.2. Measures

2.2.1. Parent-Initiated Motivational Climate. The Parent-Initiated Motivational Climate Questionnaire-2 (PIMCQ-2) was used to assess children's perceptions of the parent-initiated motivational climate. The PIMCQ-2 [39] normally provides scores on three subscales, one reflecting a mastery orientation (the learning and enjoyment-emphasis subscale) and two reflecting ego orientation (success-without-effort and worry-conducive behaviors subscales). Before using the scale in its original form, we assessed its factorial validity for our sample. Our data, based in part on an age group younger than that in which the scale was originally developed, failed to produce the three-factor solution reported by Duda and Whitehead [40]. Instead, in this younger sample, we found a 2-factor structure that was consistent with the Duda-Whitehead mastery-related factor (containing learning and enjoyment items) and a single ego factor (containing success-without-effort and worry-inducing items), with eigenvalues exceeding 1.00. Nine items with factor loadings exceeding .40 comprised the parent-initiated mastery climate scale (e.g., "is most satisfied when I learn something new") and nine items with similar loadings assessed ego climate (e.g., "looks satisfied when I win without effort"). Children responded to the stem "I feel that my mother/father/guardian..." on a 4-point scale ranging from 1 (*strongly disagree*) to 4 (*strongly agree*) for each item.

Internal consistency was acceptable at all three time points (Cronbach's *alpha* = .76 to .79 for the mastery climate scale and .83 to .85 for the ego climate scale). A Flesch-Kincaid readability analysis placed the reading level of the scale at grade 5.5 (approximately age 11). Given the relatively high socioeconomic and educational characteristics of the current sample, we judged the scale appropriate for our use.

2.2.2. Self-Esteem. Global self-esteem was measured using the Washington Self-Description Questionnaire (WSDQ). The WSDQ [31, 41] consists of 14 descriptive statements, each of which is rated on a 4-point scale ranging from 1 (*not like me*) to 4 (*very much like me*). As recommended by Wylie [6], all of the items are global evaluative in nature rather than focused on particular domains of competence, such as academics, sports, or social competencies. In this respect, the WSDQ resembles Rosenberg's (1979) scale [10], but the items are more simply worded to enhance children's comprehension. Six of the items refer to positive attributes (e.g., "I feel proud of myself"), whereas eight items relate to negative self-valuations (e.g., "I often wish I were someone else"). The scale is designed to provide a maximum range of scores (14 to 56) with a relatively small number of items. In previous research, the scale has been found to have high internal consistency (.80 to .86), good test-retest reliability in children of this age range, and validity as both a moderator and outcome variable [31, 41]. In the present sample, Cronbach's *alpha* exceeded .82 at all time periods. As in previous research with this age group, the WSDQ exhibited a low correlation (+.17) with the Children's Social Desirability Scale [42] in this sample, supporting its discriminant validity.

2.2.3. Autonomy. Swimming-related motivation was measured using an adaptation of the Self-Regulation Scale [34] used by Gagné et al. [43]. This scale consisted of 15 items designed to measure a continuum that includes intrinsic motivation, three types of extrinsic motivation that vary in terms of the degree to which they are congruent with and emanate from the self, plus amotivation. Items relevant to each type of motivation are answered in response to the question: "why do you swim?" Responses are made on a rating scale that extends from 1 (*not true at all*) to 7 (*very true*). Three items each assesses intrinsic motivation (e.g., "For the pleasure I feel when I swim") identified regulation (e.g., "It is a good way to get exercise") and introjected regulation (e.g., "I would feel bad about myself if I was not taking time to swim"), external regulation (e.g., "My parents or other family members give me money or other rewards when I do it"), and amotivation (e.g., "It is not clear to me anymore; I do not really think swimming is my sport").

In addition to providing scores on each of the subscales, a relative index of self-determined motivation, or autonomy, has been developed by Ryan and coworkers [43, 44]. This index is based on the proposition that actions governed by identified regulation share some noteworthy features of internalization and self-acceptance with intrinsic motivation. In contrast, introjected regulation involves self-esteem maintenance rather than intrinsic task involvement and is conceptually more similar to extrinsic motivation based on external contingencies. Using per item means, the relative autonomy index (RAI) is derived from the SMS subscales using the following mean-per-item formula: 2 (intrinsic motivation) + 1 (identified regulation) − 1 (introjected regulation) − 2 (external regulation). Internal consistency coefficients for the 3-item motivational subscales ranged from .62 (identified regulation) to .75 (intrinsic motivation) and averaged .69. These reliabilities are similar to those reported by Gagné and colleagues [43] and Grolnick and Ryan [44]. This single index also lent itself well to the planned mediational analysis of autonomous motivation on the relation between motivational climate and self-esteem change.

2.3. Procedure. Over a 32-week period, we administered the measures described above to groups of swimmers on three occasions (early, mid and late season). We obtained parental/guardian consent and athlete assent for all participants, trained research assistants, and conducted the data collection sessions at the respective swim clubs. Coaches were informed that our research was intended to measure influences upon athletes' attitudes and outcomes in youth sport participation, while athletes were told that the research was intended to promote greater understanding about their experiences in sport. To enhance the likelihood of valid and complete data, we told athletes prior to the season that they would be given a $4 Baskin-Robbins ice cream gift certificate after each of the three questionnaire sessions to provide a reward for their responding to each questionnaire item carefully and accurately.

3. Results

Descriptive statistics and Pearson product moment correlations among the motivational climate, self-esteem, and athlete motivational variables at each time period are presented in Table 1. As theory suggests mastery and ego climate scores, which reflect behaviors that can covary in various combinations, were negatively correlated (−.36 at Time 1, −.40 at Time 2, and −.42 at Time 3), but these correlations are not nearly as high as those reported in older athlete samples (e.g., White, 1998 [39]). Mastery climate scores averaged lower temporal stability (.55) across the season than did ego climate scores (.69) over the three 16-week measurement periods, but all stability coefficients were highly significant. The relative autonomy index demonstrated reasonably good temporal stability for the three measurement periods, averaging .69 overall.

Our analyses addressed several related empirical questions. First, we assessed the cross-sectional relations between perceived parent-initiated motivational climate and self-esteem at each of the three measurement points, allowing us to determine the replicability of relations across the season. Second, in a prospective longitudinal analysis, we examined the extent to which early-season motivational climate predicted changes in self-esteem over the course of the season after controlling for early-season self-esteem. Finally, we conducted a meditational analysis to assess the potential role of changes in autonomy as a mediator of self-esteem change over the course of the season.

We first carried out a cross-sectional analysis of the relations between motivational climate and self-esteem over the course of the season. Correlational analyses, shown in Table 1, revealed a clear pattern of relations between perceived parental motivational climate and self-esteem at all three time points. As predicted on the basis of previous research, mastery climate scores were positively associated with self-esteem scores, whereas ego climate scores were negatively correlated with self-esteem. Although autonomous motivation was studied as a possible mediator, it is worth noting that the relative autonomy index was correlated not only with self-esteem but also with motivational climate in a theoretically predicted manner. On average across the time periods, RAI correlated positively with mastery climate scores (mean $r = .43$, $P < .01$) and negatively with ego climate scores (mean $r = -.43$, $P < .01$).

TABLE 1: Descriptive statistics and bivariate correlations among motivational climate, self-esteem, and autonomy scores at each measurement period.

	Self-esteem[1]	Self-esteem[2]	Self-esteem[3]	Autonomy[1]	Autonomy[2]	Autonomy[3]	Mean (SD)
Mastery climate[1]	.31*	.28*	.28*	.36*	.38*	.37*	30.31 (3.61)
Mastery climate[2]	.31*	.36*	.36*	.32*	.42*	.43*	30.15 (3.65)
Mastery climate[3]	.26*	.34*	.45*	.26*	.24*	.41*	30.43 (3.81)
Ego climate[1]	−.37*	−.38*	−.36*	−.41*	−.43*	−.43*	15.99 (4.94)
Ego climate[2]	−.31*	−.40*	−.37*	−.35*	−.42*	−.42*	15.12 (4.87)
Ego climate[3]	−.20*	−.29*	−.40*	−.28*	−.33*	−.48*	14.90 (4.78)
Self-esteem[1]	—	.69*	.55*	.34*	.23*	.34*	46.58 (6.14)
Self-esteem[2]	—	—	.82*	.40*	.39*	.33*	46.53 (7.26)
Self-esteem[3]	—	—	—	.34*	.31*	.40*	47.03 (7.00)
Autonomy[1]	.34*	.40*	.34*	—	.68*	.62*	20.72 (13.80)
Autonomy[2]	.23*	.39*	.33*	—	—	.76*	20.81 (13.80)
Autonomy[3]	.24*	.31*	.40*	—	—	—	23.69 (13.43)

*$P < .01$, [1]early season, [2]mid season, [3]late season.

To assess the combined role of mastery and ego scores, we computed regression analyses in which the two scores predicted self-esteem at the same time period. At all three time points, we obtained significant effects for perceived parent-initiated motivational climate, $F(2,301) = 31.64$, $R = .42$, $B_{\text{mastery}} = .35$, $B_{\text{ego}} = -.37$, $P < .01$, $F(2,294) = 38.62$, $R = 46$, $B_{\text{mastery}} = .48$, $B_{\text{ego}} = -.45$, $P < .01$, and $F(2,226) = 37.30$, $R = .50$, $B_{\text{mastery}} = .64$, $B_{\text{ego}} = -.36$, $P < .01$, respectively. Thus, the combined motivational climate predictor variables accounted for 17% to 25% of the self-esteem variance.

We then examined relations between motivational climate and self-esteem change over the course of the season. As the correlations in Table 1 indicate, motivational climate exhibited a moderate level of consistency between the measurement intervals, with the relations being somewhat higher (.60 to .80) for the ego climate scores than for the mastery climate scores (.50 to .60). Given the relative stability of climate scores, we used Time 1 motivational climate scores to predict changes in self-esteem scores across the season from Time 1 to Time 3. In these analyses, we took into account the fact that the individual climate scores do not capture the potential interactions between perceived mastery- and ego-oriented parental behaviors. The moderate correlation between the two scales (around −.40) indicates that the motivational climate behaviors do not represent ends of a bipolar continuum. Rather, it is not only possible, but virtually certain that parents can exhibit both types of behaviors to varying degrees. To take into account the combined roles of mastery and ego climate behaviors, we therefore utilized a regression-based approach recommended by J. B. Cohen and P. Cohen [45] and Aiken and West [46] to clarify relations between continuous predictor and criterion variables. This procedure involves using an empirically derived regression equation to calculate predicted criterion variable scores (in this case, Time 3 minus Time 1 self-esteem change scores) within the multidimensional space representing theoretically relevant combinations of predictor variable (in this case, climate) scores. Using SPSS version 18.0, we first conducted a linear regression analysis, entering Time 1 mastery and ego climate scores as predictor variables and self-esteem change as the outcome variable. To capture four theoretically relevant patterns of mastery and climate scores, we then entered into the regression equation climate scores that were (a) high (+1 SD) above the mastery climate mean and low (−1 SD) below the ego climate mean (i.e., high mastery, low ego), (b) high mastery and mean-level ego climate scores, (c) high ego and mean-level mastery climate scores, and (d) high ego and low mastery climate scores. This procedure generated predicted self-esteem change scores for four different theoretically relevant patterns of mastery and ego behaviors, allowing a conservative assessment of the effects of each motivational climate combination.

Figure 2 shows the predicted self-esteem change scores. Mastery climate scores at Time 1 predicted a modest increase in self-esteem over the course of the season, particularly in combination with low ego climate scores. Conversely, high ego scores (particularly when combined with low mastery scores) were associated with reductions in self-esteem, particularly in combination with low levels of mastery-oriented parental behaviors. Although the mean changes were modest in magnitude, some athletes, however, exhibited notable changes across the season. The SD of self-esteem change scores exhibited by the athletes (5.94 points) spanned nearly 1 SD in the Time 1 self-esteem distribution.

To test the significance of the longitudinal pattern represented in Figure 1, we carried out a hierarchical regression analysis in which we used Time 1 motivational climate scores to predict self-esteem change scores between Time 1 and Time 3, controlling for Time 1 self-esteem level. In a hierarchical regression model, we first entered Time 1 self-esteem as a control variable then entered the two motivational climate scores at step 2. Not surprisingly, given its relative stability, Time 1 self-esteem was a significant predictor of self-esteem change, F *change* $(1,214) = 31.08$, $P < .001$, $R^2 = .127$. The motivational climate scores accounted for a

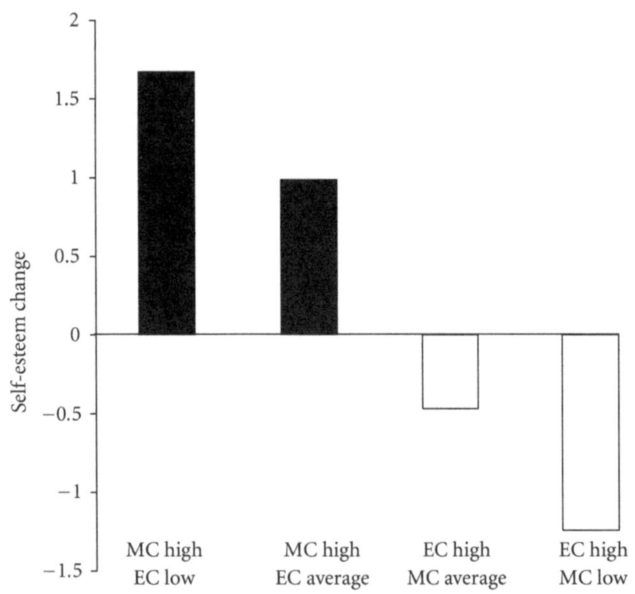

FIGURE 2: Predicted self-esteem change from early to late season, controlling for early season self-esteem, as a function of early season parent-initated motivational climate. MC = mastery climate, EC = ego climate.

modest but statistically significant increment in self-esteem change variance, *F change* (2, 212) = 4.12, $R^2 = .033$, $P < .02$, $b_{\text{mastery}} = .21$, $b_{\text{ego}} = -.14$.

A final analysis assessed the possibility that motivational climate-related changes in self-esteem were, at least in part, mediated by changes in autonomy (controlled versus autonomous motivation), as shown by López-Walle and colleagues [18] and Standage and Gillison [14], who studied coach-initiated motivational climate. Mediation requires that (a) motivational climate be related to self-esteem change (already established in previous analyses), (b) that autonomy change be significantly related to both the predictor (motivational climate) and criterion (self-esteem change) variables, and (c) the relation between motivational climate and self-esteem change is attenuated or eliminated when autonomy change is statistically controlled. Accordingly, using the meditational analytic strategy described by Baron and Kenny [47], we first regressed self-esteem change on motivational climate, controlling for self-esteem scores at Time 1, in the analysis described above, revealing a significant predictive relation. Second, we regressed Time 1–Time 3 autonomy change on motivational climate scores, controlling for autonomy level at Time 1 in a hierarchical model. This analysis revealed a significant relation, *F change* (2, 221) = 12.51, R^2 change = .08, $b_{\text{mastery}} = .45$, $b_{\text{ego}} = -.59$, $P < .001$. Third, we regressed self-esteem change on autonomy change, controlling for Time 1 autonomy and Time 1 motivational climate, again revealing a significant relation, *F change* (1, 212) = 10.25, R^2 change = .046, $B_{\text{mastery}} = .06$, $B_{\text{ego}} = -.09$, $P < .01$. Finally, to test mediation, we regressed self-esteem change on Time 1 motivational climate while controlling for autonomy change. This step eliminated the previously obtained significant relation between motivational climate and self-esteem change, *F change* (2, 212) = 0.44, R^2 change = .004, $B_{\text{mastery}} = .10$, $B_{\text{ego}} = -.06$, $P = .65$, supporting the proposition that self-esteem change was mediated by autonomy change linked to the impact of perceived parental motivational climate.

4. Discussion

The two motivational theories, AGT and SDT, that provided the conceptual framework for the present study, complement one another in important ways [13, 32]. Both focus on important aspects of motivation. AGT addresses differences in conceptions of success in the form of achievement goal orientations and the motivational climates that help establish, maintain, and change them. SDT focuses on a broader set of basic psychological needs and their links to psychological well-being, with special emphasis on the relative autonomy dimension of motivational regulation. Within the AGT framework, firm empirical linkages have been established between motivational climate and achievement goal orientations, and both variables have been related to important indices of enjoyment, achievement behaviors, and well-being, including self-esteem [28, 32, 48]. SDT-inspired research has established links between motivational autonomy and psychological well-being, including self-esteem [5]. Finally, empirical relations have been demonstrated between motivational climate, achievement goal orientations, autonomy, and self-esteem [14, 17, 27, 33]. Additional linkages between the two theories have been forged through evidence that intrinsic motivation (the strongest representation of autonomous motivation) helps mediate the effects of motivational climate on indices of psychological well-being, including self-esteem [14, 18]. Much of this work has been conducted within the sport environment, known to be an engaging and important setting for psychological development [49].

This study advanced previous findings in several ways. Virtually all of the research cited above has focused on the coach-initiated motivational climate, while none would deny that coaches play a central role in this environment, so also do parents, and the values they transmit both in the sport domain and in everyday life exert a strong influence on children's psychosocial development [37]. We therefore focused on the perceived parent-initiated motivational climate. Moreover, virtually all previous research has been cross-sectional in nature. Our study provides not only three replicated cross-sectional analyses but also an assessment of both autonomy and self-esteem change over time. The latter provided an opportunity to test the meditational hypothesis in a manner not previously reported.

At a cross-sectional level, results strongly supported hypothesized relations between the perceived parent-initiated motivational climate and both self-esteem and autonomy at all three measurement periods, with a mastery climate being positively related and an ego climate being negatively related to both variables. There is little existing evidence for the relation between perceived parent-initiated motivational climate and autonomy, making this an important finding in its own right. Moreover, in accordance with SDT, autonomy and self-esteem were positively and significantly related at all three time periods. Additionally, the longitudinal analysis revealed that a mastery motivational climate was related to positive changes in both autonomy and self-esteem and provided strong evidence that changes in autonomy mediated self-esteem changes. This finding provides additional support for previous cross-sectional evidence for a meditational role of autonomy in self-esteem enhancement [14, 18], but extends it by virtue of assessing change in both the outcome variable and the hypothesized mediator.

The fact that we studied global self-esteem (rather than sport-specific evaluations) is important because our findings indicate that sport-related experiences result in psychosocial effects that generalize beyond the sport domain [24, 49]. This is not surprising, for sports are an important and engaging aspect of most children's lives. Research has shown that mean ratings of intrinsic motivation and focused attention in sports exceed those obtained for classroom activities and interactions with friends [50, 51]. For parents as well, sports are a significant aspect of family life, and their influences on children often are focused on this aspect of the child's experience [49]. Therefore, it is not surprising that a core personality variable such as global self-esteem could be influenced in a domain of such high significance for many children and parents.

Although self-esteem scores changed in accordance with motivational climate over the course of the season, the mean score changes shown in Figure 2 appear quite modest. However, it is worth noting that an inspection of the distribution of self-esteem change scores revealed appreciable changes in many athletes over the 32-week sport season, as indicated in the aforementioned finding that the SD of the change scores nearly equaled the SD of the distribution of self-esteem scores at Time 1. A decrease representing −1 SD of scores in the Time 1 distribution was exhibited by 15.3% of the athletes, whereas 11.1% of the athletes showed an increase of similar magnitude from Time 1 to Time 3. Likewise, the stability coefficients over the three time periods indicate not only a reasonable level of stability but also the capacity for change. These findings support the contention of theorists that the late childhood-early adolescence period is one in which self-evaluations are malleable and subject to important developmental experiences [6, 8].

Our findings reinforce the conclusion, drawn from many previous studies, that the motivational climate established by significant others within the sport environment has important psychosocial consequences for young athletes. Not surprisingly, therefore, attempts have been made to develop coach- and parent-focused interventions designed to promote a mastery climate, such as the Mastery Approach to Coaching [23, 25, 52] and the Mastery Approach to Parenting in Sports [53]. These empirically supported interventions (materials related to the Mastery Approach to Coaching and the Mastery Approach to Parenting in Sports interventions can be accessed at http://www.y-e-sports.com/), which communicate specific empirically based behavioral guidelines for promoting a mastery climate, have been shown to change the motivational climate in the direction of a stronger mastery orientation and to have salutary effects on outcome variables such as athletes' achievement goal orientations and performance anxiety. The future is certain to see additional attempts to utilize basic research to intervene within the youth sport environment in ways that promote positive psychosocial development in children and youth.

Acknowledgments

This paper was supported in part by Grant 1529 from the William T. Grant Foundation awarded to R. E. Smith and F. L. Smoll. The authors wish to acknowledge the input of two anonymous reviewers who contributed to the paper's clarity.

References

[1] C. H. Cooley, *Human Nature and the Social Order*, Scribner, New York, NY, USA, 1902.

[2] S. Epstein, "The self-concept revisited. Or a theory of a theory," *The American psychologist*, vol. 28, no. 5, pp. 404–416, 1973.

[3] S. Harter, "Developmental perspectives on the self-system," in *Handbook of Child Psychology: Social and Personality Development*, E. M. Hetherington, Ed., vol. 4, pp. 275–385, John Wiley & Sons, New York, NY, USA, 1973.

[4] E. L. Deci and R. M. Ryan, "Human autonomy: the basis for true self-esteem," in *Efficacy, Agency, and Self-Esteem*, M. Kernis, Ed., pp. 31–49, Plenum, New York, NY, USA, 1995.

[5] E. L. Deci and R. M. Ryan, "The "what" and "why" of goal pursuits: human needs and the self-determination of behavior," *Psychological Inquiry*, vol. 11, no. 4, pp. 227–268, 2000.

[6] R. C. Wylie, *The Self-Concept*, vol. 2, University of Nebraska Press, Lincoln, Neb, USA, 1979.

[7] C. R. Rogers, "A theory of therapy, personality and interpersonal relationships, as developed in the client-centered framework," in *Psychology: A Study of a Science*, S. Koch, Ed., vol. 3, pp. 184–246, McGraw-Hill, New York, NY, USA, 1959.

[8] S. Coopersmith, *The Antecedents of Self-Esteem*, Freeman, San Francisco, Calif, USA, 1967.

[9] J. R. Whitehead, "A study of children's physical self-perceptions using an adapted physical self-perception profile questionnaire," *Pediatric Exercise Science*, vol. 7, no. 2, pp. 132–151, 1995.

[10] M. Rosenberg, *Conceiving the Self*, Basic Books, New York, NY, USA, 1979.

[11] W. B. Swann Jr., "To be known or to be adored? The interplay of self-enhancement and self-verification," in *Handbook of Motivation and Cognition: Foundations of Social Behavior*, R. M. Sorrentino and E. T. Higgins, Eds., vol. 2, pp. 408–488, Guilford Press, New York, NY, USA, 2009.

[12] G. R. Coudevylle, C. Gernigon, and K. A. Martin Ginis, "Self-esteem, self-confidence, anxiety and claimed self-handicapping: a mediational analysis," *Psychology of Sport and Exercise*, vol. 12, no. 6, pp. 670–675, 2011.

[13] V. Hein and M. S. Hagger, "Global self-esteem, goal achievement orientations, and self-determined behavioural regulations in a physical education setting," *Journal of Sports Sciences*, vol. 25, no. 2, pp. 149–159, 2007.

[14] M. Standage and F. Gillison, "Students' motivational responses toward school physical education and their relationship to

general self-esteem and health-related quality of life," *Psychology of Sport and Exercise*, vol. 8, no. 5, pp. 704–721, 2007.

[15] K. R. Fox, "The physical self and processes in self-esteem development," in *The Physical Self: From Motivation to Wellbeing*, K. R. Fox, Ed., pp. 111–139, Human Kinetics, Champaign, Ill, USA, 1997.

[16] J. G. Nicholls, "Achievement motivation: conceptions of ability, subjective experience, task choice, and performance," *Psychological Review*, vol. 91, no. 3, pp. 328–346, 1984.

[17] I. Balaguer, I. Casdllo, and J. L. Duda, "Apoyo a la autonomía, sadsfacción de las necesidades, motivación y bienestar en deportistas de competición: Un análisis de la teoría de la autodeterminación," *Revista de Psicología del Deporte*, vol. 17, pp. 123–139, 2008.

[18] J. López-Walle, I. Balaguer, I. Castillo, and J. Tristán, "Perceived motivational climate, self-determined motivation and self-esteem in young mexican athletes," *Revista de Psicologia del Deporte*, vol. 20, no. 1, pp. 209–222, 2011.

[19] C. Ames, "Classrooms: goals, structures, and student motivation," *Journal of Educational Psychology*, vol. 84, no. 3, pp. 261–271, 1992.

[20] J. L. Duda, "Motivation in sport: the relevance of competence and achievement goals," in *Handbook of Competence and Motivation*, A. J. Elliot and C. S. Dweck, Eds., pp. 313–385, Guilford Press, New York, NY, USA, 2005.

[21] G. C. Roberts, "Understanding the dynamics of motivation in physical activity," in *Advances in Motivation in Sport and Exercise*, G. C. Roberts, Ed., pp. 1–50, Human Kinetics, Champaign, Ill, USA, 2001.

[22] D. C. Treasure, "Enhancing young people's motivation in youth sport: an achievement goal approach," in *Advances in Motivation in Sport and Exercise*, G. C. Roberts, Ed., pp. 79–100, Human Kinetics, Champaign, Ill, USA, 2001.

[23] R. E. Smith, F. L. Smoll, and S. P. Cumming, "Effects of a motivational climate intervention for coaches on young athletes' sport performance anxiety," *Journal of Sport and Exercise Psychology*, vol. 29, no. 1, pp. 39–59, 2007.

[24] R. E. Smith, F. L. Smoll, and S. P. Cumming, "Motivational climate and changes in young athletes' achievement goal orientations," *Motivation and Emotion*, vol. 33, no. 2, pp. 173–183, 2009.

[25] F. L. Smoll, R. E. Smith, and S. P. Cumming, "Effects of a psychoeducational intervention for coaches on changes in child athletes' achievement goal orientations," *Journal of Clinical Sport Psychology*, vol. 1, pp. 23–46, 2007.

[26] D. J. O'Rourke, R. E. Smith, F. L. Smoll, and S. P. Cumming, "Trait anxiety in young athletes as a function of parental pressure and motivational climate: is parental pressure always harmful?" *Journal of Applied Sport Psychology*, vol. 23, no. 4, pp. 398–412, 2011.

[27] M. Kavussanu and G. C. Roberts, "Motivation in physical activity contexts: the relationship of perceived motivational climate to intrinsic motivation and self-efficacy," *Journal of Sport and Exercise Psychology*, vol. 18, no. 3, pp. 264–280, 1996.

[28] C. S. Dweck, *Self-Theories and Goals: Their Role in Motivation, Personality, and Development*, Taylor & Francis, Philadelphia, Pa, USA, 1999.

[29] M. Reinboth and J. L. Duda, "Perceived motivational climate, need satisfaction and indices of well-being in team sports: a longitudinal perspective," *Psychology of Sport and Exercise*, vol. 7, no. 3, pp. 269–286, 2006.

[30] D. E. Conroy and J. D. Coatsworth, "Coach training as a strategy for promoting youth social development," *Sport Psychologist*, vol. 20, no. 2, pp. 128–144, 2006.

[31] F. L. Smoll, R. E. Smith, N. P. Barnett, and J. J. Everett, "Enhancement of children's self-esteem through social support training for youth sport coaches," *Journal of Applied Psychology*, vol. 78, no. 4, pp. 602–610, 1993.

[32] J. L. Duda and D. C. Treasure, "Motivational processes and the facilitation of quality engagement in sport," in *Applied Sport Psychology: Personal Growth to Peak Performance*, J. M. Williams, Ed., pp. 59–80, McGraw-Hill, New York, NY, USA, 2010.

[33] L. Kipp and A. J. Amorose, "Perceived motivational climate and self-determined motivation in female high school athletes," *Journal of Sport Behavior*, vol. 31, pp. 108–129, 2008.

[34] L. G. Pelletier, M. S. Fortier, R. J. Vallerand, K. M. Tuson, N. M. Briere, and M. R. Blais, "Toward a new measure of intrinsic motivation, extrinsic motivation, and amotivation in sports: the sport motivation scale (SMS)," *Journal of Sport and Exercise Psychology*, vol. 17, no. 1, pp. 35–53, 1995.

[35] M. M. Georgiadis, S. J. H. Biddle, and N. L. D. Chatzisarantis, "The mediating role of self-determination in the relationship between goal orientations and physical self-worth in Greek exercisers," *European Journal of Sport Science*, vol. 1, no. 5, pp. 1–9, 2001.

[36] M. L. Babkes and M. R. Weiss, "Parental influence on children's cognitive and affective responses to competitive soccer participation," *Pediatric Exercise Science*, vol. 11, no. 1, pp. 44–62, 1999.

[37] T. S. Horn and J. L. Horn, "Family influences on children's sport and physical activity participation, behavior, and psychosocial responses," in *Handbook of Sports Psychology*, G. G. Tenenbaum and R. C. Eklund, Eds., pp. 685–711, John Wiley & Sons, Hoboken, NJ, USA, 2007.

[38] E. M. Pomerantz and R. A. Thompson, "Parents' role in children's personality development: the psychological resource principle," in *Handbook of Personality: Theory and Research*, P. John, R. W. Robins, and L. A. Pervin, Eds., pp. 351–374, Guilford Press, New York, NY, USA, 2007.

[39] S. A. White, "Adolescent goal profiles, perceptions of the parent-initiated motivational climate, and competitive trait anxiety," *Sport Psychologist*, vol. 12, no. 1, pp. 16–28, 1998.

[40] J. L. Duda and J. Whitehead, "Measurement of goal perspectives in the physical domain," in *Advances in Sport and Exercise Psychology Measurement*, J. L. Duda, Ed., pp. 21–48, Fitness Information Technology, Morgantown, WVa, USA, 1998.

[41] R. E. Smith and F. L. Smoll, "Self-esteem and children's reactions to youth sport coaching behaviors: a field study of self-enhancement processes," *Developmental Psychology*, vol. 26, no. 6, pp. 987–993, 1990.

[42] V. C. Crandall, V. J. Crandall, and W. Katkovsky, "A children's social desirability questionnaire," *Journal of Consulting Psychology*, vol. 29, no. 1, pp. 27–36, 1965.

[43] M. Gagné, R. M. Ryan, and K. Bargmann, "Autonomy support and need satisfaction in the motivation and well-being of gymnasts," *Journal of Applied Sport Psychology*, vol. 15, no. 4, pp. 372–390, 2003.

[44] W. S. Grolnick and R. M. Ryan, "Autonomy in children's learning: an experimental and individual difference investigation," *Journal of Personality and Social Psychology*, vol. 52, no. 5, pp. 890–898, 1987.

[45] J. B. Cohen and P. Cohen, *Applied Multiple Regression/Correlation Analysis for the Behavioral Sciences*, Lawrence Erlbaum Associates, Hillsdale, NJ, USA, 1983.

[46] L. S. Aiken and S. G. West, *Multiple Regression: Testing and Interpreting Interactions*, Sage, Newbury Park, Calif, USA, 1991.

[47] R. M. Baron and D. A. Kenny, "The moderator-mediator variable distinction in social psychological research. Conceptual, strategic, and statistical considerations," *Journal of Personality and Social Psychology*, vol. 51, no. 6, pp. 1173–1182, 1986.

[48] S. McArdle and J. K. Duda, "Implications of the motivational climate in youth sports," in *Children and Youth in Sport: A Biopsychosocial Perspective*, F. L. Smoll and R. E. Smith, Eds., pp. 409–434, Kendall/Hunt, Dubuque, Iowa, USA, 2002.

[49] M. R. Weiss, *Developmental Sport and Exercise Psychology: A Lifespan Perspective*, Fitness Information Technology, Morgantown, WVa, USA, 2002.

[50] M. Csikszentmihalyi and R. W. Larson, *Being Adolescent*, Basic Books, New York, NY, USA, 1984.

[51] R. W. Larson and D. Kleiber, "Daily experience of adolescents," in *Handbook of Clinical Research and Practice With Adolescents*, P. Tolan and B. Cohler, Eds., pp. 125–145, John Wiley & Sons, New York, NY, USA, 1993.

[52] R. E. Smith and F. L. Smoll, "Cognitive-behavioral coach training: a translational approach to theory, research, and intervention," in *Behavioral Sport Psychology: Evidence-Based Approaches to Performance Enhancement*, J. K. Luiselli and D. D. Reed, Eds., pp. 227–248, Springer, New York, NY, USA, 2011.

[53] F. L. Smoll, R. E. Smith, and S. P. Cumming, "Effects of coach and parent training on performance anxiety in young athletes: a systemic approach," *Journal of Youth Development*, vol. 2, Article ID 0701FA002, 2007, http://nae4a.memberclicks.net/assets/documents/JYD_070201_final.pdf.

13

Beliefs, Anxiety, and Avoiding Failure in Mathematics

Steve Chinn

Faculty of Education, Health and Sciences, University of Derby, Derby DE22 1GB, UK

Correspondence should be addressed to Steve Chinn, steve.chinn@btinternet.com

Academic Editor: Ann Dowker

Mathematics anxiety has been the subject of several books and numerous research papers, suggesting that it is a significant issue for many people. Children and adults develop strategies to cope with this anxiety, one of which is avoidance. This paper presents data taken from over 2500 mathematics test papers in order to compare the levels of accuracy and the frequency of the use of the "no attempt" strategy, that is, avoidance, for arithmetic problems given to children aged from 10 years to adults aged up to 49 years from across the UK.

1. Introduction

The difficulties in learning mathematics are a fascinating and complex area for study. The interactions between factors that can be attributed to the cognitive domain and those that can be attributed to the affective domain are many and varied. For example, anxiety has a negative influence on working memory [1]. Skemp ([2], page 127) suggested that the reflective activity of intelligence is most easily inhibited by anxiety. Lundberg and Sterner [3] claim that "over and above common cognitive demands and neurological representations and functions, performance in reading and arithmetic is influenced by a number of motivational and emotional factors such as need for achievement, task orientation, helplessness, depression, anxiety, self-esteem, self-concept…" Hattie [4] selects a pithy quote from O'Connor and Paunonen [5], "Whereas cognitive ability reflects what an individual can do, personality traits reflect what an individual will do."

The implications on learning of anxiety, motivation, self-worth, self-efficacy and attributional style are significant (e.g., [6–8]) particularly in mathematics where a curriculum may make inappropriate assumptions about how some children learn. Those assumptions may be rooted in beliefs about mathematics and how it can be taught and learnt.

There are a number of beliefs about mathematics that are long established and embedded in its culture. This does not necessarily make them helpful in creating a positive student attitude to mathematics, especially for those who have difficulties with learning mathematics or, indeed, mathematics learning difficulties. For example, Mtetwa and Garofalo [9] discuss five beliefs, which include "mathematics problems have only one correct answer" and "computation problems must be solved by using a step-by-step algorithm." The first belief leads children to perceive of mathematics as highly judgmental, that answers are right or they are wrong. The second belief leads children and their teachers to perceive of mathematics as a series of procedures which have to be memorised and not necessarily understood. Ernest [10] reviews the literature on beliefs in his book, "*The Psychology of Learning Mathematics*." Three examples from his review are "some people have a mathematics mind and some do not," "mathematicians do problems quickly in their head," and "mathematics requires a good memory." The first belief permits people to rationalise their inabilities in mathematics and to protect their feelings of self-worth. The second belief sets up children who process some information more slowly, for example dyslexic children, for failure. The last belief is pervasive, for example, Porkess et al. [11] claims that "As with any language, the fundamentals of mathematics (e.g., multiplication tables and number bonds) are most easily learnt when you are young." Unfortunately the reliance on memorising facts and procedures does not stop there.

It could be hypothesised that these beliefs have been, and still are, influential in the way mathematics' curricula are designed and in the way mathematics is taught. For example, the beliefs that surround the task of learning times table facts, where the primary belief is that, providing the child practises enough, then the learning is guaranteed and achieved early in the child's life. Informal surveys of teachers across the UK by the author lead to an estimate of somewhere around 50% of ten-year-old students failing to achieve this goal. Evidence on levels of achievement in retrieving basic facts acquired from a large sample of pupils from across the UK can be found in Chinn [12].

The implications of the experience of failure in learning are succinctly described in the back-cover summary of Covington's [13] book on motivation:

"Achievement behaviour in schools can best be understood in terms of attempts by students to maintain a positive self-image. For many students, trying hard is frightening because a combination of effort and failure implies low ability, which is often equated with worthlessness. Thus many students described as unmotivated are in actuality highly motivated—not to learn, but to avoid failure."

The experience of failure is a consequence of the inherently judgmental nature of arithmetic. For example, the answer for 8×7 is 56. Giving an answer of 54 is rarely judged empathetically as, "That was close. Well done." The "54" answer generates the response, "Wrong." Arithmetic is, unavoidably, the dominant experience of mathematics for young pupils.

Failure and the judgmental nature of mathematics contribute to anxiety. In Chinn's [14] survey of mathematics anxiety in over 2500 secondary students (ages 11 to 15 years) in England, the item "waiting to hear your score on a maths test" was ranked high for anxiety, that is, from second to 6th out of 20 items for all ages and both genders of mainstream students. "Having to take a written maths test" was ranked from second to 4th and "taking an end of term maths exam" was ranked first out of 20 items for all pupils.

The mathematics task which ranked highest was, "doing long division questions without a calculator", ranking from second to 5th. "Long multiplication without a calculator" was ranked less highly, between 9th and 13th for ten of the fifteen subgroups of students.

The ranking of the item, "having to work out the answers to maths questions quickly," which reflects the mathematics belief that computations have to be done quickly, was also ranked high, for both the dyslexic (442 males) and the mainstream school students (2084 male and female) in the sample. The anxiety generated by having to attempt a problem that is a threat to the pupil's confidence is often exacerbated by the need to work out an answer quickly, that is, within an arbitrary time limit.

Studies from many countries over many years have shown that performance in mathematics is related negatively to mathematics anxiety ([15, page 249], [16, page 334], and [17, 18]).

Failure can motivate or undermine ([6, page 5]) depending on whether students' reactions are mastery-oriented or helpless. Dweck uses the term "helpless" to include all the reactions that some students show when they meet failure, including plunging expectations, negative emotions, and deteriorating performance. It seems that the consequence of failure in mathematics is to undermine.

One reaction, or strategy, to deal with failure that Chinn [19] observed in a classroom study on errors in arithmetic is to avoid the challenge and use the "no attempt" [20] error. The study was set up to compare both the performance and the errors for pupils in mainstream schools to those for dyslexic pupils in specialist schools (ages 11 to 13 years). There appeared to be no difference in the frequency of occurrence of any of Engelhardt's other categories of errors, but the one outstanding exception was the "no attempt" error. For example, for 37.6–4, 14.0% of the dyslexic pupils did not attempt the item compared to 2.2% of the mainstream pupils. This compared to the addition item, $12.3 + 5$ (where finger counting forwards is a strategy that is accessible to almost all children) where the no attempt percentages were 2.5% and 0%, respectively. For division the contrast was greater, for the item, $6040 \div 10$, 39.7% of the dyslexic cohort did not attempt the problem in comparison to 5.8% of the mainstream cohort. The study suggested that children with specific learning difficulties, even if of above average intelligence, or perhaps because they are of above average intelligence, will use avoidance rather than risk failure. Data from a 15-minute mathematics test [12], the source of the data for this paper, is given for the bottom and top quartiles of performers to support this conjecture.

Hadfield and McNeil [21] proposed a model of mathematics anxiety, centred on three factors. Environmental factors include classroom issues and the perception of mathematics as a rigid set of rules. Intellectual variables include a mismatch of learning styles and self-doubt. Personality factors include a reluctance to ask questions in class and low self-esteem. Any or all of these three factors could influence a learner and generate a "no attempt" or avoidance attitude.

It is unlikely that this reaction is confined solely to the special needs population, nor just to avoidance of individual questions. Ashcraft and Krause [17] note that "Mathematics anxiety leads to a global avoidance pattern—whenever possible, students avoid taking math classes and avoid situations in which math will be necessary..."

The problem of avoidance begins when some children are quite young. An informal survey by the author, taken over the past ten years, of hundreds of teachers from across the UK and abroad indicates that enough children at age 7 years are withdrawing from and giving up on maths for classroom teachers to notice.

The English Government ([22], page 17) has noted that a "minority of pupils" who were making less than expected progress in mathematics shared certain characteristics, including the following.

They would work if the task was straightforward, but would get distracted and might behave badly if they decided they could not do the work.

They did not want to be told they had got something wrong—they were likely to give the impression that they did not care and give up.

They were concerned about how their peers viewed them—for some it was a risk to be seen to try and fail.

Table 1

		$34 = 4 + —$	
Age	Sample	Percentage of correct answers	Percentage of "no attempts"
8 y	225	62.2	10.2
10 y	220	77.7	5.5
12 y	173	84.4	2.9
40–49 y	129	92.2	1.6

Table 2

		$9 = — - 4$	
Age	Sample	Percentage of correct answers	Percentage of "no attempts"
8 y	225	36.9	22.2
10 y	220	72.3	9.5
12 y	173	71.1	9.2
14 y	225	81.3	5.3
40–49 y	129	82.9	4.7

These observations were personalised by a quote (p18) from a Year 9 (13 years old) girl:

> *"I don't get stuck in other subjects—only maths. When I'm doing English, I can always get on with my work. If I'm not sure about a spelling, I can just have a go and still get my work done. But I can't do that in maths. If I'm stuck I can't do anything but wait for help. Then I don't get anything done."*

2. The Sample

1783 school children from age 7 years to 15 years old. 792 people from age 16 years to 59 years old.

The sample was collected from across the UK from over 50 sources, including state schools, independent schools, colleges, a prison, postal workers, and college students. The majority of the data was collected over a period of twelve months, mid 2010 to mid 2011. Only one of the schools that participated was a special school (for dyslexic pupils).

3. The Test/Survey

The data was collected as a consequence of setting up a 15-minute norm-referenced test/survey of mathematics [12]. The "test" was renamed for adults as a "survey" in an attempt to lower anxiety levels and thus to encourage more of them to take part. The tactic was marginally successful.

The test consists of 44 items, ranging from $2 + 5 = —$, to "Write forty thousand and seventy as a number," to 20% of 140, to $2y + 5 = 31$. It is, however, primarily a test of arithmetic.

4. The Results

A number of hypotheses follow, stimulated by the analysis of the data collected for the standardising procedure combined with reflections on the author's previous research and thirty years of teaching experience with students with specific learning difficulties. This analysis of the data is in terms of the percentage of correct answers and the percentage of "no attempts." A "no attempt" may have been caused by the subject having not yet reached the relevant stage in the curriculum. The National Numeracy Strategy for England was referred to in order to ascertain at what age a topic is included in the curriculum in order to minimise this problem.

4.1. Hypothesis 1. Addition is the default operation. The other operations create less success, more insecurity and more "no attempt" errors (see Table 1).

This item is testing knowledge of place value at a basic level of two-digit numbers. It is less about testing addition skills, although a + sign is present. The percentage of correct answers grows steadily between 8 years and 12 years old and is at a slightly higher level for the 40 to 49 years old group. The percentage of "no attempts" is marginal at 12 years and older.

The problem in Table 2 is a basic fact presented as a subtraction with a missing number and in the reverse order to basic fact format, that is, $— - 4 = 9$. For those pupils who are heavily dependent on consistency, even this simple change in order may be a challenge. The percentage of pupils aged 10 and 12 years who did not get a correct answer was high at 27.7% and 28.9%, respectively. Almost 1 in 10 pupils of these ages did not attempt the question. This dropped to almost 1 in 20 at 14 years old. These figures suggest that subtraction is perceived as being more difficult than addition.

An item, which requires the subject to cross the tens (see Table 3), provides further evidence to suggest that addition is believed to be easier than subtraction. The percentages of

Table 3

36 +54 Age	Sample	Percentage of correct answers	Percentage of "no attempts"
8 y	225	71.6	7.6
10 y	220	92.7	1.0
13 y	191	92.7	1.6
14 y	225	92.4	0.9
40–49 y	129	94.6	0.8

Table 4

103 −96 Age	Sample	Percentage of correct answers	Percentage of "no attempts"
8 y	225	29.3	34.7
10 y	220	63.6	7.7
13 y	191	69.6	8.9
14 y	225	79.6	5.8
40–49 y	129	93.0	1.6

correct answers are higher and the percentages of "no attempts" are lower than for the subtraction item, 103 − 96, particularly for the school pupils (see Table 4).

The National Numeracy Strategy includes subtraction problems of the type HTU-TU in Year 4 (8 years old).

The results shown in Table 4 indicate that around one-third of pupils aged from 10 to 13 years old cannot obtain a correct answer to this question. A number of the answers given, for example 193, were manifestly incorrect.

The problem shown in Table 5 is about the commutative property. If that is recognised, then the answer is achieved quickly and accurately. If it is not recognised then the method is to add 534 and 185, giving an interim answer of 719, followed by subtracting 185. The item uses three-digit numbers and thus may be perceived as more challenging. Even though the item uses the low anxiety inducing + sign, the percentage of "no attempts" is the highest for the examples listed so far which incorporate the + symbol. It is noteworthy that the percentage of "no-attempts" is now higher than for other addition problems in the test for the 40 to 49 year olds, who may not have the frequent exposure to the commutative property of numbers that schoolchildren do.

The hypothesis may require a caveat, in that once the addition problem becomes more challenging or is perceived as more challenging, the security of "doing" addition is weakened. This caveat may be required for other hypotheses.

It can be tempting for teachers who feel that a lesson is going well to push the concept a step beyond the comfort zone of some learners.

4.2. Hypothesis 2. Multiplication is not widely understood and is judged as difficult, so more learners avoid the risk of being wrong.

Caveat: simply learning the times table facts by rote may not help in building an early understanding of the concepts of multiplication (or division).

The multiplication item in Table 6 was designed to not require the retrieval of any of the basic multiplication facts that are often perceived as difficult (to retrieve). It requires only a retrieval of 2x and 3x facts. Thus, the item is testing the ability to use a procedure. The procedures that can be used all require the ability to organise, spatially and cognitively, a relatively large amount of information on the page.

The percentage of correct answers increases from age 13 years to age 16–19 years old, but remains well under 50%. The percentage of "no attempts" is around 34% for ages 16 to 39 years and then drops to around 15% for ages 40 to 59 years. This could suggest that whatever the methods taught, the "traditional long multiplication" or the more recently favoured grid method, they are not creating enduring security and efficacy for people after-school. Even methods that resulted in a correct answer sometimes indicated a rigid adherence to procedure, for example, a 15 y 9 m student wrote:

$$\begin{array}{r} 541 \\ \underline{\times 203} \\ 1623 \\ 0000 \\ \underline{108200} \\ 109823 \end{array} \tag{1}$$

However, among 15-year-old students this method, which uses partial products selected via the place values of the digits in the multiplying number, was the preferred

TABLE 5

Age	Sample	534 + 185 = 185 + __ Percentage of correct answers	Percentage of "no attempts"
10 y	220	52.7	12.3
13 y	191	70.7	12.7
15 y	220	82.3	10.0
40–49 y	129	77.5	15.5

TABLE 6

541 ×203 Age	Sample	Percentage of correct answers	Percentage of "no attempts"
13 y	191	15.2	40.8
14 y	225	27.1	22.2
15 y	220	38.2	16.8
16–19 y	307	33.2	32.6
20–29 y	160	33.1	34.4
30–39 y	108	32.4	33.3
40–49 y	129	57.4	16.3
50–59 y	88	52.3	13.6

TABLE 7

Age	Sample	$2\overline{)38}$ Percentage of correct answers	Percentage of "no attempts"
10 y	220	59.1	30.5
13 y	191	60.7	27.2
15 y	220	75.0	13.2
16–19 y	307	67.8	20.8
40–49 y	129	86.0	8.5

method and usually led to a correct answer. Place value and partial product-based errors included

$$\begin{array}{r} 541 \\ \underline{\times 203} \\ 1043 \end{array} \quad \begin{array}{r} 541 \\ \underline{\times 203} \\ 1003 \end{array}$$

$$\begin{array}{r} 541 \\ \underline{\times 203} \\ 10820 \\ 0000 \\ \underline{1623} \\ 11443 \end{array} \quad \begin{array}{r} 541 \\ \underline{\times 203} \\ 1623 \\ 000 \\ \underline{1082} \\ 2705 \end{array} \qquad (2)$$

The insecurity, fear of failure, and anxiety created by multiplications that are perceived of as complex and demanding are likely to contribute significantly to the high percentage of "no attempts". A 59-year-old, successful, business man who scored 39/44 simply wrote "too hard" next to this item and moved on.

The percentages for correct answers suggest that whatever is happening to teach multiplication in many mathematics classrooms is not successful for a large proportion of learners.

4.3. Hypothesis 3. Division is even less understood than multiplication (and is rarely linked to multiplication in learners' minds) and is judged by learners as being even more difficult, so that more children and adults will avoid the risk of being wrong (see Table 7).

This item is at a low level of complexity. It could be viewed as "halving 38."

The percentage of "no attempts" is high for the 10 years and 13 years cohorts, representing between a third and a quarter who did not take the risk of attempting this item. Even at 40 years, the "no attempt" percentage showed that approximately 1 in 12 did not attempt a division by 2 (see Table 8).

Even though this item is still a division by a single digit number, it did create high percentages of "no attempts" and low percentages of correct answers, data that, when compared with the 541 × 203 item shows that the percentages of "no attempts" for this division item were higher than for the multiplication item (see Tables 9 and 10).

For the latter two items the percentages of "no attempts" are high. Both items could be considered to be, fundamentally, about place value. The "rules" about moving the decimal place when multiplying and dividing by powers of

TABLE 8

Age	Sample	9)927 Percentage of correct answers	Percentage of "no attempts"
13 y	191	41.9	36.1
14 y	225	47.6	29.8
15 y	220	45.5	32.3
16–19 y	307	38.1	46.0
20–29 y	160	31.2	45.6
40–49 y	129	55.8	26.4

TABLE 9

Age	Sample	$10\overline{)6030}$ Percentage of correct answers	Percentage of "no attempts"
10 y	220	44.5	31.4
11 y	200	44.5	23.0
13 y	191	48.7	27.2
15 y	220	62.3	14.5
16–19 y	307	56.5	22.8
40–49 y	129	77.5	7.8

TABLE 10

Age	Sample	$23 \div 1000$ Percentage of correct answers	Percentage of "no attempts"
13 y	191	31.4	38.7
14 y	225	42.2	30.2
15 y	220	46.8	23.6
16–19 y	307	46.9	29.3
40–49 y	129	45.0	20.2

TABLE 11

Age	Sample	1 km = ___ metres Percentage of correct answers	Percentage of "no attempts"
13 y	191	37.7	34.0
14 y	225	50.7	23.1
15 y	220	56.4	20.5
16–19 y	307	53.7	27.0
40–50 y	129	69.0	19.4

10 are still promoted as, for example, in a revision book for mathematics at Key Stage 3 ([23], p 30). Rules and procedures that bypass understanding are less likely to be remembered accurately.

Many procedures that are taught for mathematics are very unforgiving on faulty memories. Often, even one small error in the application of a procedure is enough to generate failure.

Recent research by Siegler et al. [24] found that knowledge at age 10 of division was consistently related to later mathematics proficiency. This is not happy news for the UK, if over 30% of 10-year-old pupils do not attempt to divide 38 by 2 or 6030 by 10.

4.4. Hypothesis 4. Problems that involve the application of multiplication and division generate more "no attempts" than those that are simply computations (see Tables 11 and 12).

The two items mix arithmetic and measurement. Over one-third of 13-year-old pupils and one-fifth of 15-year-old pupils did not attempt to divide a kilometre by 5. The item which involves conversion of a quantity in kilometres to metres, illustrated, via the type of errors it generated, the implications of a partial recall of the rules about "moving the decimal point and adding zeros." The most frequently occurring error was 5067 metres.

4.5. Hypothesis 5. The percentage of pupils using the "no attempt" avoidance strategy is greatest for the bottom quartile of achievers.

Caveat: as questions become "harder" more of the high achievers use the "no attempt" strategy.

Table 12

		5.67 km = __ metres	
Age	Sample	Percentage of correct answers	Percentage of "no attempts"
13 y	191	36.6	43.5
14 y	225	44.4	32.4
15 y	220	50.9	25.5
16–19 y	307	45.0	39.4
40–50 y	129	54.3	27.9

Table 13

	All	BQ	TQ	BQ/All	PC
10 years					
2)38	30.5	18.2	1.0	60.0	59.1
10)6030	31.4	18.2	1.0	58.0	44.5
13 years					
2)38	27.2	17.3	0.5	63.5	60.7
10)6030	27.2	17.8	0	65.4	48.7
15 years					
2)38	13.2	8.2	0	62.1	75.0
10)6030	14.1	10.0	0	71.0	62.3
4.8 + 5.21 + 6	12.3	9.1	0	74.0	55.4
541 × 203	17.3	8.6	1.8	49.7	38.2
(2/5) + (3/8)	29.1	13.2	0.5	45.4	37.3
9)927	33.6	17.7	0.5	52.7	45.5

All: for all students.
BQ: for the bottom quartile of total score.
TQ: for the top quartile of total score.
BQ/All: percentage of no attempts for the bottom quartile compared to all no attempts (for example, for 2)38 for pupils of 10 years, 60.0% of the "no attempts" were from the bottom quartile of students).
PC: percentage of correct answers.

The "no attempts" for two items from the 15-minute test were analysed for the bottom quartile of scores, the top quartile, and for all scores. The main focus was on the division items 2)38 and 10)6030.

The students in the bottom quartile of achievers were contributing a high proportion of the no attempts (see Table 13). When the percentage of that contribution drops below 50% the questions generate correct scores below 40%, suggesting that a larger number of the more able children are being dragged into the "no attempt" behaviour when questions become less straightforward. A related conclusion was reached by Ashcraft and Krause [17] in a study on 80 undergraduates, which investigated the correlation between math performance and math anxiety. The lower achievement of the undergraduates who were math-anxious seemed limited to more difficult math which is described as math taught at or after late elementary school.

5. Summary

Poor achievement levels in mathematics for a significant percentage of the population have been an issue in the UK for decades [25]. The data presented in this paper supports a number of hypotheses, which combine to suggest a final hypothesis, that is, that too many children and adults give up on mathematics learning by withdrawing from any task that is perceived as likely to result in failure, which in turn becomes a pervasive attitude. The withdrawal strategy avoids the learner being judged as wrong and thus adding to their sense of helplessness. Some of the demands of mathematics that contribute to a sense of failure, anxiety, and helplessness are based on beliefs, rather than academic necessity. These beliefs also have an effect on the way mathematics is taught with a focus on the curriculum whilst overlooking the characteristics of the learners.

The combination of "no attempts" and incorrect answers for many of the examples used above is not indicative of a successful outcome for the mathematics curriculum and how it is taught in the UK.

Finally, a 12-year-old student summed up his experiences of mathematics teaching as, "All I hear is talking, talking. It's a river." Perhaps it is time to challenge some of the mathematics beliefs that have a profound influence on the way the subject is perceived and taught and give more focus to how learners learn.

References

[1] M. Ashcraft, E. P. Kirk, and D. Hopko, "On the cognitive consequences of mathematics anxiety," in *The Development of Mathematical Skills*, C. Donlan, Ed., Hove, The Psychological Corporation, 1998.

[2] R. R. Skemp, *The Psychology of Learning Mathematics*, Penguin, Hardmondsworth, UK, 1971.

[3] I. Lundberg and G. Sterner, "Reading, arithmetic, and task orientation—how are they related?" *Annals of Dyslexia*, vol. 56, no. 2, pp. 361–377, 2006.

[4] J. Hattie, *Visible Learning: A Synthesis of over 800 Meta-Analyses Relating to Achievement*, Routledge, Abingdon, UK, 2009.

[5] M. C. O'Connor and S. V. Paunonen, "Big Five personality predictors of post-secondary academic performance," *Personality and Individual Differences*, vol. 43, no. 5, pp. 971–990, 2007.

[6] C. S. Dweck, *Self-Theories*, Psychology Press, Philadelphia, Pa, USA, 2000.

[7] M. Seligman, *Learned Optimism*, Vintage Books, New York, NY, USA, 2006.

[8] S. Chinn, *The Trouble with Maths: A Practical Guide to Helping Learners with Numeracy Difficulties*, Routledge, Abingdon, UK, 2nd edition, 2012.

[9] D. Mtetwa and J. Garofalo, "Beliefs about mathematics: an overlooked aspect of student difficulties," *Academic Therapy*, vol. 24, no. 5, pp. 611–618, 1989.

[10] P. Ernest, *The Psychology of Learning Mathematics*, Lambert Academic Publishing, Saarbrucken, Germany, 2011.

[11] R. Porkess et al., "A world-class mathematics education for all our youngpeople," 2011, http://www.conservatives.com/.../Vorderman%20maths%20report.ashx .

[12] S. Chinn, *More Trouble with Maths: A Complete Guide to Identifying and Diagnosing Mathematical Learning Difficulties*, Routledge, Abingdon, UK, 2012.

[13] M. V. Covington, *Making the Grade: A Self-Worth Perspective on Motivation and School Reform*, CUP, Cambridge, UK, 1992.

[14] S. Chinn, "Mathematics anxiety in secondary students in England," *Dyslexia*, vol. 15, no. 1, pp. 61–68, 2009.

[15] A. Dowker, *Individual Differences in Arithmetic*, Hove, Psychology Press, 2005.

[16] M. H. Ashcraft, J. A. Krause, and D. R. Hopko, "Is math anxiety a mathematical learning disability?" in *Why is Math so Hard for Some Children? The Nature and Origins of Mathematical Learning Difficulties and Disabilities*, M. M. M. Mazzocco and D. B. Berch, Eds., Brookes, Baltimore, Md, USA, 2007.

[17] M. H. Ashcraft and J. A. Krause, "Working memory, math performance, and math anxiety," *Psychonomic Bulletin and Review*, vol. 14, no. 2, pp. 243–248, 2007.

[18] R. Hembree, "The nature, effects and relief of mathematics anxiety," *Journal for Research in Mathematics Education*, vol. 21, pp. 33–46, 1990.

[19] S. J. Chinn, "A pilot study to compare arithmetic skill," *Dyslexia Review*, vol. 4, pp. 4–7, 1995.

[20] J. M. Engelhardt, "Analysis of childrens' computational errors: a qualitative approach," *British Journal of Educational Psychology*, vol. 47, pp. 149–154, 1977.

[21] O. D. Hadfield and K. McNeil, "The relationship between Myers-Briggs personality type and mathematics anxiety among pre-service elementary teachers," *Journal of Instructional Psychology*, vol. 21, no. 4, pp. 375–384, 1994.

[22] Department for Children, Schools and Families, "Getting back on track—pupils who make slow progress in Key Stage 3," Ref. 00654-2007BKT-EN, 2007, http://www.tsm-resources.com/pdf/VordermanMathsReport.pdf.

[23] M. Chester, K. Manson, S. Little, K. Redmond et al., *KS 3 Mathematics: Complete Revision and Practice*, Kirkby-in-Furness, Coordination Group Publications, 2004.

[24] R. S. Siegler, G. J. Duncan, P. E. Davis-Kean et al., "Early predictors of high school mathematics achievement," *Pyschological Science*, vol. 23, no. 7, pp. 691–697.

[25] S. Rashid and G. Brooks, "The levels of attainment in literacy and numeracy of 13- to 19-year olds in England, 1948–2009," *Literacy Today*, vol. 32, no. 1, pp. 13–24, 2010.

14

Children's Tolerance of Word-Form Variation

Paul R. Bruening,[1] Patricia J. Brooks,[1] Louis Alfieri,[2] Vera Kempe,[3] and Ineta Dabašinskienė[4]

[1] *Department of Psychology, College of Staten Island, City University of New York, 2800 Victory Boulevard, 4S-108, Staten Island, NY 10314, USA*
[2] *Learning Research and Development Center, University of Pittsburgh, 3939 O'Hara Street, Pittsburgh, PA 15260, USA*
[3] *Division of Psychology, University of Abertay Dundee, Bell Street, Dundee, Scotland DD1 1HG, UK*
[4] *Division of Humanities, Vytautas Magnus University, Donelaicio 58, 44248 Kaunas, Lithuania*

Correspondence should be addressed to Patricia J. Brooks, patricia.brooks@csi.cuny.edu

Academic Editor: Annie Vinter

How much morphological variation can children tolerate when identifying familiar words? This is an important question in the context of the acquisition of richly inflected languages where identical word forms occur far less frequently than in English. To address this question, we compared children's ($N = 96$, mean age 4;1, range 2;11–5;1) and adults' ($N = 96$, mean age 21 years) tolerance of word-onset modifications (e.g., for *stug: wug* and *wastug*) and pseudoaffixes (e.g., *kostug* and *stugko*) in a label-extension task. Word-form modifications were repeated within each experiment to establish productive inflectional patterns. In two experiments, children and adults exhibited similar strategies: they were more tolerant of prefixes (*wastug*) than substitutions of initial consonants (*wug*), and more tolerant of suffixes (*stugko*) than prefixes (*kostug*). The findings point to word-learning strategies as being flexible and adaptive to morphological patterns in languages.

1. Children's Tolerance of Word-Form Variation

In language development, an important question is how young children go about the task of acquiring and correctly associating new words with their referents, a process sometimes referred to as word-to-world mapping. This process has mainly been investigated in English, a language, where word forms tend to be identical or very similar across different contexts, due to the impoverished inflectional morphology of English. In this study, we explore the question of how morphological changes impact the interpretations of new words for novice language learners.

Children have been shown to have a strong bias toward mapping unfamiliar words onto unfamiliar objects [1]. They also are capable of learning new words after only a few exposures [2], an ability known as "fast mapping." In perhaps the earliest study of fast mapping, Carey and Bartlett [2] asked children to select a "chromium" tray (olive green in color) when given two choices, an object with a color (red) that they already had a name for and one they did not. They found that children were highly biased to select the nonprimary color item. To test if the child had actually learned the new color term, children were retested a year later and half of the children demonstrated retention. This fast-mapping tendency has proven to be a robust and reproducible phenomenon across many studies (e.g., [3–5]): when given an object that is familiar and one that is unfamiliar, children associate a new name with the unfamiliar object at levels far above chance. Markman and her colleagues have interpreted this bias as reflecting an innate word-learning constraint, the mutual exclusivity (ME) principle [6]. Other theorists have sought to explain this rather robust finding by proposing that children utilize a novel name for a nameless category (the Novel-Name-Nameless-Category principle (N3C) [7]) or utilize pragmatic reasoning to contrast the meanings of words in their developing vocabularies (the Principle of Contrast (PoC) [8, 9]). All of these theories explain the fast-mapping tendency by suggesting that children have learning strategies or biases that help them to identify the referents of new words. What is unclear, however, is how such learning strategies interact with morphophonological variants of familiar words. For instance, the diminutive derivation is quite common in child-directed speech across many languages [10] and children appear to successfully map both *dog* and *doggie* onto the same entity with little confusion.

It should be noted that some languages have an especially high rate of diminutive usage in child-directed speech, for example, Russian [11], Spanish [12], Dutch [13], and Lithuanian [14]; diminutives are quite common in child speech as well as child-directed speech and are the first morphological derivation that children acquire in the Baltic and Slavic languages [15]. Importantly, diminutives are not used primarily to mark a contrast between small and large objects in child-directed speech, but are instead used to convey the intimate, affectionate, and playful mood of child-focused interactions [15]. Moreover, caretakers will flexibly alternate between the diminutive and simplex forms of a noun to refer to the same referent within a conversational interaction [16, 17], and there is no evidence to suggest that this word-form variation negatively impacts on children's word learning. Thus, children's tolerance of diminutives as alternative labels would seem to indicate that there is a limit to the extent with which children conform to word-learning constraints such as ME. It further suggests that children have to adapt their word-learning strategies flexibly in response to recurrent morphological patterns. To explore the extent of children's tolerance for word-form variation we adopted a label-extension task that probes the mapping of nonwords onto familiar and novel images.

1.1. The Label-Extension Task and Children's Tolerance of Word-Form Variants. The label-extension task involves presentation of an altered word-form to investigate whether this word-form variant is extended to the familiar object or to a different object. After being introduced to the name of an object, participants are presented with a modification of that word, or a different word entirely, and asked to map this target word onto one of two objects. For example, Hupp and colleagues ([18], Experiment 1) presented adults with a novel word (e.g., *ta-te*) as the name of an object (a heart), and then asked them to identify which of two objects would be a *ta-te-be*, with the choice being a heart or a star. They reported that adults selected the same object (the heart) 17.5% of the time when given a word-form variant involving a suffix, but only 9.5% when it involved a prefix (e.g., *be-ta-te*). Thus, adults showed an overwhelming tendency to reject any word-form variant as an alternative label for a previously named object but also displayed a slight preference for suffixed words as alternative labels.

The label-extension task contrasts with a more widely used procedure in which children are given a choice between a familiar and an unfamiliar object. Merriman and Schuster [19] asked 2- and 4-year-old children to decide between a familiar or unfamiliar object after hearing a nonce word that sounded similar to the name of the familiar object. At both ages, children mapped the name-similar nonce word (e.g., *japple*) onto the familiar object (e.g., an apple) about 60% of the time. In contrast, when the nonce word (e.g., *firsh*) did not bear any similarity to the name of the familiar object, 4-year-olds (and to a much lesser extent 2-year-olds) engaged in the predictable fast mapping of the name to the unfamiliar object. Merriman and Schuster [19] introduced a wide variety of word-form modifications across items, with some items having onset-consonant additions or substitutions (e.g., *japple* for *apple*, *sagon* for *wagon*, *bruck* for *truck*), other items with suffixes added (e.g., *cardle* for *car*, *housler* for *house*, *pantiffs* for *pants*), and others having word-internal changes (e.g., *firsh* for *fish*, *lote* for *light*, *colck* for *clock*). Merriman and Schuster failed to detect any difference in how children responded to the items with onset modifications versus the items with suffixes added (i.e., they selected the familiar object with the similar sounding name 70% of the time when the nonce noun had an onset modification versus 71% of the time when it had a suffix added). However, modifications that changed the rime (i.e., items with word-internal changes involving vowels) were less likely to be treated as alternative labels.

Jarvis et al. [20] explored whether training altered how children treated word-form modifications similar to those used by Merriman and Schuster [19]. They hypothesized that the children in Merriman and Schuster [19] may have formed a response set that altered their pattern of responding over the course of testing. In particular, Merriman and Schuster's inclusion of trials with two familiar objects (e.g., an apple paired with a salamander) may have led the children to assume that *japple* referred to the apple as opposed to the salamander because *japple* sounded more like *apple* than *salamander.* Consequently, Jarvis et al. tested whether the inclusion of training trials with two familiar objects and a similar-sounding nonce word would lead children to be more accepting of word-form modifications in a posttest with a familiar object paired with an unfamiliar object. They found that prior to training (i.e., in a pretest), the children were highly biased to treat any word-form modification as a new word, but were significantly more accepting of the similar-sounding words as alternative labels of familiar objects in the posttest. Adults, in contrast to children, did not alter their response patterns after training, and selected the familiar object on only 14% of posttest trials. This high degree of resistance to any word-form modification in adult English-speakers matches the findings of Hupp et al. [18].

Importantly, Jarvis et al.'s results confirmed Merriman and Schuster's [19] finding that children did not treat all word-form modifications equivalently. However, the exact pattern of responding was not identical to that reported in Merriman and Schuster. In Jarvis et al. ([20], Experiment 1), word-form modifications involving replacements of word initial consonant(s) (e.g., *bruck* for *truck*) were associated with the familiar object (e.g., a truck) only 8% of the time in the pretest, whereas end modifications (e.g., *shoeler* for *shoe*) were associated with the familiar object (e.g., a shoe) 42% of the time. In both Merriman and Schuster [19] and Jarvis et al. [20], the word-ending modifications involved adding an unstressed final syllable to the word, whereas the word-onset manipulations involved an addition or substitution of a consonant to alter the word onset, rather than the addition of an unstressed prefix. This leaves open the question of whether children would treat prefixed versus suffixed words differently.

The research reported in this paper expands the previous findings in various ways: we investigate (1) whether affixed forms are tolerated more readily as alternative labels than stem modifications like the substitution of a word onset, (2) whether prefixed forms are tolerated differently than suffixed forms, and (3) whether tolerance for modified word forms is generally higher when those modifications are systematic as is characteristic for productive morphological patterns, rather than idiosyncratic and random. Before describing our methodology in detail, we briefly summarize considerations that suggest differences in tolerance between prefixed and suffixed forms.

1.2. The Role of Prefixes and Suffixes in Language Learning. The statistical distribution of inflections across human languages is a widely discussed topic among linguists interested in morphology [21–23]. Across languages, there appears to be a preference for suffixes over prefixes [24]; prefixing-only languages are rare in comparison to those with only suffixes [25]. However, exceptions to this asymmetry can be found in some of the world's languages such as the prefix-dominant Bantu languages, which feature a variety of prefixes including a diminutive prefix [26].

Prefixes and suffixes may be treated differently because modifications of beginnings versus ends of words differ in their impact on lexical processing. In one of the earliest studies on this topic, Bagley [27] presented adults with word-initial and word-final mispronunciations of consonants and found word-initial mispronunciations to be more disruptive to word recognition. Marslen-Wilson's Cohort model of word recognition [28, 29] proposed that the initial phoneme(s) of a word activate a cohort of words bearing the same sounds. As subsequent phonemes of the word are processed and a "uniqueness point" for the word is reached, the word is selected from the lexicon. In support, Nooteboom [30] found that adult Dutch speakers succeeded 95% of the time in identifying the word *Kannibal* when presented with initial fragments compared to only 60% of the time when presented with final fragments. The aforementioned findings by Hupp et al. [18] also confirm this asymmetry: adults judged the suffixed word-form variants (e.g., *ta-te-be*) as more similar to the target words (e.g., *ta-te*) than the prefixed forms (e.g., *be-ta-te*).

Similar results have been reported with 4- and 5-year-old children: Walley [31] examined the influence of word-initial input on children's recognition of spoken words through a mispronunciation detection task. She manipulated the position of the mispronounced phoneme (i.e., onset versus offset of the word) and, additionally, whether the word was presented within a sentence context (i.e., in a story) or in isolation (with or without an accompanying picture). When the mispronounced word occurred within a story, children were more successful at detecting mispronunciations involving word onsets than offsets. However, the children did not show this position effect when the words were presented in isolation, without accompanying pictures.

Another reason for the asymmetry between prefixes and suffixes with respect to tolerance of word-form variation may be that suffixes are more informative with respect to grammatical category information (e.g., information about parts of speech or noun gender). This is reflected in Slobin's [23] operating principle A_1: "grammatical realizations in the form of suffixes of postpositions will be acquired earlier than realizations in the form of prefixes or prepositions." This, in addition to Slobin's [23] operating principle A: "pay attention to the ends of words," acknowledges that the ends of words are more salient to early language learners than the beginnings. Clair et al. [32] explored to what extent prefixes and suffixes are differentially helpful in marking the grammatical categories of words. They conducted a corpus analysis of child-directed speech in English using the CHILDES database. For each affix, they calculated the frequency with which it pointed to a specific grammatical category and found that suffixes contained more consistent category information than prefixes. In a subsequent experiment, adults exposed to an artificial language were more accurate in identifying the grammatical categories of suffixed words than of prefixed words. Based on these findings, Clair et al. concluded that there are multiple advantages in learning and processing suffixes over prefixes, including faster processing time, greater facilitation, and lower interference with category identification.

In sum, initial segments of a word might facilitate word identification whereas final segments of a word might facilitate grammatical categorization leading to the hypothesis that children display greater tolerance for modifications involving suffixes than prefixes in the label-extension task.

1.3. The Present Study. To examine children's tolerance for various word-form modifications we conducted two experiments using the label-extension task. We also tested adults in addition to the children to provide a comparison group. Experiment 1 tested whether participants treated variants of novel words with substitutions of word-initial consonants (e.g., *wug* for *stug*) differently than word-form variants with prefixes (e.g., *wastug* for *stug*). Experiment 2 tested whether participants treated prefixes differently than suffixes. Both experiments used a label-extension task similar to that of Hupp et al. ([18], Experiment 1). However, in contrast to previous label-extension studies, all of which utilized nonproductive word-form variation, our experiments presented the same morphophonological modifications across all novel words. This allowed us to examine how children treat word-form variation that is systematic and productive, as opposed to idiosyncratic and apparently random. As noted above, input to language learners can include many productive word-form variations, such as diminutives in English or inflectional morphemes in highly inflected languages. Following Jarvis et al. [20], participants in both experiments received filler trials consisting of familiar words presented with two familiar objects in order to discourage a response set where the child selected the unfamiliar object on every single trial. However, these filler trials did not constitute a meaningful extension contrast and will therefore not be analyzed.

Table 1: Stimulus words for Experiment 1.

Introductory (simplex) word	Similar word trials			Dissimilar word trials		
	Diminutive	Onset modification		Diminutive	Onset modification	
Practice trials						
Horse	Horsy			Doggy		
Dog	Doggy			Horsy		
Pig	Piggy			Fishy		
Fish	Fishy			Piggy		
		Substitution	Prefix		Substitution	Prefix
Test trials						
Geck	Gecky	Weck	Wageck	Kazy	Waze	Wakaze
Kaze	Kazy	Waze	Wakaze	Gecky	Weck	Wageck
Tuz	Tuzzy	Wuz	Watuz	Dibby	Wib	Wadib
Dib	Dibby	Wib	Wadib	Tuzzy	Wuz	Watuz
Terp	Terpy	Werp	Waterp	Vikey	Wike	Wavike
Vike	Vikey	Wike	Wavike	Terpy	Werp	Waterp
Stug	Stuggy	Wug	Wastug	Mansey	Wanse	Wamanse
Manse	Mansey	Wanse	Wamanse	Stuggy	Wug	Wastug
Pabble	Pabbley	Wabble	Wapabble	Rutchery	Wutcher	Warutcher
Rutcher	Rutchery	Watcher	Warutcher	Pabbley	Wabble	Wapabble
Dappo	Dappoee	Wappo	Wadappo	Chitoffy	Witoff	Wachitoff
Chitoff	Chitoffy	Witoff	Wachitoff	Dappoee	Wappo	Wadappo
Burble	Burbley	Wurble	Waburble	Spirteny	Wirten	Waspirten
Spirten	Spirteny	Wirten	Waspirten	Burbley	Wurble	Waburble
Hacket	Hackety	Wacket	Wahacket	Jerpery	Werper	Wajerper
Jerper	Jerpery	Werper	Wajerper	Hackety	Wacket	Wahacket

2. Experiment 1: Tolerance of Different Types of Word-Onset Modification

2.1. Method. Experiment 1 involved a between-subjects manipulation of changes involving word onsets: in the onset substitution condition, participants heard word-onset modifications that involved substitution of /w/ for the word onset (e.g., *wanse* for *manse*). In the prefix condition, onsets were altered through the addition of a prefix *wa-* (e.g., *wamanse* for *manse*). In both conditions, participants were also presented with a diminutive derivation; due to its prevalence in natural language and child-directed speech, we anticipated that children and adults would readily tolerate the diminutive as an alternative name for the object. Thus, the inclusion of diminutives served as a manipulation check to determine whether the task made sense to the participants and whether they were detecting any relationship between the animal name provided on the introductory page and the test noun. We used animate targets throughout the experiment to comply with the constraint that the diminutive derivation in English applies predominantly to animal names. For the diminutive trials we used the most productive diminutive derivation in English (i.e., the suffix/I/).

2.1.1. Participants. Sixty-four children (mean age 4;0, range 2;11–4;11; 38 boys and 26 girls) were recruited and tested at several urban and rural preschools. The children came from predominantly white, middle-class communities and were monolingual speakers of American English. Each child received a child-study *t*-shirt for their participation. Sixty-four adult native speakers of English (mean age 21 years, range 18–40, 21 males and 43 females) were recruited from psychology classes at a large urban public university and received research participation credits. Half of the participants in each age group were assigned to the onset substitution condition and half were assigned to the prefix condition. For each age group, the numbers of male and female participants, and their ages, were matched across conditions.

2.1.2. Materials and Design. We created 8 monosyllabic and 8 bisyllabic pseudonouns like *stug* and *manse*, see Table 1 for a list of stimuli. These pseudo-nouns were combined with a diminutive suffix (e.g., *stuggy*) to create the diminutive control items. For participants in the prefix condition, pseudo-nouns were combined with the unstressed prefix *wa-* (e.g., *wastug*). For participants in the onset substitution condition, the first consonant was replaced with the phoneme /w/ as in *wug* for *stug*. Half of the trials per condition (i.e., "similar word" trials) presented a word-form modification that sounded similar to the name of the animal presented on the introductory page (e.g., for *manse*: *wanse* or *wamanse*), and the other half (i.e., "dissimilar word" trials) presented word-forms that were entirely unrelated to the name of the animal presented on the introductory page (e.g., for *manse*: *wug* or *wastug*). Note that the "dissimilar word" trials did not

Table 2: Examples of stimuli for novel animal trials in Experiments 1.

Picture	Simplex name	Onset modification		Offset modification
		Onset substitution	Prefix	Diminutive
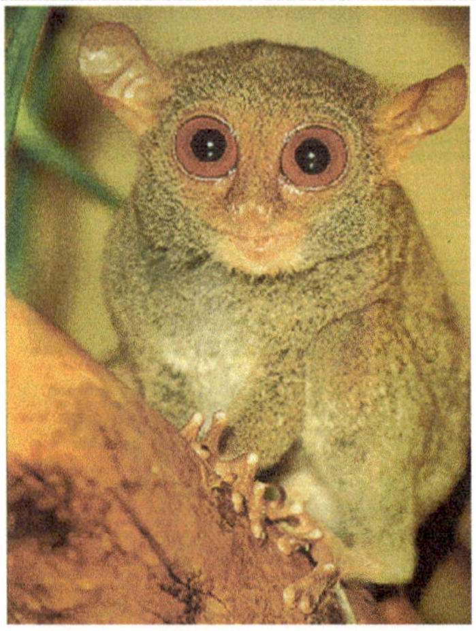	*Manse*	*Wanse*	*Wamanse*	*Mansey*
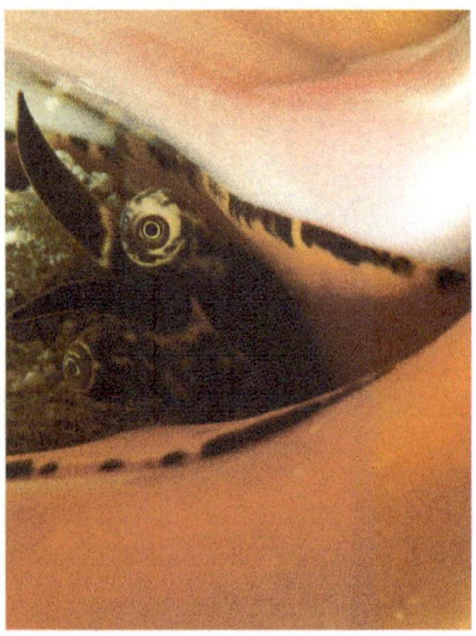	*Stug*	*Wug*	*Wastug*	*Stuggy*

constitute a word-form modification from the point of view of the participants, but rather served as a control for whether the children engaged in fast mapping of novel items to novel referents.

Novel target words and familiar fillers were combined with 6" x 4" pictures of novel and familiar animals, respectively. Examples of novel animal stimuli are shown in Table 2. The pictures were collected from nature publications, websites, and other sources. Each trial consisted of an introductory page containing a single image of an animal and a second test page containing the introductory image next to one of a different animal. The introductory page was used to establish the name of the animal, using its simplex form, by saying, for example, "I call this animal a *stug.*" The test page was used for the forced-choice probe described below. An example trial is depicted in Figure 1.

Assignment of items to conditions (similar versus dissimilar word trials; onset versus end modification) was counterbalanced across participants, yielding 8 unique lists. At the beginning of the task, participants received two practice trials consisting of familiar words and their diminutive derivations to ensure comprehension of the instructions.

2.1.3. Procedure. Each participant was tested individually in a single session of approximately 10 minutes duration. Participants were tested by one of two male research assistants: one research assistant was involved in the preparation of stimulus materials and the other was blind to the research hypotheses. Comparison of data across research assistants yielded essentially identical results.

Participants were seated in front of a binder and were invited to play a game of pointing to the picture of the animal that was named. Participants were told that some of the animals might have made-up names they had never heard before and that they should try their best to figure out which animal might be called by the given name.

Two training trials were used to ensure understanding of the task. Each trial began with the introduction of the first animal photo labeled using the simplex form of the animal name (e.g., "I call this animal a *horse*. Can you say *horse*?"). Children were asked to repeat the simplex name to confirm that they had heard it and were paying attention. This was followed by the presentation of the two photos on the test page and the probe (e.g., "now can you tell me which animal is a *horsey*?"). Children were instructed to point to a picture,

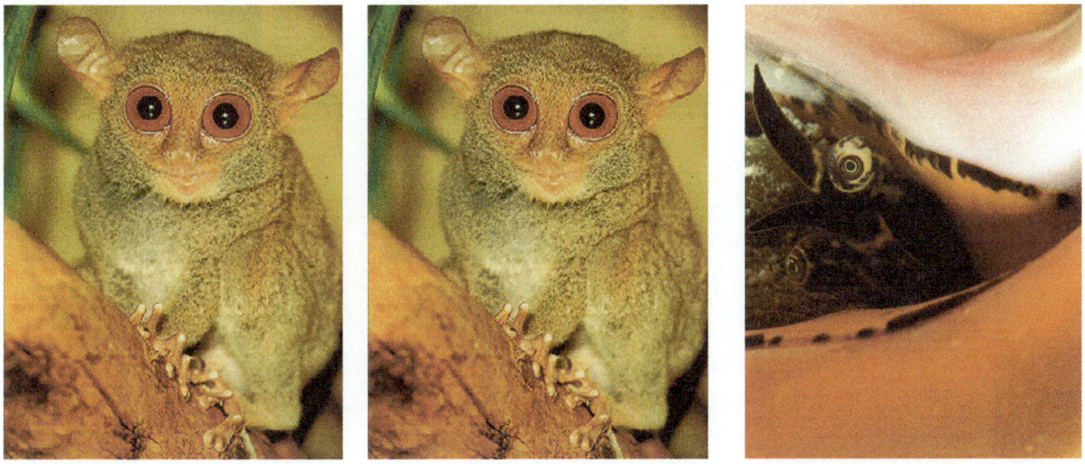

(a) Introductory page. "I call this a *manse*. Can you say *manse*?"

(b) Test page. "Now can you tell me which animal is a *wanse*?"

FIGURE 1: Example of a trial in the onset substitution condition of Experiment 1.

and their responses were recorded out of sight on a tally sheet. The tally sheets were used to record whether the children selected the picture on the left or right side of each page and were scored at the end of the testing.

The first two trials were used to train the participant on how the game was played. One of the initial trials probed for the same animal that was introduced on the initial page and the other trial probed for the other animal, with the order of "similar word" and "dissimilar word" trials counterbalanced. After these two initial training trials the experiment proceeded with the test trials, which were interspersed with filler trials using familiar animals. In both the onset substitution and the prefix conditions, the test trials were presented in a quasirandom order, with no more than three "similar word" or "dissimilar word" trials occurring consecutively, and position of word-form modification (onset versus ending) randomized across trials. To illustrate the conditions, for "similar word" trials, children heard a modification of the previously introduced name: introduced to a *stug*, they were asked "which animal is a *stuggy*?" (diminutive control condition) or "which animal is a *wug*?" (onset substitution condition) or "which animal is a *wastug*?" (prefix condition); for "dissimilar word" trials, children heard an entirely different word: introduced to a *stug*, they were asked "which animal is a *mansey*?" (diminutive condition) or "which animal is a *wanse*?" (onset substitution condition) or "which animal is a *wamanse*?" (prefix condition). No corrective feedback was given during the test.

2.2. Results. Table 3 presents mean percentages of trials in which participants selected the same animal as the one previously labeled on the introductory page in Experiment 1. Choice of same animal indicates tolerance of a word-form modification. We first examine "dissimilar word" trials to ascertain whether children understood the task, and then we focus on the "similar word" trials, which contain the main manipulation of interest. Responses for "similar word" trials and for "dissimilar word" trials were analyzed in the following way: because the factor of onset modification type (onset substitution versus prefix) was nested within position of modification in the "similar word" trials (i.e., participants in both onset modification conditions also were exposed to diminutive derivations) we performed a set of planned comparisons. We first examined whether there were differences due to position of modification (onset versus ending) and effects of age for "similar words" and "dissimilar words" separately. We then performed the critical analyses just for the onset-modified "similar word" trials to examine whether there were differences due to onset modification type (onset substitution versus prefix).

As is evident in Table 3, participants rarely chose the same animal on the "dissimilar word" trials, in which the noun was entirely different from the name of the animal on the introductory page. That is, when introduced to a *manse*, and asked for a *wug* or a *wastug* or a *stuggy*, participants avoided the picture associated with *manse*. For "dissimilar word" trials, a mixed-design ANOVA with age group as a between-subjects factor, and position of modification (onset versus ending) as a within-subjects factor yielded a significant main effect of position of modification, $F(1, 126) = 4.59$, $P = 0.034$, partial $\eta^2 = 0.04$, with participants (children and adults) selecting the "same" picture somewhat more often when faced with an onset modification (10.9%), as opposed to a diminutive (6.2%). No other effects approached significance.

For "similar word" trials, the same mixed-type ANOVA yielded only a main effect of position of modification, $F(1, 126) = 27.78$, $P = 0.0001$, partial $\eta^2 = 0.16$, with more "same" picture choices for diminutive modifications (84.0%) than for onset modifications (65.6%). However, examination of the means in Table 3 indicates that this effect of position was primarily due to a large difference between the onset substitution condition and the diminutive

Table 3: Mean percentages of selections of the same animal as on the introductory page, as a function of group (onset substitution versus prefix), trial type (dissimilar versus similar word), and modification (onset versus diminutive) in Experiment 1. $N = 32$ in each group (Standard deviations in parentheses).

		Onset substitution group		Prefix group	
		Onset substitution (e.g., *wug*)	Diminutive (e.g., *stuggy*)	Prefix (e.g., *wastug*)	Diminutive (e.g., *stuggy*)
Dissimilar word trials (*manse* on introductory page)	Children	10.9 (21.0)	6.2 (16.8)	15.6 (32.2)	10.9 (21.0)
	Adults	7.8 (18.4)	4.7 (14.8)	9.4 (19.8)	3.1 (12.3)
Similar word trials (*stug* on introductory page)	Children	40.6 (41.0)	73.4 (33.6)	82.8 (32.7)	85.9 (31.7)
	Adults	57.8 (42.3)	90.6 (23.5)	81.2 (30.5)	85.9 (22.8)

condition. Whereas participants chose fewer "same" pictures in the onset substitution condition than in the diminutive condition, $F(1,62) = 36.799$, $P = 0.0001$, partial $\eta^2 = 0.37$; the prefix and the diminutive conditions did not differ, $F(1,62) < 1$.

To compare the effects of different types of onset modifications on "similar word" trials, we conducted a two-way ANOVA with age group and onset modification type as between-subjects factors. This ANOVA yielded a main effect of onset modification type, $F(1,124) = 25.20$, $P = 0.0001$, partial $\eta^2 = 0.17$, with the prefix group (82.0%) selecting more "same" pictures for "similar word" trials with onset modifications than the onset substitution group (49.2%). Age group did not show any significant effects in any of the analyses. Still, to confirm that participants at each age distinguished the two types of onset modification, we conducted analyses of "similar word" trials with onset-modifications for each age group separately. These additional analyses confirmed an effect of onset modification type for children, $F(1,124) = 20.71$, $P = 0.0001$, partial $\eta^2 = 0.25$, and for adults, $F(1,124) = 6.46$, $P = 0.014$, partial $\eta^2 = 0.09$, with both groups selecting more "same" pictures in the prefix condition. To explore a possible developmental trend within the group of children, we calculated the correlation between children's age in months and the number of selections of the "same" picture on "similar word" trials with onset modifications. The correlation did not approach statistical significance for children in either group (onset substitution condition, $r(N = 32) = -0.06$, prefix condition, $r(N = 32) = -0.11$), which indicates that preschool children across ages responded similarly.

2.3. Discussion. The main goal of Experiment 1 was to determine whether children would distinguish different types of word-onset modifications that involved (1) substitution of initial consonants or (2) the addition of a prefix. The children's performance was contrasted with adults to explore the extent to which learners of different ages show flexibility in adapting to morphophonological changes that are systematic in the sense that they apply across different nouns, as in the case of the English diminutive derivation.

Across all analyses, children and adults responded similarly to the different experimental conditions: Onset modifications involving novel prefixes were tolerated to a much greater extent than those involving consonant substitutions. That is, *wastug* was a more acceptable variant of *stug* than was *wug*, and it was equally acceptable to the diminutive *stuggy*. This result suggests that children are able to keep track of the underlying base forms (e.g., *stug*), and treat variants that preserve the base forms (e.g., *wastug*, stuggy) differently from those that do not (e.g., *wug*). Thus, both children and adults exposed to the prefixed and suffixed words generally treated both as acceptable variations of the targets, with only a nonsignificant trend favoring the diminutives. The overwhelming tolerance for the prefixed forms suggests that acquisition of morphological knowledge may be achieved after only a short training session (cf. [33], for further evidence of rapid learning of affixes in a study with adults). The lack of a difference in tolerance for prefixed versus suffixed forms was unexpected given findings of Hupp and colleagues [18], where adults judged suffixed word-forms (e.g., *ta-te-be*) to be more similar to targets (e.g., *ta-te*) than the prefixed forms (e.g., *be-ta-te*). To further explore this issue, in Experiment 2 we held constant the morphophonological segment added to the beginning versus the end of a word, to test the effect of position more directly.

3. Experiment 2: Tolerance of Prefixes versus Suffixes

3.1. Method

3.1.1. Participants. Thirty-two children (mean age 4;3, range 3;2–5;1, 17 boys and 15 girls) were recruited and tested at the same schools as in Experiment 1. All of the children were monolingual speakers of English, and none had participated in Experiment 1. Each child received a child-study *t*-shirt for their participation. Thirty-two adult native speakers of English (mean age 22 years, range 18–43 years, 12 men, 20 women) were recruited from psychology classes at a large public university and received research participation credits for their participation.

3.1.2. Materials and Design. The materials and design of the experiment were identical to Experiment 1, with the exception that different novel word-form modifications were introduced. For the word-onset modification, the unstressed, nonce prefix *ko-* was added to the beginning of each noun, and for the word ending modification, the unstressed, nonce suffix, *-ko*, was added to the end of each noun. These modifications were manipulated within participants.

TABLE 4: Examples of stimuli for novel animal trials in Experiment 2.

Picture	Simplex name	Word-form modification	
		Prefix	Suffix
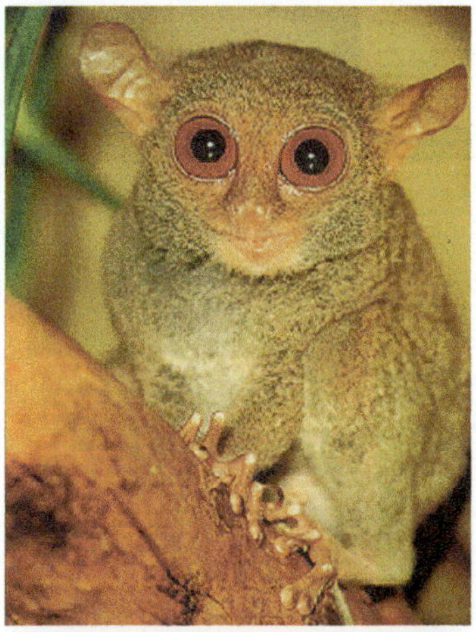	*Manse*	*Komanse*	*Manseko*
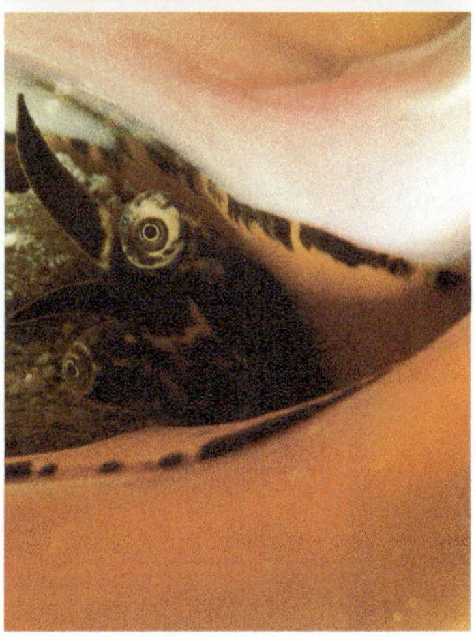	*Stug*	*Kostug*	*Stugko*

Examples of stimuli for the novel animal trials are shown in Table 4. Table 5 provides the complete list of stimuli.

3.1.3. Procedure. The procedure was the same as Experiment 1.

3.2. Results. Table 6 presents mean percentages of trials in which participants selected the same animal as the one previously labeled on the introductory page. We analyzed the selection of "same" pictures in "dissimilar word" and "similar word" trials separately, using mixed-type ANOVAs with age group as between-subjects factor and position of modification as a within-subjects factor. The analysis of "dissimilar word" trials (e.g., for *manse*: hearing *kostug* or *stugko*) produced no significant effects. Both age groups rarely selected the "same" animal for the "dissimilar word" trials (see Table 6 for means).

For "similar word" trials involving word-form modifications of previously introduced nouns (e.g., for *stug*: hearing *kostug* or *stugko*), only the main effect of position of modification was significant, $F(1,62) = 10.19$, $P = 0.002$, partial $\eta^2 = 0.14$. Participants selected the "same" animal more often when *ko* was a suffix (e.g., *stugko*) than when it was a prefix (e.g., *kostug*), 76.6% versus 67.2%. Age group did not show any significant effects in any of the analyses. Nevertheless, to confirm the effect of position of modification at each age we conducted separate analyses: for the children, the effect of position of modification was significant, $F(1,31) = 6.36$, $P = 0.017$, partial $\eta^2 = 0.17$, whereas for the adults, the effect of position of modification was marginally significant, $F(1,31) = 3.89$, $P = 0.057$, partial $\eta^2 = 0.11$. Finally, to explore a possible developmental trend within the group of children, we calculated the correlation between children's age in months and the number of selections of the "same" picture on "similar word" trials. A negative correlation approached statistical significance for the prefix condition, $r(N = 32) = -0.31$, $P = 0.08$, and the suffix condition, $r(N = 32) = -0.33$, $P = 0.06$. This pattern of results indicates that older children were somewhat more likely than younger children to select the "different" picture across trials, perhaps due to their greater reliance on a word learning strategy such as ME or N3C.

TABLE 5: Stimulus words for Experiment 2.

Introductory (simplex) word	Similar word trials		Dissimilar word trials	
	Suffix	Prefix	Suffix	Prefix
Practice trials				
Horse	Horsy		Doggy	
Dog	Doggy		Horsy	
Pig	Piggy		Fishy	
Fish	Fishy		Piggy	
Test Trials				
Gep	Gepko	Kogep	Kazeko	Kokaze
Kaze	Kazeko	Kokaze	Gepko	Kogep
Tuz	Tuzko	Kotuz	Dibko	Kodib
Dib	Dibko	Kodib	Tuzko	Kotuz
Terp	Terpko	Koterp	Vikeko	Kovike
Vike	Vikeko	Kovike	Terpko	Koterp
Stug	Stugko	Kostug	Mansko	Komanse
Manse	Mansko	Komanse	Stugko	Kostug
Pabble	Pabbleko	Kopabble	Rutcherko	Korutcher
Rutcher	Rutcherko	Korutcher	Pabbleko	Kopabble
Dappo	Dappoko	Kodappo	Chitofko	Kochitoff
Chitoff	Chitofko	Kochitoff	Dappoko	Kodappo
Burble	Burbleko	Koburble	Spirtenko	Kospirten
Spirten	Spirtenko	Kospirten	Burbleko	Koburble
Hacket	Hacketko	Kohacket	Jerperko	Kojerper
Jerper	Jerperko	Kojerper	Hacketko	Kohacket

TABLE 6: Mean percentages of selections of the same animal as on the introductory page, as a function of trial type (dissimilar versus similar word) and condition (prefix versus suffix) in Experiment 2. $N = 32$ in each group (standard deviations in parentheses).

		Prefix (e.g., *kostug*)	Suffix (e.g., *stugko*)
Dissimilar word trials (*manse* on introductory page)	Children	10.9 (27.6)	12.5 (28.4)
	Adults	6.2 (16.8)	6.2 (21.1)
Similar word trials (*stug* on introductory page)	Children	60.9 (41.6)	71.9 (38.0)
	Adults	73.4 (40.1)	81.2 (35.4)

3.3. Discussion. Experiment 2 contrasted children's tolerance of word-form modifications involving prefixes versus suffixes, using the same affix in both positions across nouns. These affixed forms were predominantly interpreted as referring to the same animals as the uninflected introductory forms. Despite this overall bias to accept word-form modifications, participants were more accepting of *ko* when it was a suffix than when it was a prefix. This bias favoring suffixes matches the position effect reported by Hupp et al. ([18], Experiment 1) despite large differences in adults' overall tolerance of the word-form variants across the two studies. In Hupp et al., each word was altered with a unique prefix or suffix, whereas we used the same affix across all items. Our participants picked up on the productive usage of the experimental affix seemingly right away, as we failed to find any effect of trial position in follow-up analyses.

Although Jarvis and colleagues [20] also reported a position effect in a word-learning task, this study compared children's tolerance of word-form variants that had onset-substitutions (e.g., *japple*) with their treatment of suffixed nouns (*shoeler*). To our knowledge, our study is the first to test for a position effect, holding constant the complexity of the affixed material. Our results complement the word recognition studies of Walley [31] that showed that children were more sensitive to modifications involving word onsets than word offsets.

4. General Discussion

This study examined how systematic patterns of word-form variation influence children's ability to map words onto referents. It addressed the question as to whether children and adults treat words with onset substitutions differently from prefixed words, and whether they treat prefixed words differently from suffixed words, using an established experimental framework, a forced-choice label-extension task.

To confirm that children understood the task, a familiar word-form variation (i.e., the diminutive derivation common in child-directed speech) provided the necessary comparison in the first Experiment 1. If the participants rejected the diminutives, it would suggest that the task was not making sense to them. Also, following Jarvis and colleagues [20], on half of the trials, children heard a word totally dissimilar to the previously introduced animal name, in order to establish that the fast mapping mechanism was present. In this respect, the "dissimilar word" condition served as an additional manipulation check that the task was understood. In the "dissimilar word" condition, children were observed to fast map novel word forms onto previously unseen novel animals, in agreement with predictions of ME [6] or N3C [7].

Although English is a language with a relatively impoverished inflectional morphology, the children and adults in our study appeared to readily accept the novel prefixes or suffixes after very limited exposure to the recurring affixes. This result confirms other findings [34–36] that children show some tolerance for multiple words referring to the same referent. Our study adds to these findings by suggesting that language learners are able to track systematic and productive word-form variation across words, and adjust their word-learning strategies to accommodate recurring affixes (see also [33]). In contrast to previous studies using the label-extension task [18, 20], which presented a wide variety of word-form modifications making it impossible to systematically compare the impact of prefixes versus suffixes, or of affixes versus onset substitutions, we observed that adults, as well as children, were able to parse a nonce prefix or suffix from a word and map the stem onto the same referent. This indicates that systematic word-form variation invites greater tolerance than idiosyncratic, random variation.

At the same time, our participants were much less accepting of modifications that involved replacements of word-initial consonants. Previous research [19, 20] has shown that children do not treat words with onset modifications as alternative labels of previously named objects (e.g., *japple* does not mean *apple*), even after training. Our Experiment 1 replicated this general finding that children are more likely to choose a novel object when the initial phoneme was altered than when the word form involved the addition of an affix. Again, the stimuli used in Jarvis et al. [20] used a wide variety of word-form modifications which prevented systematic comparisons of the impact of prefixes versus suffixes, or of affixes versus onset substitutions. Our study provides new insights into this question. Experiment 1 showed that adding a separate syllable to the beginning of the word did not have the same effect as changing the initial consonant. Words with onset substitutions were generally treated as novel nouns, whereas children showed the ability to parse the prefix *wa-* from the word stem and treated the prefixed word as a word form variant just like the diminutive. Thus, in accordance with the cohort model [28], the process of elimination of lexical candidates with shared word beginnings prevents participants from activating lexical items with different word beginnings such as *weetle* as a competitor for *beetle* or, as in this study, *wanse* as a competitor for *manse.* In contrast, in the prefix condition, participants appeared to have been able to parse the prefixes from the word stems which enabled them identify the similar sounding target word. Children's apparent ability to recognize the base forms (stems) of words in variants such as *wastug* or *stuggy* suggests sensitivity to the fact that, in English, stems can occur in multiple positions within complex words. Position-independent identification of word stems has been demonstrated in adults in visual-word recognition tasks [37], but has yet to be demonstrated in children. Representations of suffixes, in contrast to stems, appear to be position (or context) specific, such that interference effects on visual word recognition vary in accordance with the position of a suffix, for example, *shootment* is harder to reject as a nonword than *mentshoot* [38].

Experiment 2 showed that suffixed words were more likely to be accepted as word-form variants than prefixed words, although a similar trend in Experiment 1 failed to reach statistical significance. As discussed earlier, suffixes may create more acceptable word-form variants than prefixes due to their universal tendency to provide cues to grammatical categories, and this may be reflected in the universal "operating principles" that the ends of words are more salient than the beginnings, which have been postulated to guide early language learners [23]. Those principles were supported by the observation that case marking seems to be learned earlier in languages that use suffixes compared to those that use articles to mark case. An alternative to a universal bias is the idea that children's experience with the distributional characteristics of their native language leads them to adapt their word-learning strategies to the morphological and grammatical properties of the language input. Specifically, in English, the native language of our participants, suffixes are more frequent comprising 181 different forms [39] and have broader productivity than prefixes, which comprise only 56 forms and modify a smaller set of word types. Thus, the present results do not allow us to decide whether the observed preference for suffixed over prefixed word-form variants represents a universal word-learning bias or the product of language-specific learning. In future research, the asymmetry between acquisition and acceptance of prefixes versus suffixes should be tested crosslinguistically by examining languages with different distributions of prefixes and suffixes (e.g., Bantu languages). In addition, cross-linguistic comparison should address whether having been exposed to a morphologically rich language is associated with different patterns of word-form tolerance than exposure to morphologically more impoverished languages such as Chinese or, in our case, English. Finally, to test the generality of these findings, future studies should also vary the phonological complexity of the prefixes and suffixes.

The findings presented here suggest that native English-speaking preschool age children and adults tolerate prefixed and suffixed words as labels for familiar referents when the introduced morphological variants are used consistently, as is the case with morphologically productive changes in natural languages. One possibility is that children simply learn to tolerate word-form variants that preserve the base forms of words (e.g., *stug* embedded in *kostug or stugko*) over those that do not (e.g., *wug*)—this possibility requires further testing to determine whether children can readily learn morphological patterns that involve stem changes as well as affixation. Children and adults are much less tolerant of modifications involving initial phonemes, which suggests that the emergence of sensitivity to the structure of words leads to the appropriate adjustment of word learning strategies.

Acknowledgments

This paper includes data from the first author's doctoral dissertation. The project was supported by a PSC-CUNY Award to P. J. Brooks and a Fulbright Fellowship to I. Dabašinskienė. A portion of the work was presented at the biennial meeting of the *Society for Research in Child Development*.

References

[1] S. A. Graham, D. Poulin-Dubois, and R. K. Baker, "Infants' disambiguation of novel object words," *First Language*, vol. 18, no. 53, pp. 149–164, 1998.

[2] S. Carey and E. Bartlett, "Acquiring a single new word," *Papers and Reports on Child Language Development*, vol. 15, pp. 17–29, 1978.

[3] E. M. Markman, "Constraints children place on word meanings," *Cognitive Science*, vol. 14, no. 1, pp. 57–77, 1990.

[4] A. E. Booth and S. R. Waxman, "Shape bias special section: taking stock as theories of word learning take shape," *Developmental Science*, vol. 11, no. 2, pp. 185–194, 2008.

[5] E. M. Markman, J. L. Wasow, and M. B. Hansen, "Use of the mutual exclusivity assumption by young word learners," *Cognitive Psychology*, vol. 47, no. 3, pp. 241–275, 2003.

[6] E. M. Markman, *Categorization and Naming in Children: Problems of Induction*, MIT Press, Cambridge, Mass, USA, 1989.

[7] R. M. Golinkoff, K. Hirsh-Pasek, L. M. Bailey, and N. R. Wenger, "Young children and adults use lexical principles to learn new nouns," *Developmental Psychology*, vol. 28, no. 1, pp. 99–108, 1992.

[8] E. V. Clark, "On the pragmatics of contrast," *Journal of child language*, vol. 17, no. 2, pp. 417–431, 1990.

[9] G. Diesendruck and L. Markson, "Children's avoidance of lexical overlap: a pragmatic account," *Developmental Psychology*, vol. 37, no. 5, pp. 630–641, 2001.

[10] D. Jurafsky, "Universal tendencies in the semantics of the diminutive," *Language*, vol. 72, no. 3, pp. 533–578, 1996.

[11] V. Kempe, P. J. Brooks, and L. Pirott, "How can child-directed speech facilitate the acquisition of morphology?" in *Research on Child Language Acquisition: Proceedings of the 8th conference of the International Association for the Study of Child Language*, M. Almgren, A. Barrena, M. J. Ezeizabarrena, I. Idiazabal, and B. MacWhinney, Eds., pp. 1237–1247, Cascadilla Press, Medford, Mass, USA, 2001.

[12] G. Melzi and K. A. King, "Spanish diminutives in mother-child conversations," *Journal of Child Language*, vol. 30, no. 2, pp. 281–304, 2003.

[13] S. Gillis, "The acquisition of diminutives in Dutch," in *Studies in Pre- and Protomorphology*, W. Dressler, Ed., pp. 165–179, Verlag der Österreichischen Akademie der Wissenschaften, Vienna, Austria, 1997.

[14] I. Savickienė, *The Acquisition of Lithuanian Noun Morphology*, Verlag der Österreichschen Akademie der Wissenschaft en, Wien, Austria, 2003.

[15] I. Savickienė and W. U. Dressler, *Acquisition of Diminutives: A Cross-Linguistic Perspective*, John Benjamins, Amsterdam, The Netherlands, 2007.

[16] V. Kempe, P. J. Brooks, N. Mironova, A. Pershukova, and O. Fedorova, "Playing with word endings: morphological variation in the learning of Russian noun inflections," *British Journal of Developmental Psychology*, vol. 25, no. 1, pp. 55–77, 2007.

[17] K. King and G. Melzi, "Intimacy, imitation and language learning: Spanish diminutives in mother-child conversation," *First Language*, vol. 24, no. 2, pp. 241–261, 2004.

[18] J. M. Hupp, V. M. Sloutsky, and P. W. Culicover, "Evidence for a domain-general mechanism underlying the suffixation preference in language," *Language and Cognitive Processes*, vol. 24, no. 6, pp. 876–909, 2009.

[19] W. E. Merriman and J. M. Schuster, "Young children's disambiguation of object name reference," *Child development*, vol. 62, no. 6, pp. 1288–1301, 1991.

[20] L. H. Jarvis, W. E. Merriman, M. Barnett, J. Hanba, and K. S. Van Haitsma, "Input that contradicts young children's strategy for mapping novel words affects their phonological and semantic interpretation of other novel words," *Journal of Speech, Language, and Hearing Research*, vol. 47, no. 2, pp. 392–406, 2004.

[21] S. A. Kuczaj, "Evidence for a language learning strategy: on the relative ease of acquisition of prefixes and suffixes," *Child Development*, vol. 50, pp. 1–13, 1979.

[22] M. Mithun, "The acquisition of polysynthesis," *Journal of Child Language*, vol. 16, no. 2, pp. 285–312, 1989.

[23] D.I. Slobin, "Cognitive pre-requisites for the acquisition of grammar," in *Studies of Child Language Development*, C. A Ferguson and D. I. Slobin, Eds., Holt, Rinehart & Winston, New York, NY, USA, 1973.

[24] E. Sapir, *Language: An Introduction to the Study of Speech*, Harcourt, Brace & Co., New York, NY, USA, 1921.

[25] J. A. Hawkins and G. Gilligan, "Prefixing and suffixing universals in relation to basic word order," *Lingua*, vol. 74, no. 2-3, pp. 219–259, 1988.

[26] N. Grandi and F. Montermini, "Prefix suffix neutrality in evaluative morphology," in *Morphology and Linguistic Typology, On-line Proceedings of the Fourth Mediterranean Morphology Meeting (MMM4)*, University of Bologna, Catania, Italy, September 2003, http://morbo.lingue.unibo.it/mmm/.

[27] W. A. Bagley, "The apperception of the spoken sentence: a study in the psychology of language," *American Journal of Psychology*, vol. 12, pp. 80–130, 1900.

[28] W. D. Marslen-Wilson, "Functional parallelism in spoken word-recognition," *Cognition*, vol. 25, no. 1-2, pp. 71–102, 1987.

[29] W. D. Marslen-Wilson and A. Welsh, "Processing interactions and lexical access during word recognition in continuous speech," *Cognitive Psychology*, vol. 10, no. 1, pp. 29–63, 1978.

[30] S. Nooteboom, "Lexical retrieval from fragments of spoken words: beginnings vs. endings," *Journal of Phonetics*, vol. 9, no. 4, pp. 407–424, 1981.

[31] A. C. Walley, "Young children's detections of word-initial and -final mispronunciations in constrained and unconstrained contexts," *Cognitive Development*, vol. 2, no. 2, pp. 145–167, 1987.

[32] M. C. S. Clair, P. Monaghan, and M. Ramscar, "Relationships between language structure and language learning: the suffixing preference and grammatical categorization," *Cognitive Science*, vol. 33, no. 7, pp. 1317–1329, 2009.

[33] M. Merkx, K. Rastle, and M. H. Davis, "The acquisition of morphological knowledge investigated through artificial language learning," *Quarterly Journal of Experimental Psychology*, vol. 64, no. 6, pp. 1200–1220, 2011.

[34] G. O. Deák and M. Maratsos, "On having complex representations of things: preschoolers use multiple words for objects and people," *Developmental Psychology*, vol. 34, no. 2, pp. 224–240, 1998.

[35] G. O. Deák, L. Yen, and J. Pettit, "By any other name: when will preschoolers produce several labels for a referent?" *Journal of Child Language*, vol. 28, no. 3, pp. 787–804, 2001.

[36] C. B. Mervis, R. M. Golinkoff, and J. Bertrand, "Two-year-olds readily learn multiple labels for the same basic-level category," *Child Development*, vol. 65, no. 4, pp. 1163–1177, 1994.

[37] D. Crepaldi, K. Rastle, C. J. Davis, and S. J. Lupker, "Seeing stems everywhere: position-independent identification of stem morphemes," *Journal of Experimental Psychology: Human Perception and Performance*. In press.

[38] D. Crepaldi, K. Rastle, and C. J. Davis, "Morphemes in their place: evidence for position-specific identification of suffixes," *Memory and Cognition*, vol. 38, no. 3, pp. 312–321, 2010.

[39] E. Fudge, *English Word-Stress*, George Allen & Unwin, London, UK, 1984.

Spatial Language and Children's Spatial Landmark Use

Amber A. Ankowski,[1] Emily E. Thom,[2] Catherine M. Sandhofer,[1] and Aaron P. Blaisdell[1]

[1] *Department of Psychology, University of California, Los Angeles, CA 90095, USA*
[2] *Department of Child and Adolescent Development, California State University, Northridge, CA 91330, USA*

Correspondence should be addressed to Amber A. Ankowski, aankowski@ucla.edu

Academic Editor: Andrew N. Meltzoff

We examined how spatial language affected search behavior in a landmark spatial search task. In Experiment 1, two- to six-year-old children were trained to find a toy in the center of a square array of four identical landmarks. Children heard one of three spatial language cues once during the initial training trial ("here," "in the middle," "next to this one"). After search performance reached criterion, children received a probe test trial in which the landmark array was expanded. In Experiment 2, two- to four-year-old children participated in the search task and also completed a language comprehension task. Results revealed that children's spatial language comprehension scores and spatial language cues heard during training trials were related to children's performance in the search task.

1. Introduction

Adults are extremely adept at using landmarks to navigate space (e.g., turn left at the gas station) and to remember the location of objects (e.g., the keys are between the vase and the lamp). Yet what is easy for adults is difficult for young children. Children's ability to use landmarks develops slowly throughout the preschool years [1, 2]. During this time, children's ability to use spatial language also develops (e.g., "by," "middle") [3, 4]. The current study examines how these processes mutually influence one another by investigating how spatial language contributes to spatial learning. We examine this relationship by: (1) analyzing whether comprehension of spatial words is related to search behavior and (2) analyzing how search behavior is affected by spatial language cues. We focus our examination on the spatial concept of "middle." Middle is a particularly challenging spatial concept because it requires children to estimate location equidistant from multiple landmarks.

2. The Development of Children's Landmark Use

A central task in the development of spatial cognition is to learn to use objects as landmarks for another object's location. Initially, children's ability to use landmarks is limited, but the ability to use single and then multiple landmarks becomes gradually more sophisticated. Children learn to use single landmarks before using multiple landmarks in conjunction [2]. During the first year of life, children begin to use single landmarks as direct markers, or beacons, of an object's location (the cookie is *in* the cookie jar) [5–8]. Children later learn to use single landmarks as indirect markers of an object's location (the cookie is *next to* the cookie jar) [2, 9]. For example, Plumert and Hawkins [9] asked children to find a toy in either a direct landmark condition (e.g., "the toy is *in* the chair") or an indirect landmark condition (e.g., "the toy is *next to* the chair"). Three-year old children found the toy significantly faster in the direct landmark condition. Still a more complex way of using landmarks is to attend to the relation between multiple landmarks (e.g., the cookie is *between* the cookie jar and the blender). Using landmarks relationally requires calculating the location of an object in relation to multiple referents, a task that, like other relational tasks in the preschool years [10–12], poses a greater challenge to children than locating an object in regard to a single referent.

Typically, children do not use multiple landmarks to find a hidden object until well into their preschool years [13–15]. However, there is debate regarding at what age children acquire the ability to do so [15, 16]. In some studies, by the age of four or five years old children readily use multiple landmarks to find a hidden object [13, 15]. In other studies, four- and five-year old children fail to use multiple landmarks to find a hidden object when other methods of solving the task are possible [16]. Contradictory accounts regarding the timing of relational landmark development may suggest that children's performance is related to task-specific factors (e.g., some studies used two landmarks while others used four landmarks, some studies used an open field while other studies used a small box, etc.), or that children may favor solutions that allow attention to only one landmark when available.

Nonhuman animals also appear not to use multiple landmarks relationally [16–19]. In expansion tasks in which animals were first trained to search in the center of an array of landmarks followed by a test trial in which the landmarks were expanded, gerbils [18], pigeons [20], and primates [16, 21, 22] did not search relationally (i.e., in the center of the expanded landmark array). Instead, these species tended to search at a discrete distance and direction from one of the landmarks in the array. Though some species (e.g., Clark's nutcrackers) have been trained to use a relational strategy when a task cannot be solved in other ways [19], nonhuman animals do not readily use multiple landmarks relationally when other methods of solving the task are available [16].

The data from nonverbal animals and young children support one possible explanation for children's struggles with relational encoding at this age. It is possible that learning spatial words helps children to solve spatial landmark tasks. The current study examined how the development of spatial language relates to children's performance in relational landmark tasks. We focused on the relationship between the spatial relational word "middle" and children's ability to use the middle relation in a spatial search task, because the middle relation may be particularly challenging to children. First, middle is a viewpoint-independent term [1]. Unlike egocentric (e.g., left) or allocentric (e.g., north) spatial terms, the word "middle" does not have a reliable, unchanging referent. Instead, the word "middle" is used flexibly to refer to the relationship between any object and any of multiple landmarks of any distance apart from one another. Second, identifying the middle of multiple landmarks requires estimating distances with a fair degree of accuracy (but see [23], for a perceptual alternative used by honeybees). Previous research suggests that in nonsearch tasks in which children are habituated to spatial relationships between objects, children as young as six months old can categorize based on the *between* relation when distance calculation is not a factor [24, 25]. Yet unlike the *between* spatial relation, the *middle* relation requires children to attend to the precise distance between landmarks, which may be more challenging to children. Third, the word "middle" commonly appears in both spatial contexts (e.g., the location equidistant from multiple landmarks) and nonspatial contexts (e.g., the second of three children). Even when the word "middle" is used in a spatial context, it is often inexact. For example, phrases such as "standing in the middle of the room" only rarely indicate standing in the precise location that is equidistant from each corner of the room.

3. Spatial Language Comprehension

Children's experience with language is temporally linked with their understanding of associated concepts in the same domain [26, 27]. For example, children's acquisition of disappearance words (e.g., "gone") corresponds with their emerging skills in object permanence tasks and children's acquisition of success/failure words (e.g., "there," "uh-oh") corresponds with their emerging skills in means-end tasks [27]. Cross-cultural research shows similar ties between language experience and cognition, revealing that children develop early cognitive skills associated with word types emphasized in their native languages. For example, Korean-speaking children tend to acquire verbs earlier in language development than English-speaking children, and English-speaking children tend to acquire nouns earlier than Korean-speaking children [28–31]. Korean-speaking children also show earlier skill in verb-related means-end tasks, whereas English-speaking children show earlier skill in noun-related categorization tasks [30, 32].

Similar findings in the domain of space indicate strong ties between spatial language and spatial reasoning [26, 33]. For example, the different ways in which spatial terms are used across languages result in children's development of very different spatial categories according to the conventions of their native language [26]. Such findings have led some researchers to argue that the development of spatial language and the development of spatial cognition mutually influence one another.

Although the precise mechanisms by which spatial language and spatial cognition develop are unknown, they appear to mutually affect one another in studies of infant spatial category recognition [26, 34, 35]. By eighteen months old, children identify language-specific spatial relationships [26, 35], suggesting that spatial language input helps to construct and order children's view of space from very early in development. Casasola et al. [34] further showed that even minimal exposure to spatial language influences children's perception of spatial relationships. English-speaking children were familiarized to a novel spatial relation (i.e., the tight-fit relation) with or without a novel word. Only children who saw the spatial relation paired with the novel word learned to distinguish the tight-fit spatial relation from a contrasting loose-fit spatial relation. Because spatial language influences the way that children perceive spatial relationships, learning the word "middle" may result in a greater ability to use the middle spatial relation and thus lead to more middle search behavior in the current studies.

Other studies, however, suggest that comprehension of the term "middle" and nonverbal performance with the spatial concept may not be so closely related. In a study of English-speaking preschool-aged children, Loewenstein and Gentner [4] found that 84% of three-year old children and 100% of four-year old children comprehended the word "middle" in a spatial search task. Even though three and four year old children comprehend the word "middle," however, children at these ages (and older) do not consistently use the middle relation in spatial search tasks when other methods of solving the spatial task are available [16]. Even after the term "middle" enters children's comprehensive vocabularies, children may not apply the concept to a spatial search task when the task can be solved in simpler ways (i.e., searching a discrete distance and direction from a single landmark).

4. Spatial Language Cues

Experimenter-provided language cues can also affect children's performance during a task. In categorization studies, labeling objects during the task facilitates categorization by heightening attention to similarities between objects and aggregating discrete instances [10, 36–41]. Language cues may be particularly important for facilitating children's relational reasoning, because children show substantial difficulty acquiring relational categories across domains [11]. Unlike categories (e.g., object categories) that are defined by static, shared perceptual features, members of relational categories share little perceptual similarity. For example, there is little perceptual similarity between the middle relation depicted by a house in the *middle* of two hills and a book on the *middle* shelf in a stack of shelves. Multiple studies indicate that children match objects based on salient perceptual features well before they match objects based on relational information (see [11] for a review). Because of the lack of shared perceptual similarity between different instances of *middle*, language cues may be particularly important for helping children detect and use middle spatial relations.

5. The Current Studies

The current studies investigated the relationship between children's acquisition of the term "middle" and their performance in a landmark task. We chose a landmark task with multiple solutions (i.e., using multiple or single landmarks), and examined how comprehension of the spatial word "middle" related to use of a single-landmark strategy versus a multiple-landmark strategy. We used a modified version of MacDonald et al.'s [16] task, in which children were trained to find a goal in the center of a square array of four identical landmarks (see Figure 1(a)). After performance reached criterion, children were given a probe test trial in which the landmark array was expanded (see Figure 1(b)). There were two ways for children to approach the spatial task. For example, children could search at a location equidistant from each of the four landmarks in the expanded array (middle search), as adult humans do. Alternatively, children could search at the same absolute distance and direction from a single landmark in one of the four corners of the expanded array (corner search), as nonhuman animals do. Children could also exhibit other search behavior, including searching in random locations in or outside of the landmark array, or could fail to reach criterion for the expanded test trial. We examined whether children's comprehension of the spatial word "middle" and children's search behavior were related. Finally, we examined how different spatial word primes affected children's search behavior.

6. Experiment 1

6.1. Method

6.1.1. Participants. Thirty-six children completed the experiment (mean age = 54.4 months, SD= 16.36, range: 24.1–82.9 months): five two-year olds (mean age = 30.32 months, SD = 2.08, range: 24.1–34.4 months), nine three-year olds (mean age = 41.94 months, SD = 1.55, range: 36.9–45.1 months), seven four-year olds (mean age = 53.1 months, SD = 1.76, range: 48.1–57.1 months), nine five-year olds (mean age = 65.8 months, SD = 1.55, range: 61.1–71.9 months), and six six-year olds (mean age = 77.57 months, SD = 1.9, range: 72.5–82.9 months). All children were from native English-speaking households. An additional six children were excluded for failure to meet test criterion (mean age = 21.47 months, SD = 5.66, range: 13.2–28.8 months).

6.1.2. Materials and Apparatus. Figure 1 shows the 1.2 × 1.4 m sandbox custom-made for this study. The sandbox was placed in the center of a well-lit, 5.8 × 6.2 m classroom containing twelve standard classroom desks and a whiteboard. An overhead camera was positioned directly over the sandbox to record each trial. The walls of the sandbox were 15.2 cm high and contained approximately 8 cm of standard white sand. The bottom of the sandbox was raised 10 cm above the floor. The sandbox was dark brown and small pieces of masking tape were placed along its edge at 25 cm intervals, marking predetermined locations at which landmark arrays were placed during the experiment.

Eight identical blue wooden posts, each 2.5 cm in diameter and 15 cm in length served as landmarks. Four landmarks were configured into a 25 × 25 cm square array (Figure 1(a)), and the other four were configured into a 50 × 50 cm square array (Figure 1(b)). Wooden dowels (0.6 cm diameter) connecting the bottom of the landmarks held each array together. When placed in the sandbox, the bottom of the landmark array was buried 5 cm below the sand, leaving 10 cm of each blue post exposed above the sand. A 2.5 × 3.8 cm plastic toy monkey was used as the goal during cued and uncued training trials. During these trials, the monkey was hidden about 2.5 cm below the sand.

A parent questionnaire was used to assess children's spatial vocabularies, which included a list of spatial relational terms (e.g., "middle," "center," "by" and "near") and questions regarding children's experience with books, games and other activities in which they may have used spatial concepts (e.g., "Have you read any books to your child that may have taught him or her spatial concepts such as "middle"?").

6.1.3. Design. Children were divided into one of three between-subjects language conditions: (1) control, (2) "next to," and (3) "middle."

In order to preserve procedural details from MacDonald et al. [16], half of the children in this study heard three cued training trials. To investigate whether multiple-cued training trials influenced children's search behavior, the other half of children heard only one cued training trial. Children were

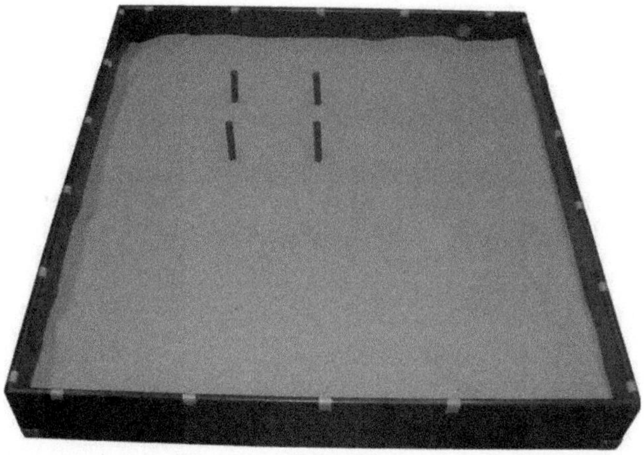

(a)

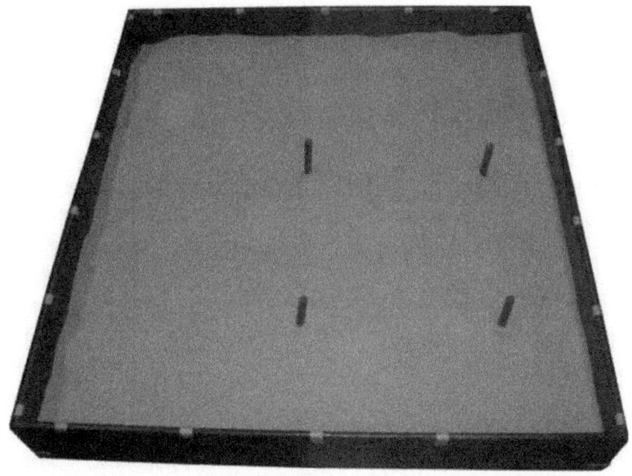

(b)

FIGURE 1: Pictures of the small and large landmark arrays in the sandbox. (a) shows the training landmark array and (b) shows the expanded landmark array.

assigned to one versus three training trials equally according to age and language condition.

6.1.4. Procedure. The experiment consisted of three phases: (1) cued training trials, (2) uncued training trials, and (3) expanded test trial. During each trial, Experimenter 1 placed landmark arrays in randomized predetermined locations, which corresponded with grid locations created by masking tape placed on the sides of the sandbox at 25 cm intervals (Figure 1). Twenty locations were possible for the small (nonexpanded) landmark array and 12 locations were possible for the large (expanded) landmark array. Landmark locations were randomly assigned per trial for each child, so no two children saw the same sequence of hiding locations. Experimenter 1 also hid the toy and timed children while they searched. Experimenter 2 distracted children and ensured that they did not observe the sandbox between trials. Because children had the option to dig from either inside or outside of the sandbox, Experimenter 2 also helped children into the sandbox when needed.

Cued Training Trials. Cued training trials served as instruction for children, allowing children to watch the object being hidden so that they would know where to retrieve it on subsequent uncued trials. Children experienced either one or three cued training trials. During these trials, children watched as Experimenter 1 hid the toy in the center of the small landmark array by pressing the toy into the sand and brushing the sand to smooth it over. Children also heard one of three language cues. Children in the control condition heard, "I am hiding the toy *here*." Children in the "next to" condition heard, "I am hiding the toy *next to this one*." Children in the "middle" condition heard, "I am hiding the toy *in the middle*." Children were given ten seconds to find the toy. If they did not do so, the experimenter uncovered the toy for the child to retrieve.

Uncued Training Trials. During uncued training trials, Experimenter 1 placed the small landmark array in a randomized predetermined location and hid the toy in the center of the landmark array while Experimenter 2 distracted the child. Children were then asked to find the toy (i.e., "The toy is hidden. Can you find it?"), but no other language cues were provided. If children retrieved the toy within ten seconds on three consecutive trials, they advanced to the test trial. Children who reached twenty trials without finding the toy within ten seconds on three consecutive trials were excluded from the experiment.

Expanded Test Trial. During the expanded test trial, Experimenter 1 placed the large landmark array in a randomized, predetermined location, while Experimenter 2 distracted the child. Children were told to look for the toy, but there was, in fact, no toy present. Children were given ten seconds to search after which the trial was terminated.

Experimenters 1 and 2 independently charted children's initial search locations. Children were also filmed during the task. For data analysis, children's search locations were determined by overhead camera footage. Children's searches were coded in two ways. First, children's searches were coded for their distance from the center of the expanded landmark array. Second, children's searches were coded as being in middle, corner, or other regions of the landmark array. Figure 2 depicts five 12.7 cm regions representing possible search locations (one center "middle" location and four "corner" locations).These locations were based on hypothetical search strategies. The middle location was determined based on the search strategy used by adults in this task [16], in which adults calculate the middle of the expanded landmark array. The corner locations were determined based on the search strategy used by pigeons and other nonverbal animals in this task [16], in which animals search the same distance and direction from a single landmark as the goal had been in the nonexpanded landmark array. Two independent coders judged the videotapes for children's initial search locations,

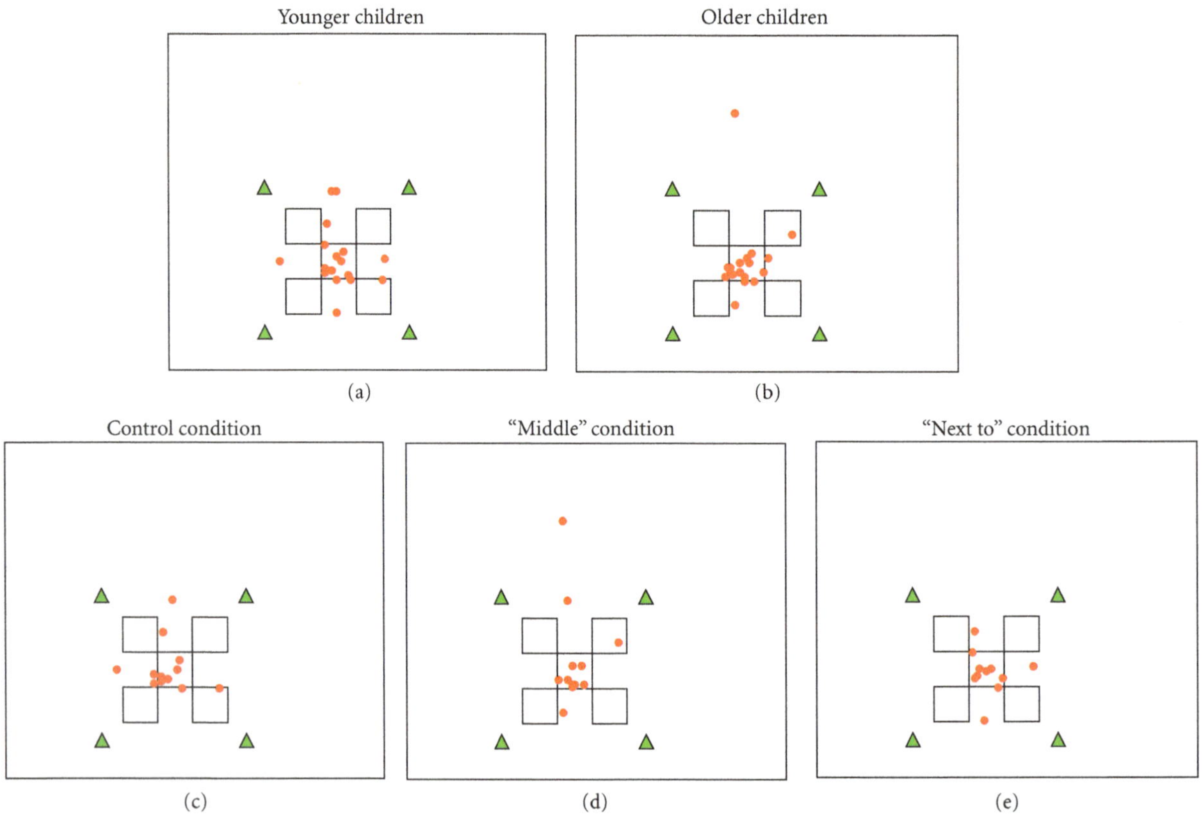

Figure 2: Experiment 1: Plots of children's initial search location during the expanded test trial by age group and language condition. Search locations are plotted according to age (younger children: $n = 18$, M age = 40.65 months, SD = 8.73, range: 24.1–54.6 and older children: $n = 18$, M age = 68.15 months, SD = 8.63, range: 55.4–82.9) and language condition (control, "middle", and "next to").

with 100% agreement between coders regarding the regions of children's searches (middle, corner, other). If children's search locations were not discernible from video footage or if footage was not available ($n = 4$), an average of the charted locations captured from the two experimenters was used to determine the child's search location. If there was disagreement between the two experimenters regarding the search location (middle, corner, other) of a child who was not videotaped, the child would be excluded from the study ($n = 0$).

6.2. Results and Discussion

6.2.1. Training Trials. Results revealed no effects of whether children were exposed to one or three cued training trials. There was no difference in the number of uncued training trials that children required ($F(1, 34) = .15$, $P = .7$, $\eta^2 = .004$) according to the number of cued training trials they heard. There was also no difference in the number of children who searched in the middle region of the landmark array ($\chi^2(1, N = 36) = .18$, $P = .67$) or in the distance children searched from the center of the landmark array ($F(1, 34) = .04$, $P = .85$, $\eta^2 = .00$) according to whether they experienced one ($M = 9.06$, SD = 7.19) or three ($M = 9.67$, SD = 10.99) cued training trials. Thus, we collapsed across this variable for the remainder of the analyses.

There was no effect of age ($F(1, 31) = .62$, $P = .65$, $\eta^2 = .07$) or gender ($F(1, 34) = .69$, $P = .41$, $\eta^2 = .02$) on the number of uncued training trials children required. On average, children required 4.97 uncued training trials to meet criterion (SD = 3.81).

6.2.2. Expanded Test Trials. Across all three language conditions, most children searched in the middle region of the expanded landmark array. Figure 2 depicts five 12.7 cm regions representing possible search locations (one center "middle" location and four "corner" locations). Chi-square analysis revealed that more children searched in the center of the expanded landmark array than searched in any other location, ($\chi^2(1, N = 36) = .16.67$, $P = .00$). Combining all three of the language-cued conditions revealed that overall 61% of children searched in the middle region of the landmark array. Only 6% of children searched in the corners of the array. The remaining 33% of children searched in locations outside of the five designated possible target regions. Of these children, only one child searched outside of the expanded landmark array. We additionally coded the distance of children's searches from the center of the landmark array. This analysis revealed that across ages and language conditions, children searched an average of 9.36 cm (SD = 9.16) from the center of the landmark array.

Across conditions, children's search strategies were not significantly related to children's age. A median split by age revealed that 67% of older children ($n = 18$, M age = 68.15 months, SD = 8.63, range: 55.4–82.9) across conditions searched in the middle, and 56% of younger children ($n = 18$, M age = 40.65 months, SD = 8.73, range: 24.1–54.6) searched in the middle, $\chi^2(1, N = 36) = .47$, $P = .49$. Analyses on distance from middle yielded similar results. An ANOVA revealed that the distance from children's searches to the center of the landmark array did not differ by whether children were from younger ($M = 10.06$, SD = 7.16) or older ($M = 8.67$, SD = 10.98) age groups, $F(1, 34) = .20$, $P = .66$, $\eta^2 = .01$. There was no correlation between the distance that children searched from the center of the array and age in months ($r = -.17$, $P = .33$) or age in years ($r = -.11$, $P = .53$). Unlike previous research citing sex differences in young children's use of landmarks [14], we did not find differences in girls' and boys' search locations ($\chi^2(1, N = 36) = .33$, $P = .56$) or in the distance that boys ($M = 7.47$, SD = 5.73) and girls ($M = 10.71$, SD = 10.92) searched from the center of the landmark array ($F(1, 34) = 1.10$, $P = .30$, $\eta^2 = .03$).

6.2.3. Spatial Language Cues. When children of all ages were combined, language cues appeared to have little effect on children's search strategies. The number of children who searched in the middle of the landmark array did not differ by language condition, $\chi^2(1, N = 36) = .94$, $P = .63$. Of children in the control language condition, 50% searched in the middle, 8% searched in a corner, and the remaining 42% searched in other locations. Of children in the "next to" condition, 67% searched in the middle, 0% searched in a corner, and the remaining 33% searched in other locations. Of children in the "middle" condition, 67% searched in the middle, 8% searched in a corner, and the remaining 25% searched in other locations. The distance that children searched from the center of the array also did not differ according to whether children heard a "middle" ($M = 11.50$, SD = 13.53), "next to" ($M = 7.42$, SD = 5.35) or control ($M = 9.17$, SD = 6.79) language cue, $F(2, 33) = 59$, $P = .56$, $\eta^2 = .03$. Overall, children's tendency to use a middle search strategy did not differ by language condition; however, analysis of individual language conditions revealed that middle language cues may have facilitated younger children's performance.

As Figure 3 shows, children in the control condition who were not prompted with a spatial language cue appeared to show increases with age in middle searches. Although 0% of two-year olds searched in the middle, 100% of six-year olds did, and by six years old children performed equivalently to adults in the same procedure [20, 42]. Performance in the "middle" and "next to" conditions, however, appeared more varied across ages.

The results of the "middle" condition suggest that prompting children with relational language may have helped younger children ($n = 18$, M age = 40.65 months, SD = 8.73, range: 24.1–54.6), but not older children ($n = 18$, M age = 68.15 months, SD = 8.63, range: 55.4–82.9) to employ a middle search strategy. A median split by children's age revealed that 80% of younger children in the "middle" language condition searched in the middle region, but less than 60% of younger children in the control or "next to" language conditions did so (Figure 4). Hearing the term "middle" did not have the same effect on older children's searches. Instead, across conditions, most older children searched in the middle of the array regardless of the language cue they heard during the experiment. Hearing relational language may not have affected older children's performance because their performance was at ceiling regardless of language condition. Older children may have been able to

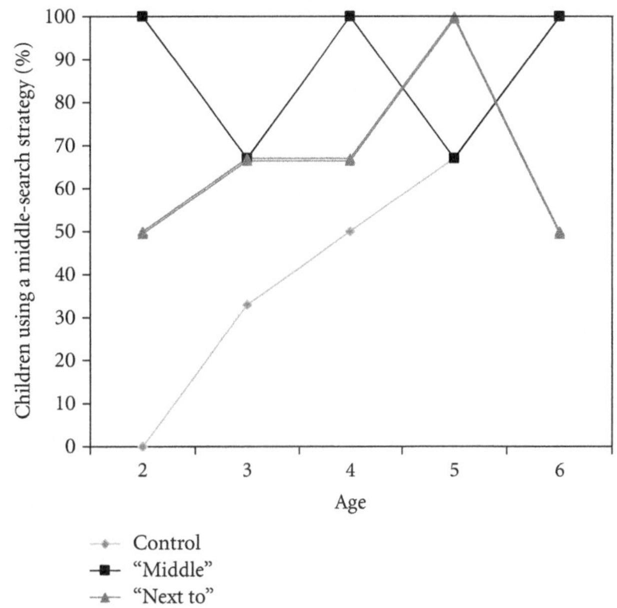

FIGURE 3: Experiment 1—percentage of middle searches by age and condition.

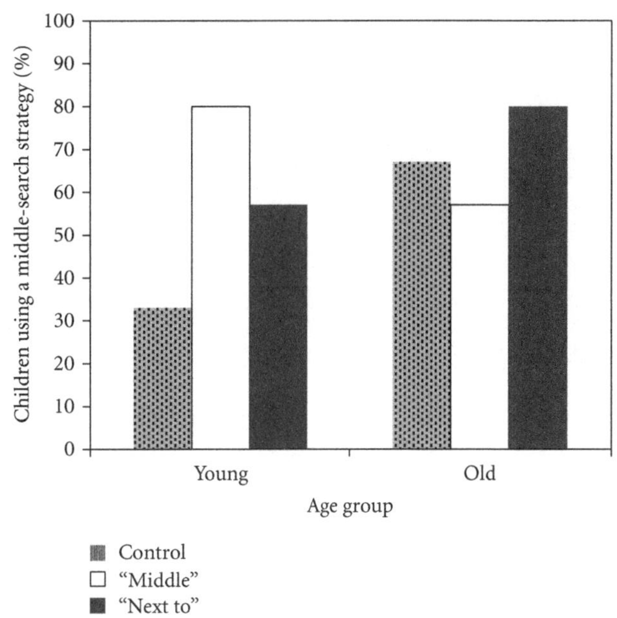

FIGURE 4: Experiment 1—percentage of middle searches by age group and language condition.

perceive and act on the middle relation without the aid of language (due to their preexisting knowledge). However, the tendency for young children to search in the middle appeared to be facilitated by spatial language cues. This finding is especially striking because half of these children heard the language cue only once. However, the sample of young children in this study was too small to determine statistical significance. Because of this, Experiment 2 focused on the younger ages of two to four years old to better examine how language cues affect search behavior in children who do not yet understand the word "middle."

Results of the "next to" language condition show that this relatively ambiguous language cue did not lead any children at any of the ages tested to search in the corner of the expanded landmark array as we expected. Indeed, children in the "next to" and "middle" language conditions searched in the middle at the same rate. One possibility is that the "next to" language cue may have increased children's attention to the landmarks. Telling children, "I'm hiding the toy *next to this one*," may have attracted attention to the landmarks, thereby also attracting attention to the relationship between the landmarks and the goal. In Experiment 2, we eliminated the "next to" condition and focused on search behavior in the middle and control conditions with young children.

6.2.4. Spatial Language Comprehension. Parent reports reflected that children's knowledge of the term "middle" increased with age, with parents reporting that 40% of two-year olds, 89% of three-year olds and 100% of four-to six-year olds understood and produced the word "middle." These reports were consistent with previous reports showing that 84% of three-year olds and 100% of four-year olds respond correctly in a "middle" comprehension test [43]. Parents in the current study reported that 89% of three-year olds and 100% of four-year olds comprehended and produced the term "middle," suggesting that our comprehension measure was valid.

Children's searches were consistent with the idea that spatial search was related to comprehension of spatial relational terms. Most children who were reported to know the word "middle" also searched in the middle of the landmark array. Of the children who were reported to understand and produce middle (n = 31), 67% searched in the middle and 33% did not. Of the children reported not to understand and produce the word "middle" (n = 5), 40% searched in the middle and 60% did not. Because only a small number of parents reported that their children did not comprehend the word "middle," there were too few children to determine whether this difference was statistically significant. Comprehending the term "middle" did not guarantee a middle search strategy. For example, although all children were reported to comprehend the term "middle" by the time they were four years old, 14% of four-year olds searched in locations other than the middle of the expanded array.

7. Experiment 2

In Experiment 2, we focused on the performance of two-, three-, and four-year old children in the middle search task for two reasons. First, the results of Experiment 1 showed that children begin to comprehend the term "middle" between two to four years of age. According to parent reports, comprehension grew from 40% of children at age two to 100% of children at age four. Experiment 2 examined how children's search behavior developed with their understanding of the spatial term "middle" during these years. Second, in Experiment 1, spatial language cues heard during the task seemed to have influenced younger children's performance, whereas older children tended to search in the middle of the expanded array regardless of the language they heard. Therefore, Experiment 2 examined searches of two-, three-, and four-year old children and compared their performance to their score on a middle comprehension test.

7.1. Method

7.1.1. Participants. Seventy-two children completed the experiment, including 24 two-year olds (mean age = 29.96 months, SD = 2.51, range: 25.03–33.4 months) 24 three-year olds (mean age = 42.32 months, SD = 2.87, range: 37.9–47.8 months), and 24 four-year olds (mean age = 53.25 months, SD = 3.48, range: 48.07–59.1 months). All children were from native English-speaking households. An additional 15 children were excluded for failure to meet test criterion (mean age = 28 months, SD = 2.9, range: 24.9–33.8 months).

7.1.2. Materials and Apparatus. The materials and apparatus were the same as those used in Experiment 1, with one minor change to the vocabulary questionnaire. Questions regarding children's experiences with the "middle" relation through books, games, etc. were eliminated from the questionnaire, because parents found the questions hard to answer and often left them incomplete.

7.1.3. Design. There were two between-subjects language conditions: (1) control and (2) "middle." Twelve two-year olds, 12 three-year olds, and 12 four-year olds participated in each language condition.

7.1.4. Procedure. There were two minor changes to the procedure used in Experiment 1. First, all children heard only one language-cued training trial (versus hearing either one or three language-cued training trials in Experiment 1). Second, children completed a forced-choice "middle" comprehension test. Six pairs of cards were used in the test (Figure 5 shows an example of the stimuli). Within each pair, one card pictured the middle relation and one card pictured a different spatial relation (e.g., "bottom," "left"). Three of the six pairs of cards pictured an array of three objects and three of the six pairs pictured an array of five objects. Children were shown two cards at a time and asked to identify the card that pictured the middle relation. For example, children saw a pair of cards, one with a cow in the middle of two horses and another with a cow below two horses. The child was asked, "Can you hand me the card with the cow in the middle?" No feedback was provided. The order of pairs and the location of the correct

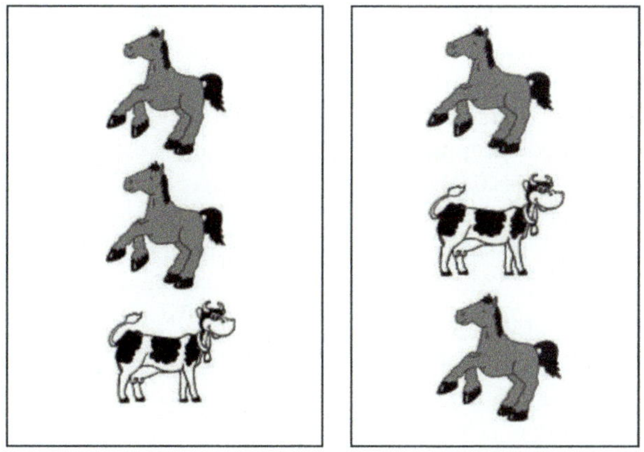

FIGURE 5: Example of the type of cards used for the comprehension test in Experiment 2.

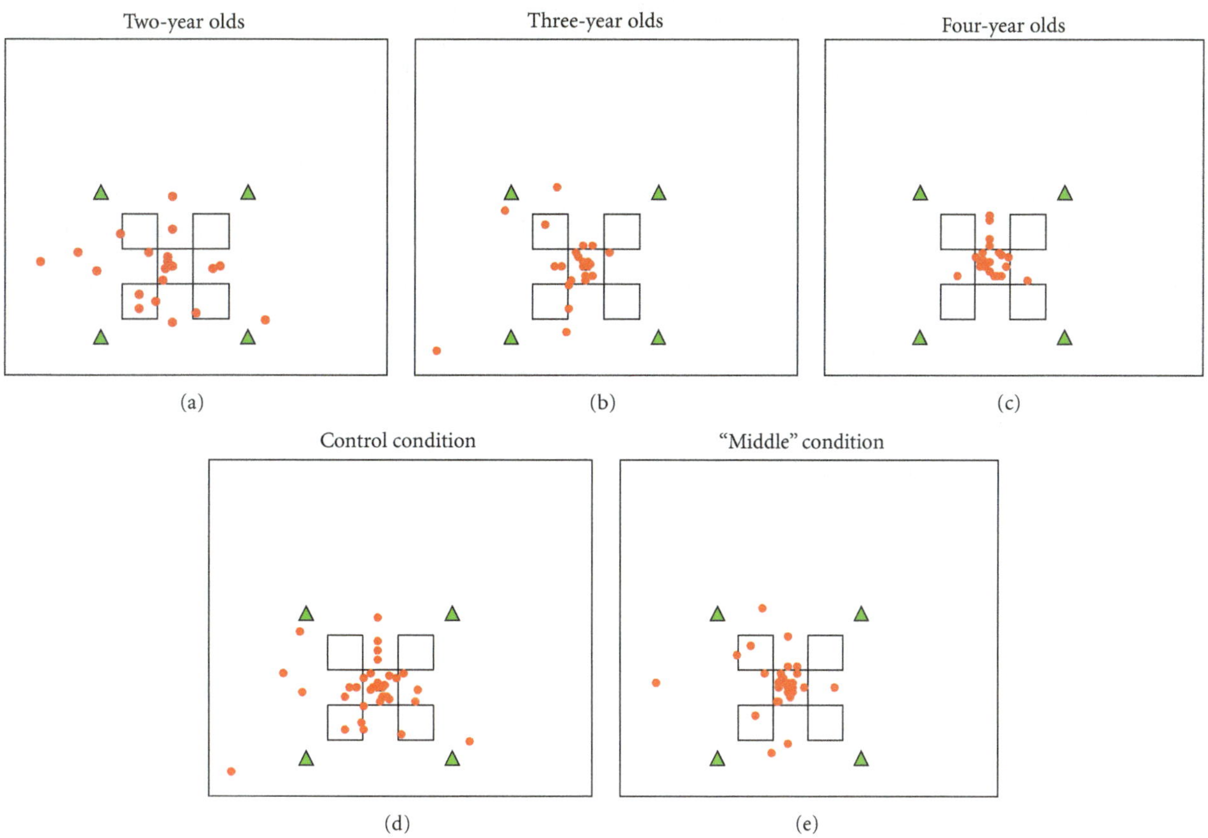

FIGURE 6: Experiment 2—children's search locations by age and language condition.

card were randomized. The comprehension test was always administered after the search task.

Children's search locations were captured via overhead camera footage. Two independent coders judged the videotapes for children's initial search locations, with 91% agreement between coders regarding the regions of children's searches (middle, corner, other). If children's search locations were not discernible from video footage or if footage was not available ($n = 7$), an average of the charted locations captured from the two experimenters was used to determine the child's search location. If there was disagreement between the two experimenters regarding the search location (middle, corner, other) of a child who was not videotaped, the child would be excluded from the study ($n = 0$).

7.2. Results and Discussion

7.2.1. Training Trials. On average, children required 5.11 uncued training trials to meet criterion (SD = 3.35). There was a significant effect of age on the number of uncued training trials that children required to reach criterion, $F(2, 69) = 15.21$, $P = .00$, $\eta^2 = .31$. Post hoc tests (Tukey's

HSD) revealed that two-year olds (M = 7.71, SD = 4.32) required significantly more search trials to reach criterion than both three-year olds (M = 4, SD = 2.13, $P < .01$), and four-year olds (M = 3.63, SD = .97, $P < .01$). There was no effect of gender on the number of uncued training trials children required ($F(3, 64) = .35$, $P = .79$, $\eta^2 = .02$) and no interaction between age and gender ($F(2, 64) = .21$, $P = .81$, $\eta^2 = .01$).

7.2.2. Expanded Test Trial. Figure 6 depicts children's initial search locations according to age and language condition. Most children used a middle-search strategy rather than a corner or other search strategy in Experiment 2, $\chi^2(2, n = 72) = 12.25$, $P = .00$. Across all ages and both of the language-cued conditions, 51% of children searched in the middle region of the landmark array, and 15% searched in a corner of the array. The remaining 34% of children searched in locations outside of the five designated targets. Of these children, only four searched outside of the expanded landmark array. Analysis of the distance of children's searches from the center of the landmark array revealed that across ages and language conditions, children searched an average of 10.69 cm (SD = 10.39) from the center of the landmark array.

A chi-square revealed that children's search behavior was significantly related to children's age ($\chi^2(2, n = 72) = 16.79$, $P = .00$), such that children's tendency to search in the middle region of the landmark array increased with age (Table 2). The distance that children searched from the center of the landmark array was also significantly correlated with age in months ($r = -.45$, $P = .00$) and age in years ($r = -.49$, $P = .00$). There was no effect of gender on the regions of children's searches. A two-way ANOVA analyzing the distance of children's searches by age and gender showed significant effects. There was a Main effect of age ($F(2, 66) = 7.95$, $P = .00$, $\eta^2 = .19$), such that two-year olds (M = 16.61, SE = 1.95) searched significantly farther from the center than three-year olds (M = 9.59, SE = 2.04; $P = .03$), and four-year olds (M = 5.79, SE = 1.95; $P = .00$). Search distance did not significantly differ between three-year olds and four-year olds ($P = .13$). Children's searches were also related to gender, such that on average girls (M = 8.13, SE = 1.62) searched closer to the center of the landmark arrays than did boys (M = 13.20, SE = 1.61), $F(1, 66) = 4.95$, $P = .03$, $\eta^2 = .07$. This was in contrast to the findings of Spetch and Parent [14] showing an advantage for boys in a similar search task. Future research should further investigate the role of gender in children's search strategies. There was no interaction between age and gender, $F(2, 66) = .80$, $P = .45$, $\eta^2 = .02$.

7.2.3. Spatial Language Cues. As Figure 7 shows, children tended to search in the middle more often if they heard the "middle" search cue. Thirty-nine percent of the children in the control condition compared to 61% of the children in the "middle" condition searched in the middle. A chi-square measuring the number of children who searched in the middle of the expanded array versus the number of children who did not search in the middle by condition found the difference to be marginally significant, $\chi^2(2, n = 72) = 2.72$, $P = .09$. The distance that children searched from the center of the landmark array did not significantly differ according to whether children heard "middle" (M = 8.94, SD = 8.63) or control (M = 12.44, SD = 11.77) language cues, $F(1, 70) = 2.07$, $P = .15$, $\eta^2 = .03$.

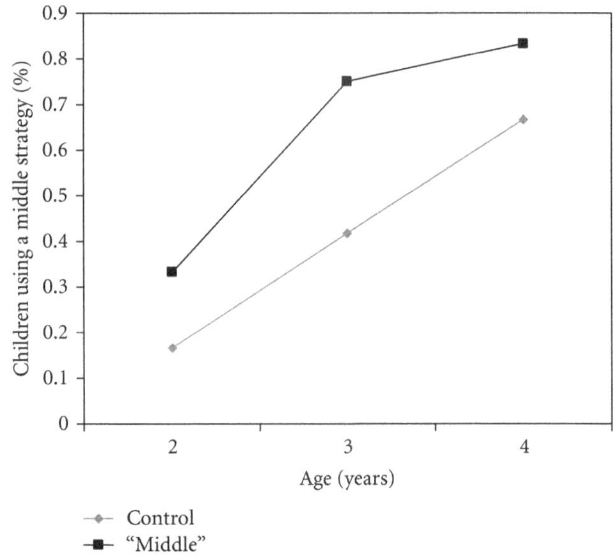

FIGURE 7: Experiment 2—children's search locations by age and language condition.

7.2.4. Spatial Language Comprehension. Most of the children in this study (68%) were reported to comprehend and produce the term "middle." However, parent reports reflected that children's knowledge of the term "middle" increased with age, $\chi^2(2, n = 72) = 24.6$, $P = .00$. According to parent reports, 38% of two-year olds, 88% of three-year olds, and 96% of four-year olds understood or produced the term. Children reported by parents to understand the term "middle" scored an average of 5.17 correct (SD = 1.23) on the middle comprehension test, whereas children reported not to understand the term averaged 2.42 correct (SD = 1.5). An ANOVA revealed that this difference was statistically significant. Parent reports of children's comprehension of the term "middle" were significantly related to children's scores on the forced-choice middle comprehension test, $F(1, 69) = 11.78$, $P = .00$, $\eta^2 = .15$.

Analysis showed that children's comprehension of the term "middle" was related to children's search behavior. Children's scores on the forced-choice middle comprehension test were significantly related to children's tendency to use middle search behavior, $F(1, 69) = 4.25$, $P = .04$, $\eta^2 = .06$. Children who searched in the middle had an average score of 4.95 (SD = 1.68) on the comprehension test, whereas children who did not search in the middle had an average score of 3.85 (SD = 1.75). Comprehension test scores were also negatively correlated with children's search distance ($r = -.27$, $P = .02$), such that children who scored higher on

TABLE 1: Experiment 1—children's "Middle" comprehension and search location by age.

Child's age (in years)	Parent reported "Middle" comprehension	Searched in middle	Searched in corner	Searched in other location
2	40%	40%	20%	40%
3	89%	56%	0%	44%
4	100%	86%	0%	14%
5	100%	56%	11%	33%
6	100%	100%	0%	0%

TABLE 2: Experiment 2—children's "Middle" comprehension and search location by age.

Child's age (years)	Parent reported "Middle" comprehension	"Middle" comprehension test score	Searched in middle	Searched in corner	Searched in other location
2	38%	47%	25%	29%	46%
3	88%	81%	54%	13%	33%
4	96%	95%	79%	4%	17%

the comprehension test tended to search closer to the center of the landmark array. Comprehension test scores were also related to age, $F(2, 69) = 30.69$, $P = .00$, $\eta^2 = .47$, such that children scored higher as a function of age. Post hoc tests (Tukey's HSD) revealed that scores of two-year olds ($M = 2.79$, SD = 1.5) were significantly lower than those of both three-year olds ($M = 4.88$, SD = 1.57, $P < .01$), and four-year olds ($M = 5.7$, SD = .63, $P < .01$). Scores of three- and four-year old children were only marginally statistically different from one another ($P = .09$). Because we tested children on their ability to identify the middle relation in arrays of both three and five objects, we analyzed whether the number of objects pictured influenced children's performance. A paired-samples t-test revealed that there was no difference in children's ability to identify the middle relation in arrays of three ($M = 2.24$, SD = .96) versus five objects ($M = 2.2$, SD = 1), $t = .43$.

Parent reports of children's comprehension were significantly related to children's search distance from the center of the array ($F(1, 70) = 6.40$, $P = .01$, $\eta^2 = .08$), but not significantly related to children's tendency to search in the middle region of the landmark array, ($\chi^2(2, n = 72) = 2.63$, $P = .10$). Children searched significantly closer to the middle when parents indicated knowledge of "middle."

Finally, two children in Experiment 2 spontaneously uttered the word "middle" during the course of the task. Both of those children met criteria for using a middle-search strategy.

8. General Discussion

Across two studies, we demonstrated that comprehension of spatial language and spatial language cues provided during the course of a spatial search task were related to children's ability to detect and use spatial relations. Our results revealed that spatial language cues for the middle relation may be particularly helpful to children between the ages of two and four years old, during the same years in which we found children's knowledge of the word "middle" to undergo the most growth. Children's ability to use the middle relation was also related to their comprehension of the associated spatial relational term "middle." Our findings contribute to current literature by showing that spatial language influences children's ability to use landmarks relationally when alternative ways of solving a search task are possible.

It could be argued that our participants searched in the middle of the landmark array simply because children are biased to search in the middle of a continuous space or because the middle location represents the central tendency [44]. If children's attention was drawn toward the center because of some natural tendency unrelated to comprehension of the middle relation, however, then all children would have searched in the center regardless of their comprehension of the term "middle" or the type of language they heard during the course of the study. This was not the case; we found that children's tendency to search in the center of the landmark array was significantly related to children's spatial language comprehension and marginally related to spatial language cues. Thus, it appears that children's middle searches were not random.

Nonhuman species, including pigeons [20], gerbils [18], and marmoset monkeys [16], consistently use the distance and direction from a single landmark to solve this task (i.e., corner search). Research shows that children begin to use single landmarks before they use multiple landmarks relationally [2, 15]. This trajectory of landmark use is in line with Gentner's [11] description of the "relational shift" wherein children initially rely on simple strategies before they develop the ability to act on complex relational information. We did not, however, observe this course of development in the current task—that is, there was no tendency for younger children to use a single landmark. Instead, children who did not search in the middle of the landmark array tended to search at some other location inside the imaginary boundary created by the array of landmarks. In fact, children only rarely used a corner strategy in this task, suggesting that young children did not favor using a single landmark over using multiple landmarks despite the fact that both methods of solving the task were possible. We suggest two possible explanations for why we did not observe a relational shift in children's landmark use. First, children's searches may have been imprecise. According to the stringent criteria used in this task, children's initial hand placement in the sand must have been within a fairly small region to count as a middle or corner search. Second, the majority of children in the current studies were reported by parents to understand the word "middle," including 40% of two-year olds. To further examine whether children initially prefer a single landmark strategy, future research should investigate children's multiple landmark use prior to two years old.

8.1. Spatial Language Comprehension. Research in other domains has revealed a temporal link between children's emerging skills and related vocabulary growth [26, 27, 33]. The current studies also reveal a temporal link between children's ability to use the middle spatial relation and the development of related spatial language. That is, children's search behavior was related to children's comprehension of the spatial term "middle." Searching in the middle of the landmark array was significantly related to children's performance on a forced-choice middle comprehension task. Previous research has described an anecdotal relationship between children's comprehension of the term "middle" and children's search behavior [13, 16]. For example, MacDonald et al. [16] reported that the two children who searched closest to the center of the expanded landmark array also spontaneously uttered the term "middle" during the task. We observed similar behavior in Experiment 2, as two children who met criteria for searching in the middle of the landmark array also spontaneously said "middle." This combined with the clear link between comprehension and searching in the current studies suggests that language was affecting children's search behavior.

Although there was a relationship between children's spatial language comprehension and children's search behavior, we cannot determine the direction of the relationship from the current study. There are competing views regarding the direction of the relationship between spatial language and spatial cognition [26, 33, 45–48]. At the extreme ends of this debate, theorists argue that: (1) language is necessary for spatial category formation and language guides children's attention to relevant spatial information [26, 33], or (2) spatial information is already nonlinguistically available to children, and language simply helps to select which of many ways of carving up space the child uses as a language convention [48]. Support for the latter viewpoint is that several habituation studies have shown that even preverbal infants can be trained to identify and categorize spatial relationships [49, 50], including those not used in their native language [51, 52]. However, this is not true for all spatial categories, such as the support "on" relation [53, 54]. In cases in which spatial relations are less easily abstracted, hearing a spatial word can facilitate category acquisition. For example, when trained with the word "on", infants were successful in learning the support relation, but without the "on" label children did not learn [53], suggesting that spatial terms may be essential for forming some spatial categories. As a whole, evidence for the direction of language and thought is mixed. One possibility is that spatial language and spatial concepts develop simultaneously and are initially contextually bound such that the precise nature of the task influences the roles of language and cognition. Future research should investigate the direction of the relationship between children's "middle" comprehension and children's landmark use.

Although there was a relationship between "middle" comprehension and searching, comprehending the term "middle" did not guarantee middle search behavior. Instead, across all ages, searching in the middle appeared to lag behind comprehension of the term "middle" (see Tables 1 and 2). We offer two possible reasons. First, children may exhibit comprehension of the term "middle" in some contexts, but not others. Dissociation between comprehension of a spatial term and the ability to use the associated concept in a search task has also been found in regard to the "left/right" relation. Well after the terms "left" and "right" enter children's productive vocabularies, children continue to experience left/right confusion [55–57]. Children may exhibit similar difficulty with the word "middle," causing an inability to accurately apply the term to a spatial task even after the term has entered a child's vocabulary. Second, children may comprehend the term "middle," but fail to see its relationship to the current spatial task. Support for this claim can be found in our finding that cueing children with the term "middle" was marginally significantly related to children's ability to use the spatial relationship in this task. Experimenter-provided spatial relational language cues appeared particularly effective for younger children, ages two to four years old, the ages at which children are gaining proficiency with the word "middle." This suggests that when children are first acquiring spatial language, they may especially benefit from being prompted with associated language when performing a spatial task. This finding also adds to a growing body of research on children's categorization (see [11] for a review), showing that relational reasoning is difficult for young children but may be aided by linguistic cues.

8.2. Spatial Language Cues. Our findings regarding experimenter-provided spatial language cues provide a possible explanation for why previous studies have shown differing results regarding children's ability to use multiple landmarks [2, 13–16]. Whereas some studies show that children can use the middle relation to find a hidden object by four or five years of age [2, 15], other studies show that children at these ages do not always use a middle search strategy when other methods of solving the task are possible [16]. Situational factors, such as experimenter-provided language input, may influence children's relational reasoning. Thus, one possibility is that the multiple differences between past investigations of the middle relation (e.g., some studies used two landmarks while others used four landmarks, some studies used an open field while other studies used a small box, etc.) differentially support children's relational reasoning.

The question of how spatial language cues may have facilitated children's relational abstraction remains unanswered. It is possible that cueing children with the term "middle" may have activated children's knowledge of the spatial term "middle." In that case, the term "middle" would prove uniquely helpful to children's performance compared to any other type of language cue. Some support for this idea can be seen in Loewenstein and Gentner's [11] study of children's ability to use the middle relation to retrieve an object on the middle shelf of a set of three shelves. Their results showed that specific spatial relational terms (i.e., top, middle, bottom) were more helpful than less specific terms (i.e., in, on, under). On the other hand, the spatial relational cue provided to children in the current study may have been helpful simply because it heightened children's attention to the relationship between the landmarks and the goal. Some evidence for this account can be found in the results of Experiment 1. We found that rather than causing children to search in the corner of the landmark array, the "next to" language cue ("I'm hiding the toy *next to this one*,") may have actually led more children to search in the middle of the landmark array. This suggests that any cue that heightens children's attention to the landmark array may also heighten children's attention to the relationship between the goal and multiple landmarks, thereby facilitating middle search behavior. In that case, heightening attention in other ways, including providing a different label ("I'm hiding the toy *in the blicket*") or manipulating landmarks themselves such that their relationship to one another is highlighted (e.g., four arrows pointing toward the center) may serve the same facilitative purpose. Future research should examine these possibilities to determine *how* middle language cues influence children's ability to act on the middle relation.

9. Conclusions

In the current studies, children's comprehension of spatial language and spatial language cues provided during the search task influenced children's use of landmarks. Children's comprehension of the word "middle" was significantly related to children's ability to perform middle searches among multiple landmarks. We also found that simply hearing the spatial term "middle" once was marginally related to increased middle searches, revealing language as one way to facilitate children's ability to notice and act on spatial relations. Because even some two-year olds in this study demonstrated comprehension of the term "middle," further research should be conducted to investigate how children search among multiple landmarks prior to the acquisition of related spatial language. Although we cannot determine the direction of the relationship between children's "middle" comprehension and increased middle searches from the current studies, these findings demonstrate the strong relationship between children's spatial vocabulary development and the ability to use multiple landmarks in conjunction. With the acquisition of spatial language children become more skilled landmark users, emphasizing the central role of language in children's developing ability to reason about relations.

Acknowledgments

Support for this research was provided by NIH Grant MH066855 (A. P. Blaisdell) and Sigma Xi Grant-In-Aid of Research (A. A. Ankowski). This research was conducted following the relevant ethics guidelines for human research. The authors would like to thank the families who participated in this research and their dedicated research assistants (Bambi DeLaRosa, Diana Escobar, Ryan Holliday, Laura Hughes, Smreeti Joshi, Elaine Kim, Grace Pagunuran, Kathleen Parker, Katerina Schenke, Abby Singla, Virginia Valle, and Isha Varma) for assistance in collecting data.

References

[1] N. Newcombe and J. Huttenlocher, *Making Space: The Development of Spatiala. Representation and Reasoning*, MIT Press, Cambridge, Mass, USA, 2000.

[2] J. E. Sutton, "The development of landmark and beacon use in young children: evidence from a touchscreen search task," *Developmental Science*, vol. 9, no. 1, pp. 108–123, 2006.

[3] A. M. Hund and A. R. Naroleski, "Developmental changes in young children's spatial memory and language in relation to landmarks," *Journal of Cognition and Development*, vol. 9, no. 3, pp. 310–339, 2008.

[4] J. Loewenstein and D. Gentner, "Relational language and the development of relational mapping," *Cognitive Psychology*, vol. 50, no. 4, pp. 315–353, 2005.

[5] L. P. Acredolo and D. Evans, "Developmental changes in the effects of landmarks on infant spatial behavior," *Developmental Psychology*, vol. 16, no. 4, pp. 312–318, 1980.

[6] E. W. Bushnell, B. E. McKenzie, D. A. Lawrence, and S. Connell, "The spatial coding strategies of one-year-old infants in a locomotor search task," *Child Development*, vol. 66, no. 4, pp. 937–958, 1995.

[7] J. S. DeLoache and A. L. Brown, "Very young children's memory for the location of objects in a large-scale environment," *Child Development*, vol. 54, no. 4, pp. 888–897, 1983.

[8] A. R. Lew, K. A. Foster, H. L. Crowther, and M. Green, "Indirect landmark use at 6 months of age in a spatial orientation task," *Infant Behavior and Development*, vol. 27, no. 1, pp. 81–90, 2004.

[9] J. M. Plumert and A. M. Hawkins, "Biases in young children's communication about spatial relations: containment versus proximity," *Child Development*, vol. 72, no. 1, pp. 22–36, 2001.

[10] D. Gentner, "Why we're so smart," in *Language in Mind: Advances in the Study of Language and Thought*, D. Gentner and S. Goldin-Meadow, Eds., pp. 195–235, 2003.

[11] D. Gentner, "The development of relational category knowledge," in *Building Object Categories in Developmental Time*, L. Gershkoff-Stowe and D. H. Rakison, Eds., pp. 245–275, 2005.

[12] D. Gentner and K. Kurtz, "Relational categories," in *Categorization Inside and Outside the Lab*, W. K. Ahn, R. L. Goldstone, B. C. Love, A. B. Markman, and P. W. Wolff, Eds., pp. 151–175, APA, Washington, DC, USA, 2005.

[13] N. Simms and D. Gentner, "Spatial language and landmark use: can 3-, 4- and 5-year-olds find the middle?" in *Proceedings of the 30th Annual Conference of the Cognitive Science Society (CogSci '08)*, 2008.
[14] M. L. Spetch and M. B. Parent, "Age and sex differences in children's spatial search strategies," *Psychonomic Bulletin and Review*, vol. 13, no. 5, pp. 807–812, 2006.
[15] D. H. Uttal, L. B. Sandstrom, and N. S. Newcombe, "One hidden object, two spatial codes: young children's use of relational and vector coding," *Journal of Cognition and Development*, vol. 7, no. 4, pp. 503–525, 2006.
[16] S. E. MacDonald, M. L. Spetch, D. M. Kelly, and K. Cheng, "Strategies in landmark use by children, adults, and marmoset monkeys," *Learning and Motivation*, vol. 35, no. 4, pp. 322–347, 2004.
[17] R. Biegler, A. McGregor, and S. D. Healy, "How do animals do geometry?" *Animal Behaviour*, vol. 57, pp. F4–F8, 1998.
[18] T. S. Collett, B. A. Cartwright, and B. A. Smith, "Landmark learning and visio-spatial memories in gerbils," *Journal of Comparative Physiology*, vol. 158, pp. 835–851, 1986.
[19] A. C. Kamil and J. E. Jones, "The seed-storing corvid Clark's nutcracker learns geometric relationships among landmarks," *Nature*, vol. 390, no. 6657, pp. 276–279, 1997.
[20] M. L. Spetch, S. E. MacDonald, K. Cheng, B. A. Linkenhoker, D. M. Kelly, and S. R. Doerkson, "Use of landmark configuration in pigeons and humans: II. Generality across search tasks," *Journal of Comparative Psychology*, vol. 111, no. 1, pp. 14–24, 1997.
[21] P. Potì, P. Bartolommei, and M. Saporiti, "Landmark use by Cebus apella," *International Journal of Primatology*, vol. 26, no. 4, pp. 921–948, 2005.
[22] J. E. Sutton, A. Olthof, and W. A. Roberts, "Landmark use by squirrel monkeys (Saimiri sciureus)," *Animal Learning and Behavior*, vol. 28, no. 1, pp. 28–42, 2000.
[23] K. Cheng, "Landmark-based spatial search in honeybees. I. Use of elements and interlandmark angles," *Animal Cognition*, vol. 2, no. 2, pp. 73–78, 1999.
[24] P. C. Quinn, A. Adams, E. Kennedy, L. Shettler, and A. Wasnik, "Development of an abstract category representation for the spatial relation between in 6- to 10-month-old infants," *Developmental Psychology*, vol. 39, no. 1, pp. 151–163, 2003.
[25] P. C. Quinn, C. M. Norris, R. N. Pasko, T. M. Schmader, and C. Mash, "Formation of a categorical representation for the spatial relation between by 6- to 7-month-old infants," *Visual Cognition*, vol. 6, no. 5, pp. 569–585, 1999.
[26] S. Choi and M. Bowerman, "Learning to express motion events in English and Korean: the influence of language-specific lexicalization patterns," *Cognition*, vol. 41, no. 1–3, pp. 83–121, 1991.
[27] A. Gopnik and A. N. Meltzoff, "Relations between semantic and cognitive development in the one-word stage: the specificity hypothesis," *Child Development*, vol. 57, pp. 1040–1053, 1986.
[28] S. Choi and A. Gopnik, "Early acquisition of verbs in Korean: a cross-linguistic study," *Journal of child language*, vol. 22, no. 3, pp. 497–529, 1995.
[29] P. M. Clancy, "The acquisition of Japanese," in *The Cross-Linguistic Study of Language Acquisition*, D. S. Slobin, Ed., vol. 1 of *The Data, Vol. 2 of Theoretical Issues*, pp. 373–524, Lawrence Erlbaum Associates, Hillsdale, NJ, USA, 1985.
[30] A. Gopnik and S. Choi, "Do linguistic differences lead to cognitive differences? A cross-linguistic study of semantic and cognitive development," *First Language*, vol. 10, pp. 199–215, 1990.
[31] A. Fernald and H. Morikawa, "Common themes and cultural variations in Japanese and American mothers' speech to infants," *Child Development*, vol. 64, no. 3, pp. 637–656, 1993.
[32] A. Gopnik, S. Choi, and T. Baumberger, "Cross-linguistic differences in early semantic and cognitive development," *Cognitive Development*, vol. 11, no. 2, pp. 197–227, 1996.
[33] M. Bowerman, "The origins of children's spatial semantic categories: cognitive versus linguistic determinants," in *Rethinking Linguistic Relativity*, J. J. Gumperz and S. C. Levinson, Eds., pp. 145–176, Cambridge University Press, New York, NY, USA, 1996.
[34] M. Casasola, M. P. Wilbourn, and S. Yang, "Can English-learning toddlers acquire and generalize a novel spatial word?" *First Language*, vol. 26, no. 2, pp. 187–205, 2006.
[35] S. Choi, L. McDonough, M. Bowerman, and J. M. Mandler, "Early sensitivity to language-specific spatial categories in English and Korean," *Cognitive Development*, vol. 14, no. 2, pp. 241–268, 1999.
[36] M. T. Balaban and S. R. Waxman, "Do words facilitate object categorization in 9-month-old infants?" *Journal of Experimental Child Psychology*, vol. 64, no. 1, pp. 3–26, 1997.
[37] V. M. Sloutsky, "The role of similarity in the development of categorization," *Trends in Cognitive Sciences*, vol. 7, no. 6, pp. 246–251, 2003.
[38] V. M. Sloutsky and A. V. Fisher, "Induction and categorization in young children: a similarity-based model," *Journal of Experimental Psychology*, vol. 133, no. 2, pp. 166–188, 2004.
[39] V. M. Sloutsky and Y. F. Lo, "How much does a shared name make things similar? Part 1. Linguistic labels and the development of similarity judgment," *Developmental Psychology*, vol. 35, no. 6, pp. 1478–1492, 1999.
[40] V. M. Sloutsky and A. C. Napolitano, "Is a picture worth a thousand words? preference for auditory modality in young children," *Child Development*, vol. 74, no. 3, pp. 822–833, 2003.
[41] L. B. Smith, "Learning to recognize objects," *Psychological Science*, vol. 14, pp. 244–250, 2003.
[42] M. L. Spetch, K. Cheng, and S. E. MacDonald, "Learning the configuration of a landmark array: I. Touch-screen studies with pigeons and humans," *Journal of Comparative Psychology*, vol. 110, no. 1, pp. 55–68, 1996.
[43] J. Loewenstein and D. Gentner, "Spatial mapping in preschoolers: close comparisons facilitate far mappings," *Journal of Cognition and Development*, vol. 2, no. 2, pp. 189–219, 2001.
[44] J. Huttenlocher, L. V. Hedges, and S. Duncan, "Categories and particulars: prototype effects in estimating spatial location," *Psychological Review*, vol. 98, no. 3, pp. 352–376, 1991.
[45] "Individuation, relativity and early word learning," in *Language Acquisition and Conceptual Development*, M. Bowerman and S. Levinson, Eds., pp. 215–256, Cambridge University Press, Cambridge, UK.
[46] M. Bowerman and S. Choi, "Space under construction: language-specific spatial categorization in first language acquisition," in *Language in Mind: Advances in the Study of Language and Thought*, D. Gentner and S. Goldin-Meadow, Eds., pp. 387–427, MIT Press, Cambridge, Mass, USA, 2003.
[47] B. Landau and R. Jackendoff, "Whence and whither in spatial language and spatial cognition?" *Behavioral and Brain Sciences*, vol. 16, pp. 255–265, 1993.
[48] J. M. Mandler, "The foundations of conceptual thought in infancy," *Cognitive Development*, vol. 7, no. 3, pp. 273–285, 1992.

[49] M. Casasola, L. B. Cohen, and E. Chiarello, "Six-month-old infants' categorization of containment spatial relations," *Child Development*, vol. 74, no. 3, pp. 679–693, 2003.

[50] P. C. Quinn, M. Cummins, J. Kase, E. Martin, and S. Weissman, "Development of categorical representations for above and below spatial relations in 3- to 7-month-Old infants," *Developmental Psychology*, vol. 32, no. 5, pp. 942–950, 1996.

[51] S. J. Hespos and E. S. Spelke, "Conceptual precursors to language," *Nature*, vol. 430, no. 6998, pp. 453–456, 2004.

[52] L. McDonough, S. Choi, and J. M. Mandler, "Understanding spatial relations: flexible infants, lexical adults," *Cognitive Psychology*, vol. 46, no. 3, pp. 229–259, 2003.

[53] M. Casasola, "Can language do the driving? the effect of linguistic input on infants' categorization of support spatial relations," *Developmental Psychology*, vol. 41, no. 1, pp. 183–192, 2005.

[54] M. Casasola and L. B. Cohen, "Infant categorization of containment, support and tight-fit spatial relationships," *Developmental Science*, vol. 5, no. 2, pp. 247–264, 2002.

[55] M. C. Corballis, "Of the right and left," *Studia Psychologica*, vol. 20, pp. 91–108, 1978.

[56] M. C. Corballis, "The left right problem in psychology," *Canadian Psychologist*, vol. 15, no. 1, pp. 16–33, 1974.

[57] C. B. Fisher and L. G. Braine, "Left-right coding in children: implications for adult performance," *Bulletin of the Psychonomic Society*, vol. 20, pp. 305–307, 1982.

16

What Grasps and Holds 8-Month-Old Infants' Looking Attention? The Effects of Object Size and Depth Cues

Yu Guan and Daniela Corbetta

Department of Psychology, The University of Tennessee, Knoxville, TN 37996-0900, USA

Correspondence should be addressed to Daniela Corbetta, dcorbett@utk.edu

Academic Editor: Jeffrey W. Fagen

The current eye-tracking study explored the relative impact of object size and depth cues on 8-month-old infants' visual attention processes. A series of slides containing 3 objects of either different or same size were displayed on backgrounds with varying depth cues. The distribution of infants' first looks (a measure of initial attention switch) and infants' looking durations (a measure of sustained attention) at the objects were analyzed. Results revealed that the large objects captured infants' attention first, that is, most of the times infants directed their visual attention first to the largest object in the scene regardless of depth cues. For sustained attention, infants preferred maintaining their attention to the largest object also, but this occurred only when depth cues were present. These findings suggest that infants' initial attention response is driven mainly by object size, while infants' sustained attention is more the product of combined figure and background processing, where object sizes are perceived as a function of depth cues.

1. Introduction

Imagine a mom reading a picture book to her baby. On one page, there are two similar dogs pictured running down an alley. Based on the perspective depth cues provided on the drawing, the leading dog appears bigger and closer to the baby looking at the book, while the other dog, following behind, appears smaller and further away. Which dog will catch the baby's attention first and at which dog will the baby look longer? And what if the depth cues were changed or the sizes of the two dogs were the same? Would the infant produce the same visual attention looking patterns? In this study, we are interested in understanding how infants direct their visual attention to scenes like the one illustrated above, when objects of different sizes are presented on backgrounds with varied pictorial depth cues. In particular, we aim to understand how infants relate object size to depth cues and gain insights on how they integrate figures with their background. By studying how infants visually process information in 2D displays, we can gain better knowledge of the mechanisms underlying infants' cognitive processes.

Visual attention is a complex phenomenon that contains several underlying processes. Cohen was one of the first to examine visual attention in infants. He identified two components of visual information processing that he called "attention getting" and "attention holding" [1]. In Cohen's original 1972 study, looking behavior was assessed while infants were exposed to pairs of checkerboards with checkers varying in size and number. Cohen found that the latency of infants' first head turn toward one checkerboard was mainly determined by the size of the checkers than by their number, while the duration of looking was more determined by the number of checkers than their size. Based on these findings, Cohen suggested a two-process model of infants' visual attention: an *attention-getting* process that determines whether and how quickly infants orient to a stimulus that has been detected, and an *attention-holding* process that determines the duration that infants look at the stimulus once fixated. These two processes can be investigated separately.

Cohen's important contribution to the field of infant visual processing revealed that infants' visual attention is not a unitary, but a dual process involving different mechanisms of attention [1, 2]. Following on Cohen's footsteps, other researchers continued to investigate different types of attention. Ruff and Rothbart [3] proposed a *visuospatial orienting* response that is specific to infants' initial head and eyes orientation to a newly appearing stimulus. Such initial response is present during most of the first postnatal year of life and is dominated by an orienting/investigative system of attention. The fast maturation in all levels of this system enables infants to deploy rapidly and flexibly their visuospatial orienting abilities to objects in their surrounding from their very early age. Because this process is a fast initial visuospatial orienting response, it requires minimal information processing and is mainly driven by obvious physical features such as salience and size that can be captured easily by a first fixation.

Another component of attention called *sustained attention* is used in contexts when information requires more prolonged scrutiny and further processing [2, 3]. Sustained attention is considered more of a controlled cognitive process dedicated to directing attention to specific object features and details. As a result, this type of attention involves a more protracted voluntary selective engagement of the behavioral system. Furthermore, sustained attention is accompanied by body changes (i.e., in posture, facial expression, and body movements), physiological changes (in heart rate), and brain changes (in EEG waveforms) [4, 5]. For instance, the heart rate drops and stays low when the infant is actively directing attention to the stimulus. Also, evidence has been provided that in sustained attention infants show greater memory encoding [6]. Finally, Colombo et al. [7] suggested that looking duration is negatively correlated with cognitive performance. For instance, short looking infants are more likely to show recognition memory than long looking infants. Also, very long looking duration is not necessary associated to information processing, but rather indicates a low ability to disengage attention [8]. In sum, these studies have demonstrated that active information processing happens during sustained attention, and that this type of attention is accompanied by physiological changes such as a drop in heart rate. Sustained attention is the product of a slower process that requires longer time and more specific information processing in order to explore and combine the details of an object or a scene. This process can be captured by the looking duration and can be influenced by the richness or complexity of the elements in the scene.

In this study, we focus on two related attention processes: the initial switch in attention to a new object on a slide after the infants have already begun orienting to the novel stimulus and the duration and location of sustained attention to a particular region of the scene. We used these two attention processes to better understand how infants visually scan 2D images containing objects of different sizes displayed on backgrounds with varying pictorial depth cues. We aimed to understand whether infants can relate object size to depth cues and whether they can integrate figures with their background. Prior research has shown that object size plays an important role in capturing infant's initial attention. Cohen's study described above showing that infants first oriented to the board with wide checkers is one example of that. A similar object size effect was reported by Newman and colleagues with 3D objects [9]. These researchers presented two cylinders of different diameters to infants to test their first fixation. They found that infants preferred to shift their first fixation toward the larger cylinder. These studies, however, focused only on the effects of the size features of objects on visual attention. They did not investigate how visual attention to object size was processed in relation to background information. Thus, how infants process visual information in more complex scenes containing multiple objects of various sizes displayed on different backgrounds is fully open to speculation. This is an important question to address as our perception of objects in our surrounding takes place in a world where objects and background provide constant information essential for body orientation and action guidance. Depth cues, in particular, represent important background information in a scene, as they directly relate to objects' size perception. A number of classic studies on size perception in adults have demonstrated that size estimation is more accurate when depth cues are present. For example, Holway's and Boring's [10] classic study showed that when depth cues were progressively removed, a regression occurred in the perceived size of objects that was approaching the visual angle of the object on the retina, not the actual physical size of the object. Other studies revealed the importance of texture gradient as another important depth cue in judging object size [11–13]. Further, a study has indicated that, the more depth cues are available, the fewer adults overestimate the size of objects [14].

We know that infants also rely on pictorial depth cues to perceive object size in 2D displays, but reports show that they do so only from about 5 or 7.5 months old. Since the 1970s, Yonas and his colleagues have systematically studied infants' depth perception using stimuli displaying different pictorial depth cues [15–18]. In one study, infants were presented with two identical 3D toy dolls of the same size suspended in front of a photo of a textured background that depicted a surface receding in depth [18]. Under monocular viewing conditions, 7-month olds reached more for the apparently nearer object, while the 5-month olds did not show any reaching preference to one of the two objects. The researchers concluded that the depth cues background affected the 7-month-old infants' perception of object size but not the 5-month olds. Similar findings were observed in a longitudinal study, confirming that the emergence of sensitivity to pictorial depth cues based on texture gradients and linear perspectives occurred between 5 and 7 months of age [19].

Our interest, in this study, is to examine infants' visual attention processes in relation to stimuli containing figure and background information as in the case of object size and depth cues. Investigating such question will provide important and novel information on how infants process and integrate figures in relation to their background. To explore this research question, we examined how infants directed their visual attention to a series of slides that displayed objects varying in sizes on backgrounds containing different linear perspective depth cues. The number of objects on the slides was always three, so that object number, which was shown by Cohen [1] to affect looking duration, was controlled. Also, we chose to begin exploring this research question with 8-month-old infants because the research reviewed above clearly indicated by that age, infants are sensitive to depth cues [15–19]. Thus, this age provided us with a good starting point to measure unambiguously how object size is perceived in relation to background depth cues. Furthermore, to specifically assess the relative impact of object size and depth cues on infants' visual-attention processes, we manipulated both the object sizes and the depth cues. Some slides had three objects of different sizes and others had three objects of the same size. We also combined object size with perspective depth cues in such a way that some slides contained depth cues while others did not. Finally, we used eye-tracking to determine on which object infants directed their visual attention first (a measure of initial fixation switch following the stimulus appearance) and on which object they maintained their visual attention the longest (a measure of sustained attention). The use of an automated corneal-reflection system provided a number of advantages: first, it provided accurate information on eye gaze at a relatively high sample rate (50 Hz) and second, it allowed us to determine objectively and accurately to which object the first shift in fixation was directed and on which object looking duration was maintained for the longest. Based on the research reviewed above, we expected that the largest object size would grasp 8-month-old infants' attention first, whether depth cues would be present or absent. Thus, in the conditions when objects are varying in size, the first shift in gaze following the appearance of the slide, should go to the largest object regardless of depth cues because the largest object is the most salient stimulus on the slide. In contrast, when objects are of the same size, we expected infants' first shift in fixation to not be linked to a particular object or location. Our expectations were also that depth cues should be playing more of a role in the sustained attention process as depth cues should be interacting with object size in driving visual attention preferences. We hypothesized that when infants have more time to explore the objects in relation to their background, they should combine object size and background information such as to "hold" their looking attention on the largest object for a longer time particularly when depth cues are present. If this assumption is correct, that the presence of depth cues matters and drives looking preferences to the largest object, then, when objects are of the same size, depth cues should continue to drive infants' looking attention to the object that would appear the largest on the depth background, consistently with Yonas et al. [18] findings on the two dolls experiments. We do not expect observing these looking preferences when depth cues are absent.

2. Method

2.1. Participants. Forty infants (20 females, 20 males) aged 8 months (±7 days) participated in the study. All infants were recruited via formal recruitment mailings and follow-up phone calls. The names and addresses of the participants were obtained through a government-supplied database of births. Additional 45 infants were brought to the laboratory but were excluded from the analyses due to fussiness ($N = 22$), improper eye movement calibration ($N = 7$), or lack of useable eye-tracking data ($N = 16$). According to previous infant studies using remote eye trackers, the attrition rate can range from 33% to 59% [20–22]. Thus the 53% attrition rate in this study is consistent with other studies that relied on this technology. Among our sample that yielded useable data, 35 participants were White and 5 were African Americans. All of them were born full term, and were free of visual impairments. All parents gave consent to have their infant participate in this study and they were given a photograph of their child and a certificate of participation.

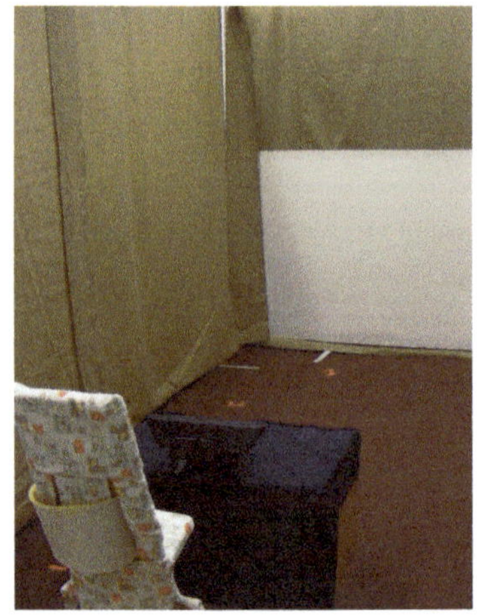

Figure 1: Experimental setup showing the infant seat, the eye-tracker, the projection screen, and the surrounding enclosure.

2.2. Materials and Stimuli. Figure 1 depicts the experimental set-up. A custom-made infant seat, reclined 10 degrees from vertical, was used to support the participants in front of the testing apparatus. A wide foam strap around their torso provided full trunk support while permitting a full range of motion of the arms and legs.

A small wooden table (64 × 38 × 38 cm, width × depth × height), supporting a remote eye-tracking device (Tobii x50, Tobii Technology, Inc., Danderyd, Sweden) was placed in front of the infant seat such that the eye tracker was located at 60 cm distance from the infant eyes. The eye-tracker used corneal reflection to record where on the slides infants directed their gaze at a frame rate of 50 Hz and with an accuracy of 0.5 degrees. A Dell 3400MP projector (Dell Inc., TX, USA), connected to a computer located in an adjacent room, was positioned under the table out of the view of the child. The projector was used to project stimuli on a large white cardboard screen (102 cm height × 151 cm width) situated at a distance of 267 cm from the participant. A speaker, connected to the same computer, was behind the projection screen.

Custom designed panels measuring 205 cm (height) × 155 cm (width) × 320 cm (length) enclosed the projection area and surrounded both the infant and the projection screen such that extraneous visual distractions were removed. The infant was seated at one end of the panel

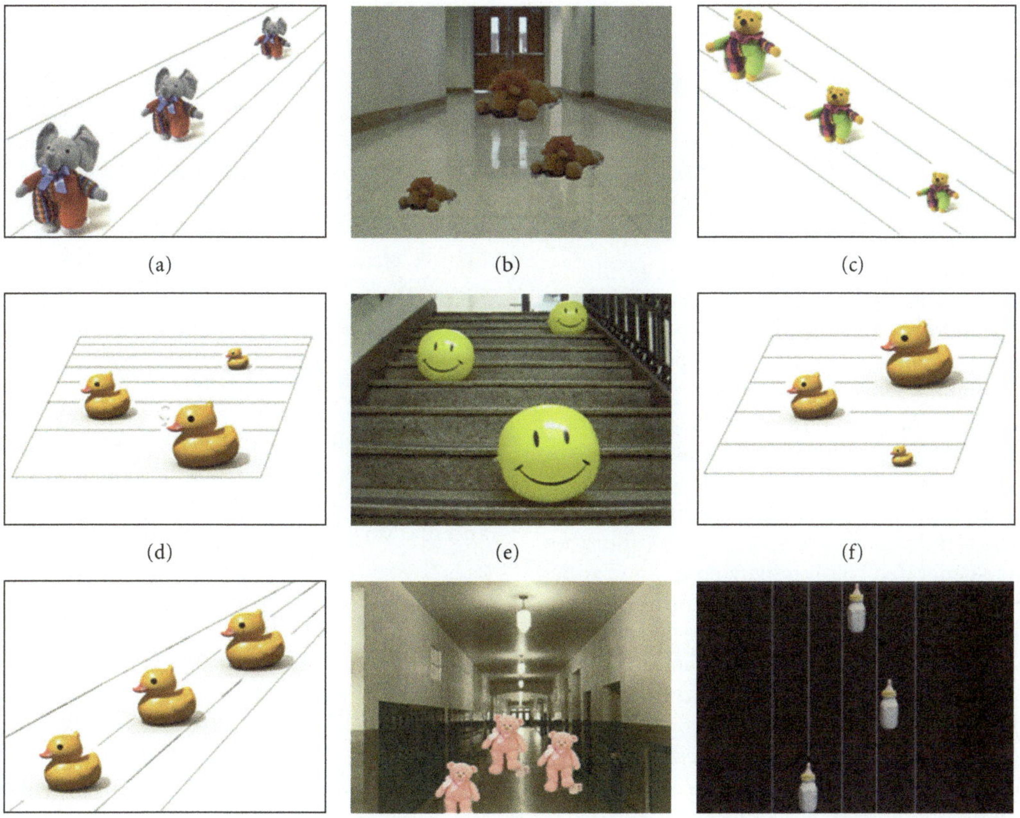

(a) (b) (c) (d) (e) (f) (g) (h) (i)

Figure 2: Example of slides used for the different conditions. (a)–(f): The 3 objects are of different sizes. (g)–(i): The 3 objects are the same sizes. Columns 1 and 2 display slide exemplars with linear pictorial depth cues and change in texture gradient for the same and different size objects conditions. Columns 3 displays slide exemplars for the no depth conditions with object of same size or different size.

enclosure and the projection screen was located at the other end.

2.2.1. Stimulus Slides. Thirty slides were used as the stimuli. Once projected on the cardboard screen, the slides were 87 cm (height) × 115 cm (width), visual angle: 20.6 degrees vertically, 27.0 degrees horizontally. The stimuli comprised five conditions which corresponded to different combinations of object size variations and depth cues.

Condition 1 (congruent depth cues) included slides that depicted scenes as infants would typically see them in the natural environment, that is, with the object sizes and depth cues being congruent with one another. Three different-size objects (large, medium, small) were scaled gradually and consistently with the background perspective depth cues. Thus, the apparent nearest object was the largest and the apparent more distant object was the smallest (see examples in Figures 2(a), 2(d), and 2(e)).

Slides in conditions 2 and 3 displayed three objects of different sizes scaled either on a background of reversed linear perspective depth cues (condition 2: reversed depth cues), such that the apparent nearest object was the smallest and the apparent furthest object was the largest (see example in Figure 2(b)), or on a background containing no depth cues (condition 3: no depth cues) so that no object appeared closer or more distant than the others based on background cues (see examples on Figures 2(c) and 2(f)).

Conditions 4 and 5 included slides that displayed three objects of the same size either arranged on a background with perspective depth cues (see examples on Figures 2(g) and 2(h)) or on a background with no depth cues (see example on Figure 2(i)).

All conditions contained a mix of real photos backgrounds and backgrounds with simple lines. The object targets were toys or other infants friendly items such as baby bottles, and the layout of the objects on the slides were also arranged in such a way that the position of certain objects (i.e., the largest object) appeared in different locations of the slides to control for directional looking biases (see Figure 2 for examples of slides used). All stimuli and overlay of the objects on the backgrounds were created in Microsoft Office PowerPoint 2003. All 30 slides were presented in a random order and for two successive rounds with a music background that was synchronized to the slide projection to help capture and maintain infants' visual attention to the slides. Each slide was projected on the screen for a 5-second duration and was immediately followed by a 2-second interslide containing a smiley face at the center of the slide displayed on a uniform black background. This intermediate slide was used to draw the infant's attention back to the center of the screen before the appearance of the next slide and to allow the researchers to monitor the continued accuracy of the eye signal throughout the entire slide show presentation.

2.3. Procedure. The participants came to the laboratory accompanied by one or two of their parents. Parents signed the consent form after they were explained the goal of the study, procedure, and their questions were answered. Then, the participants were seated in the infant seat facing the projection screen and the eye tracker. One parent was seated close to the infant, but out of his/her view.

Before the experiment started, the participant was presented with an infant video on the projection screen to capture her/his attention. When the infant was looking at the screen and the eye tracker provided a stable signal for both eyes, the video was replaced by stimuli to initiate the calibration procedure. We used a five point calibration procedure. To attract the infant's attention to each calibration point, a computer-generated colored figurine that expanded and contracted over a white background appeared on the projection screen at 5 different locations. These calibration figurines were provided by the Tobii eye-tracker software (Clearview v2.7.1). They appeared for 3 seconds at the top left, top right, bottom left, bottom right, and center of the projection screen. A calibration was considered successful if measures from at least three calibration points were obtained. Otherwise, the procedure would be repeated. The light level during the calibration and the experiment were kept constant to minimize recording errors due to differences in pupil size. The calibration procedure never lasted beyond 5 minutes. If we were unable to calibrate at least three points, the data for that participant were not used.

Once calibration was achieved, all 30 slides with inter-slides were presented to every participant on the projection screen in a random order. The entire 30 slides presentation took 3 minutes and 28 seconds to play. A second round of the same slides was presented right after the first round, thus, overall, infants saw each slide twice. No recalibration was performed between rounds. Maintenance of calibration accuracy was monitored throughout the entire experiment by checking that the infants' gaze always fell on the smiley faces during the 2-second interslides.

2.4. Data Analyses. All looking data were exported by Clearview v2.7.1 (the software provided by Tobii to run the eye-tracker and analyze the data) in three formats: videos, fixation tables, and gaze plots. We used the gaze plots and videos to identify the objects to which infants switched their visual attention first. For the looking duration analysis, we used the fixation tables.

2.4.1. Initial Attention Switch and Looking Latency to the First Object Fixated. The gaze plots on each slides revealed the order in which infants scanned and successively fixated the scenes on the slides. Because we used eye-tracking and presented a single slide stimulus (as opposed to two in prior studies) right after each interslide with a smiley face at its center, we determined the first fixation switch to the first object attended as follow. Once the stimulus slide appeared, we ignored the very first fixation point on the slide. This is because in 84.13% (sd = 1.24) of the time, the very first fixation point appeared at the center of the slide where the smiley face of the previous inter-slide was located (this very first fixation point appeared at the top of the screen only on 3.79% (sd = 0.59) of the time and at the bottom of the screen only on 2.11% (sd = 1.00) of the times). Although infants already begun orienting to the display when the stimulus slide appeared, we did not consider the very first fixation point on the stimulus slide as the product of an alert and attentive attention switching from the participant. We instead considered the very next fixation point as the infant initial attention switch to a novel object on the stimulus slide. From the gaze plots and videos, we identified the object to which that very next fixation switch was directed and we determined the time elapsed between the first fixation point and that very next object-directed attention switch (latency).

2.4.2. Sustained Attention: Looking Duration to Each of the Three Objects. The fixation table contained the looking time of each fixation as per area of interests (AOIs) defined for each slide. Each slides had 3 AOIs. Each were determined by one object surface and contour, plus an added 1 cm margin surrounding the edges of that object. The looking duration was the accumulated fixations durations within each of these AOIs. Thus, this measure provided the amount of time infants spent looking at each object individually during each 5 seconds slide presentation time.

2.4.3. Criterion for Selection of Useable Data. We only analyzed data from infants who yielded at least 3 seconds of useable eye-tracking data per slides across the two rounds. The looking durations at each object were then normalized by the total looking time at the slide.

3. Results

Our first questions were to determine (1) to which object infants initially switched their visual attention and (2) the time it took infants to direct their attention to such object (latency).

3.1. First Object Visually Attended. Figures 3(a) and 3(b) display the average proportion of times each object was first visually attended after visual attention was switched from its initial center position on the slide. Analyses were performed as a function of object group type (same size versus different sizes) and depth condition. Because these data were frequencies and did not follow a normal distribution, we performed independent non parametric repeated measures ANOVAs on ranks (Friedman tests) on the different groups and conditions to assess specifically whether one object on the slides was first attended visually more frequently than the two others.

3.1.1. Objects of Different Sizes. Figure 3(a) shows that the patterns of initial attention switch to one of the three objects

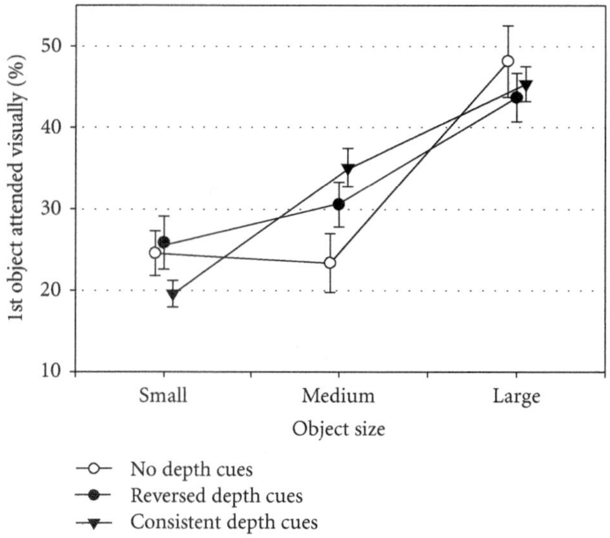

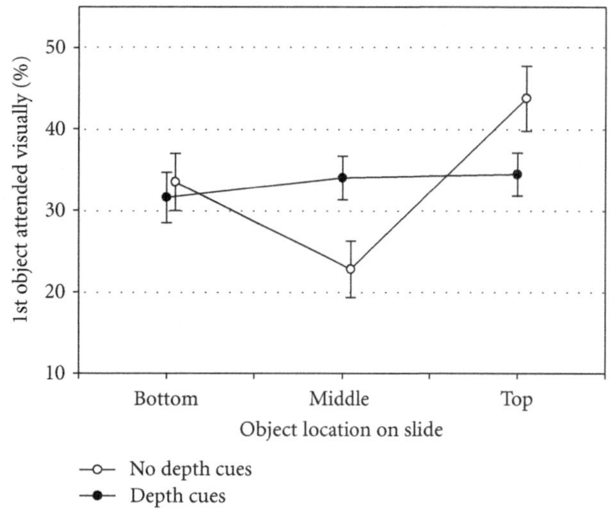

FIGURE 3: Mean percentages (and error bars) of object first visually attended plotted as a function of object type ((a) different size objects; (b) same size objects) and depth cue condition.

on the slides were scaled as a function of the sizes of the object. All infants tended to direct their gaze significantly first and most frequently to the largest object in all three different-size conditions (congruent depth cues: Friedman's $\chi^2(2) = 31.36$, P (exact) $= .0001$; reversed depth cues: Friedman's $\chi^2(2) = 10.38$, P (exact) $= .006$; no depth cues: Friedman's $\chi^2(2) = 11.14$, P (exact) $= .004$).

3.1.2. Objects of Same Sizes. When the three objects were of the same size (Figure 3(b)), only one statistical test led to significant differences in initial direction of visual attention between objects. This was for the no depth cues condition (Friedman's $\chi^2(2) = 11.31$, P (exact) $= .004$). Figure 3(b) shows that in that condition, when the slide appeared, infants initially switched their gaze more frequently to the objects located at either the top or bottom of the slides, than the object located in the middle of the slide. This result is not surprising. Since the first fixation was in most cases located at the middle of the slide and we removed it, in the absence of size differences between objects, infants were more likely to move their gaze next to one of the two other objects locations on the slide. For the depth cues condition, there was no statistical significant effect.

3.2. Latency to the First Object Visually Attended. This measure captured the time (in msec) infants took to direct their gaze from their first fixation at the center of the slide, when the slide appeared, to the first object attended. These data were averaged as a function of object size and type of depth cues. Because these data met normal distribution and equal variance, they were analyzed using repeated measures General Linear Models. When sphericity assumptions were not met, we used the P values provided by the Greenhouse-Geisser or Huynh-Feldt corrections, depending on whether the Epsilon value was greater or lower than 0.75.

3.2.1. Objects of Different Sizes. When objects on the slides were of different sizes, we ran a 3 depth cues (congruent, reversed, no depth cues) $\times$ 3 object sizes (small, medium, large) GLM with repeated measures on the depth and object size factors. Results revealed no main effects of depth cues ($F(2,76) = 2.747$, $P = .07$), or object size ($F(2,76) = 1.764$, $P = .178$) on visual latency. Overall, the average looking latency for all objects and depth cues conditions was 632 ms (sd = 34.63).

3.2.2. Objects of Same Sizes. When objects on the slides were of identical sizes, we ran a 2 depth cues (depth cues, no depth cues) $\times$ 3 object locations (bottom, middle, top) GLM with repeated measures on the depth and object location factors. Results only revealed a main effect of object location ($F(2,76) = 5.59$, $P < .005$). There was no main effect of depth cues ($F(1,38) = 0.001$, $P = .974$). Repeated measure contrasts on object location revealed that infants had greater latencies when directing their gaze to the bottom object first (764 ms) compared to latencies to the middle or top objects first (701 ms and 707 ms, resp., $P < .013$).

3.3. Looking Duration to the Different Objects. Our next question was to determine whether, after the first look at one object, accumulated visual attention was maintained toward that object or directed toward another object (measure of sustained attention). We also wanted to determine whether sustained attention to one object was modulated by background depth cues (a measure of figure/ground integration). Looking durations to each of the 3 objects on the slides were averaged by depth cues condition and were entered into 2 separate repeated measures GLMs depending on the type of object presented (same sizes versus different sizes) after verifying that the data met the requirements of normal

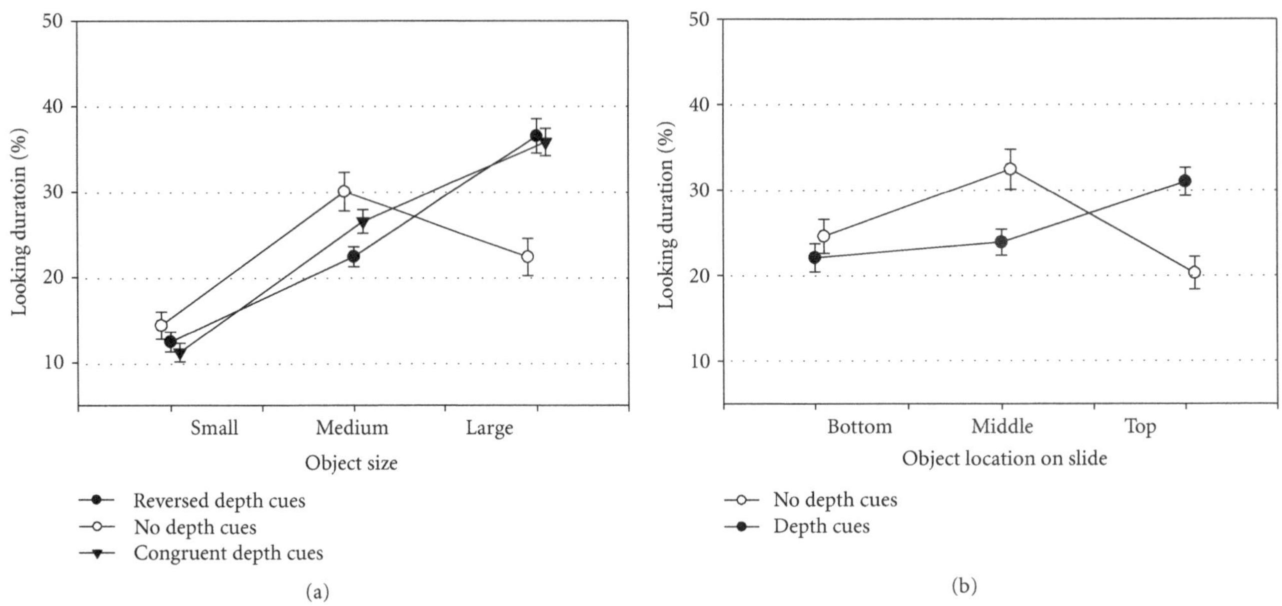

Figure 4: Mean percentages (and error bars) of looking duration on each object plotted as a function of object type ((a) different size objects; (b) same size objects), and depth cue conditions.

distribution and equal variance. Again, when sphericity assumptions were not met, we used the P values provided by the Greenhouse-Geisser or Huynh-Feldt corrections, depending to whether the Epsilon value was greater or lower than 0.75.

3.3.1. Objects of Different Sizes. A 3 depth conditions (congruent, reversed, no depth cues) × 3 object sizes (small, medium, large) GLM with repeated measures on the two last factors revealed a main effect of depth cues ($F(2,76) = 8.066$, $P < .001$), a main effect of object size ($F(2,76) = 65.082$, $P < .0001$), and a significant depth × object size interaction ($F(4,152) = 15.236$, $P < .0001$). Figure 4(a), displaying these results, shows that on average, infants looking duration increased with the size of the object attended. Pairwise comparisons revealed that infants looked significantly longer at the medium object compared to the smaller objects ($P < .0001$) and that they looked longer at the largest object compared to the medium one ($P < .002$), but this object effect was moderated by the presence or absence of depth cues ($P < .0001$). Interestingly, sustained attention to the largest object occurred only when there were depth cues in the background (congruent and reversed depth cues). When background depth cues were absent (no depth condition), infants no longer displayed sustained attention to the largest object. This result is particularly notable, because it indicates that the observed looking durations were not purely a proportional response to the size of the object attended, but rather were the combined product of attending the objects in relation to their background.

3.3.2. Objects of Same Sizes. Figure 4(b) displays the average looking duration at each object as a function of depth cues. A 2 depth conditions (depth cues, no depth cues) × 3 object locations (bottom, middle, top) GLM with repeated measures on the two last factors revealed no main effect of depth cues ($F(1,38) = .015$, $P < .905$) and no main effect of object size ($F(2,76) = 2.757$, $P < .07$), but a significant depth × object location interaction ($F(2,76) = 20.180$, $P < .0001$). As for the initial attention switch, this data show that once variations in object size were removed, infants did not display a strong looking preference for any of the objects in particular, but the significant interaction with depth cues adds an interesting twist to these results. Follow-up contrasts revealed that the significant interaction rested right in between the middle and top object. When depth cues were present, infants looked significantly longer at the top object compared to the middle object ($P < .0001$), whereas when depth cues were absent they did not. Interestingly, in the depth cues condition, the top object was the one close to the receding lines or the one located where increased texture gradient depth cues were present. This finding may suggest that infants may have spent more time looking at that object in that condition, because it may have appeared larger to them given the depth cues present. The fact that infants did not show the same looking trend in the no-depth condition suggests again that infants did not just process object and their location in their looking patterns, but integrated figure/ground information.

4. Discussion

According to Cohen's [1] and others [2–8], infants' visual attention of 2D displays contains two distinct processes. First, a visuospatial orienting response which is a fast initial orienting response that requires little information processing and is measured by the direction and latency of the first fixation. Second, sustained attention which is a slower process that requires some information processing time and is measured by looking duration. Although past research on infants' visual attention has emphasized the roles of object's properties (i.e., size) and scene complexity (i.e., object number) on these attention processes, they did not measure the individual and interrelated effects of object size and depth cues on these two processes. This is the first study assessing the roles of object size and depth cues in 8-month-old infants' orienting response and sustained attention using eye-tracking technology.

Because we used eye-tracking and therefore a method that differed from prior studies that assessed orientation and looking preference between two adjacent slides, our measure of attention orientation was more a measure of attention switching from an initial central position on the slide to a new one where an object was located. We considered that switch as our measure of first fixation. Results showed that, when the three objects were of *different sizes*, infants tended to shift their first fixation toward the largest object no matter where it was located on the slide or whether depth cues were present or not. In contrast, when the three objects were of the *same size*, infants did not reveal a significant preference in attention direction in relation to their first fixation. For the results on looking duration, when the three objects were of *different sizes*, infants spent longer time looking at the largest object on the slide, but they did this only when depth cues were provided in the background. When depth cues were absent, infants' looking preferences for the largest object or any object disappeared. Furthermore and interestingly, in the *same size* conditions, when the depth cues were provided, infants' revealed a looking preference for the object located at the converging/texture gradient receding side of the depth cues. However, again, when depth cues were absent, infants did not display such looking preference for any of the three objects.

Our results on the first fixation switch are in agreement with findings from several prior developmental studies that showed that infants usually tend to direct their visual attention first to the larger objects, because larger objects are more effective attention grabbers [1, 9]. Thus, consistent with Ruff's and Rothbart's [3] suggestion, infants in the first postnatal year will respond to object salience quickly. Such rapid visuospatial orienting response requires little information processing.

The novel aspect of this research resided mostly in extending our understanding of the sustained attention in infants' visual exploration. According to early reports of attention development during the first year, the maturation of the posterior and anterior attention systems increase infants' visual ability such that they can begin to respond to other objects properties, and not just object salience [3]. Furthermore, behavioral research has suggested that attention holding is particularly the product of information processing, and, therefore, can be directly influenced by the richness, details, or complexity of the patterns [23, 24]. For instance, Cohen's finding revealed that the number of checkers determined looking duration [1]. The more checkers were provided in the scene, the longer time infants spent looking at them because infants required longer time to process the rich information. In our study, we controlled the richness of the foreground information by providing an equal numbers of objects in all slides but we varied the depth cues background information. Interestingly, using these stimuli, our findings demonstrated that the depth information in the background can also influence infants' looking duration preferences in a dynamic way. For instance, when the slides contained objects of *different sizes*, infants' looking patterns preferences were altered depending on whether there were depth cues or not in the background. Specifically, when depth cues were present, they spent longer time looking at the largest object, but this effect dissipated when the depth cues were removed. We think this result is linked to the time infants had to explore and process the information on the slides visually. When depth cues were present in the background, they came into play in the perception process and interacted with object size information. In other words, the longer looking duration enabled infants to combine the size and depth cues information in the scene so as to hold their visual attention on one object only when depth cues were present. Yet, even though during the initial orienting response infants looked first at the largest object in the scene, we found that object size alone could not continue to hold infants' looking attention on the largest object during continued exploration of the slide. Only the interaction of both size and depth cues could hold infants' attention to that more salient object. Thus, the novelty of this study helps us further understand the sustained attention process by showing that richness and complexity of foreground patterns are not the only factors that can hold infants' visual attention. As this study shows, foreground patterns with similar richness, but placed on backgrounds containing varying depth cue information can also contribute to "hold" 8-month-old infants visual attention discriminately.

Another interesting issue that emerged from these data on looking duration concerns the possibility that infants may have been responsive to a certain kind of 2D visual illusion that involved object size and depth cues. The Ponzo illusion has been widely studied in adults and findings have shown that linear perspective depth cues in the background have a powerful effect on size perception. In the Ponzo illusion, two rods of the same size are scaled with linear perspective depth cues, the rod on the converging sides (usually on the top part of the slide) looks larger because the scaling mechanism corrects for the apparently increased depth [25]. In this study, the same object size condition with depth cues background created a similar Ponzo illusion visual effect, that is, the object that was located at the converging/receding side of lines/texture gradient could have been perceived to be larger than the other two objects (see Figures 2(g) and 2(h)). When infants were presented with these particular types of slides (objects same size with background depth cues), we found that their fixation time was longer on the object that was located on the converging texture gradient receding side of the depth cues. In contrast, when depth cues were absent (object size was still the same), infants did not show any looking preference for any given object. These findings share some similarities to the way adults perceive the Ponzo illusion. Although adult research has indicated that the

Ponzo illusion has a powerful effect on adults' perception of size, no developmental study so far has investigated this effect with infants. We believe the findings from this study may provide the first evidence that infants as young as 8-month old can respond to such illusion. The fact that they spent more time looking at the object that should appear larger in the illusion could suggest that they were able to detect the effects created by the depth cues on the object size.

An alternate possible explanation for this particular finding in the same object size condition could be that infants examined more the object near the greater gradient receding lines when depth cues were present because that area contained more information and therefore was more complex to explore. To investigate that possibility, we examined whether infants spent some time looking at the background lines surrounding the different objects on the slides. First, we found that infants hardly explored the lines on the slides background; they spent most of their looking time on the objects *per se*, not the background. Second, their little exploration of the lines was no greater at their receding point than at any other locations on the slides. This suggests that background depth cues were not processed by the infants through the direct perception of the specific depth cues provided on the slides (i.e., lines and other cues) but rather were gathered peripherally as they were directing their attention on the object targets. A recent study has demonstrated indeed that infants are capable of processing peripheral information even when their visual attention is attracted to somewhere else in the visual filed neighborhood [26]. The results of this analysis on the amount of looking directed specifically at the background lines would lead us to infer again, that infants possibly directed greater attention to the top object when objects were of the same size and depth cues were provided because that object may have appeared larger due to the Ponzo illusion, and not necessarily because there was more information to explore in that area of the slide in that condition. But more investigations will be necessary to examine this issue more in depth.

We used 8-month-old infants in this study mainly because previous literature demonstrated that infants become sensitive to pictorial depth cues between 5 to 7.5 months old [15–19]. Thus, the age of 8-month old provided us with a good starting point to measure unambiguously how object size is perceived in relation to background depth cues. And as we expected, infants of this age group were able to combine depth cues information with object size so that their attention was "held" longer by the depth cues on the largest object. In future studies, we are planning to investigate these effects with younger infants to establish the developmental trajectory of these orienting responses and looking durations to figure-ground perception. Particularly, we are interested in assessing whether depth cues will lead to similar looking trends in younger infants and whether younger-aged infants can also show some form of sensitivity to what might be the Ponzo illusion. We speculate that infants younger than 4-month old might not be able to fully integrate figure/ground perception and thus may not respond differentially to the varied pictorial depth cues as the 8 months old in this study did. In addition, infants aged between 5 and 7.5 month might show some variations in their responses to depth cues since this is a transition period in the development of sensitivity to pictorial depth cues. But on average, we anticipate that the influence of the depth cues on object size during sustained attention should become progressively stronger during the first year of life as a result of infants' increased information processing ability.

In conclusion, this research expanded our understanding of infants' initial attention direction and sustained attention when processing a scene visually. We have shown that these attention processes go beyond object salience and complexity and apply to figure/ground perception. We also have shown that 8-month-old infants are well capable of integrating and combining efficiently the foreground and background elements of a scene. Indeed, in our task, infants responded differentially to our 2D picture stimuli depending on whether objects had similar or different sizes but also, and more importantly, whether the background depth cues were present or not.

References

[1] L. B. Cohen, "Attention-getting and attention-holding processes of infant visual preferences," *Child Development*, vol. 43, no. 3, pp. 869–879, 1972.

[2] J. E. Richards, "Infant attention, arousal, and the brain," in *Infant Perception and Cognition: Recent Advances, Emerging Theories, and Future Directions*, L. M. Oakes, C. Cashon, M. Casasola, and D. H. Rakison, Eds., Oxford University Press, New York, NY, USA, 2011.

[3] H. A. Ruff and M. K. Rothbart, *Attention in Early Development: Themes and Variations*, Oxford University Press, New York, NY, USA, 2001.

[4] J. E. Richards and B. J. Casey, "Development of sustained visual attention in the human infant," in *Attention and Information Processing in Infants and Adults*, B. A. Campbell, H. Hayne, and R. Richardson, Eds., Lawrence Erlbaum Associates Press, Hillsdale, NJ, USA, 1992.

[5] G. D. Reynolds and J. E. Richards, "Infant heart rate: a developmental psychophysical perspective," in *Developmental Psychophysiology: Theory, Systems, and Applications*, L. A. Schmidt and S. J. Segalowitz, Eds., Cambridge University Press, Cambridge, UK, 2007.

[6] J. E. Richards, G. D. Reynolds, and M. L. Courage, "The neural bases of infant attention," *Current Directions in Psychological Science*, vol. 19, no. 1, pp. 41–46, 2010.

[7] J. Colombo, D. W. Mitchell, J. T. Coldren, and L. J. Freeseman, "Individual differences in infant visual attention: are short lookers faster processors or feature processors?" *Child Development*, vol. 62, no. 6, pp. 1247–1257, 1991.

[8] J. Colombo, "On the neural mechanisms underlying individual differences in infant fixation duration: two hypotheses," *Developmental Review*, vol. 15, no. 2, pp. 97–135, 1995.

[9] C. Newman, J. Atkinson, and O. Braddick, "The development of reaching and looking preferences in infants to objects of different sizes," *Developmental Psychology*, vol. 37, no. 4, pp. 561–572, 2001.

[10] A. H. Holway and E. G. Boring, "Determinants of apparent visual size with distance variant," *The American Journal of Psychology*, vol. 54, pp. 21–37, 1941.

[11] J. C. Hull, R. T. Gill, and S. N. Roscoe, "Locus of the stimulus to visual accommodation: where in the world, or where in the eye?" *Human Factors*, vol. 24, no. 3, pp. 311–319, 1982.

[12] J. H. Iavecchia, H. P. Iavecchia, and S. N. Roscoe, "The moon illusion revisited," *Aviation Space and Environmental Medicine*, vol. 54, no. 1, pp. 39–46, 1983.

[13] L. Kaufman and I. Rock, "The moon illusion, I," *Science*, vol. 136, no. 3520, pp. 953–961, 1962.

[14] J. W. Meehan and T. J. Triggs, "Magnification effects with imaging displays depend on scene content and viewing condition," *Human Factors: The Journal of the Human Factors and Ergonomics Society*, vol. 30, pp. 487–494, 1988.

[15] A. Yonas, W. T. Cleaves, and L. Pettersen, "Development of sensitivity to pictorial depth," *Science*, vol. 200, no. 4337, pp. 77–79, 1978.

[16] A. Yonas, L. Pettersen, and C. E. Granrud, "Infants' sensitivity to familiar size as information for distance," *Child Development*, vol. 53, no. 5, pp. 1285–1290, 1982.

[17] C. E. Granrud, A. Yonas, and L. Pettersen, "A comparison of monocular and binocular depth perception in 5- and 7-month-old infants," *Journal of Experimental Child Psychology*, vol. 38, no. 1, pp. 19–32, 1984.

[18] A. Yonas, C. E. Granrud, M. E. Arterberry, and B. L. Hanson, "Infants' distance perception from linear perspective and texture gradients," *Infant Behavior and Development*, vol. 9, no. 3, pp. 247–256, 1986.

[19] A. Yonas, C. A. Elieff, and M. E. Arterberry, "Emergence of sensitivity to pictorial depth cues: charting development in individual infants," *Infant Behavior and Development*, vol. 25, no. 4, pp. 495–514, 2002.

[20] D. Amso and S. P. Johnson, "Learning by selection: visual search and object perception in young infants," *Developmental Psychology*, vol. 42, no. 6, pp. 1236–1245, 2006.

[21] D. Corbetta, Y. Guan, and J. L. Williams, "Infant eye-tracking in the context of goal-directed actions," *Infancy*, vol. 17, no. 1, pp. 102–125, 2012.

[22] P. C. Quinn, M. M. Doran, J. E. Reiss, and J. E. Hoffman, "Time course of visual attention in infant categorization of cats versus dogs: evidence for a head bias as revealed through eye tracking," *Child Development*, vol. 80, no. 1, pp. 151–161, 2009.

[23] M. L. Courage, G. D. Reynolds, and J. E. Richards, "Infants' attention to patterned stimuli: developmental change from 3 to 12 months of age," *Child Development*, vol. 77, no. 3, pp. 680–695, 2006.

[24] L. B. Cohen, J. S. DeLoache, and M. W. Rissman, "The effect of stimulus complexity on infant visual attention and habituation," *Child Development*, vol. 46, no. 3, pp. 611–617, 1975.

[25] H. W. Leibowitz and H. A. Pick, "Cross-cultural and educational aspects of the Ponzo perspective illusion," *Perception & Psychophysics*, vol. 12, no. 5, pp. 430–432, 1972.

[26] F. Farzin, S. M. Rivera, and D. Whitney, "Spatial resolution of conscious visual perception in infants," *Psychological Science*, vol. 21, no. 10, pp. 1502–1509, 2010.

17

Children's Use of Arithmetic Shortcuts: The Role of Attitudes in Strategy Choice

Katherine M. Robinson and Adam K. Dubé

Department of Psychology Campion College at the University of Regina, 3737 Wascana Parkway, Regina, SK, Canada S4S 0A2

Correspondence should be addressed to Katherine M. Robinson, katherine.robinson@uregina.ca

Academic Editor: Ann Dowker

Current models of strategy choice do not account for children's attitudes towards different problem solving strategies. Grade 2, 3, and 4 students solved three sets of three-term addition problems. On inversion problems (e.g., $4 + 8 - 8$), if children understand the inverse relation between the operations, no calculations are required. On associativity problems (e.g., $5 + 27 - 23$), if children understand the associative relation between the operations, problem solving can be facilitated by performing subtraction before addition. A brief intervention involving demonstrations of different problem solving strategies followed the first problem set. Shortcut use increased after the intervention, particularly for students who preferred shortcuts to the left-to-right algorithm. In the third set, children were given transfer problems (e.g., $8 + 4 - 8$, $4 - 8 + 8$, $27 + 5 - 23$). Shortcut use was similar to first set suggesting that transfer did occur. That shortcut use increased the most for students who had positive attitudes about the shortcuts suggests that attitudes have important implications for subsequent arithmetic performance.

1. Children's Use of Arithmetic: The Role of Preference in Strategy Choice

Children's understanding of the relations between addition and subtraction is considered integral for later mathematical skills [1]. Part of the research agenda needs to understand and account for the large individual differences in children's conceptual knowledge [2]. While many researchers have focussed on factors such as general mathematics skills [3] or working memory [4] to account for individual differences in understanding the relationship between addition and subtraction, one overlooked factor may be students' attitudes and beliefs towards mathematics. Attitudes are positive or negative evaluations (e.g., "I like addition") and beliefs are "thoughts" based on experience (e.g., "division is difficult") [5] and both are considered to be integral in determining success in mathematics [6]. These attitudes and beliefs could be integral in the conceptual knowledge that children use and understand when making problem solving strategy choices.

Researchers have often considered children's use of the inversion shortcut strategy on inversion problems of the form $a + b - b$ as an indicator of understanding of the inverse relation between the two operations [3]. The inversion shortcut involves stating that the answer is a without performing any calculations as the two b terms cancel each other out. Children's understanding of the relationship between addition and subtraction can also be assessed via children's use of the associativity shortcut on problems of the form $a + b - c$, which were originally included in studies of children's inversion as control problems [7]. When children understand that addition and subtraction are associative, they can use that information to simplify and speed up problem solving by first subtracting and then adding (e.g., $3 + 29 - 27$ would be solved by calculating $29 - 27$ and then adding 3) [4]. Both inversion and associativity three-term problems are novel and therefore children must implement spontaneous problem solving strategies [8]. Researchers have taken advantage of this novelty to gain an understanding of children's knowledge of the relations between addition and subtraction by utilizing children's use of conceptually-based shortcuts as an indicator of conceptual understanding because understanding the inverse or associative relations between addition and subtraction is required to implement the inversion and associativity shortcuts [9].

Given the importance of understanding the relations between addition and subtraction, some studies have gone beyond assessing children's spontaneous use or evaluation of the inversion shortcut by trying to promote conceptually-based shortcut use focussing exclusively on inversion problems. In these studies, 8-year-old children's conceptual understanding of the inverse relation between addition and subtraction, as assessed via shortcut use, increased after either 2 or 3 training sessions with concrete objects [10, 11] or after repeated weekly exposure to inversion problems [12].

A possible alternative to the longer interventions used in previous studies comes from a study with Grade 2, 3, and 4 students by Robinson and Dubé [13] who asked children to solve inversion and associativity problems and then had the children complete an evaluation of procedures task [9] as a second measure of conceptual understanding. In the task, for both inversion and associativity problems, the shortcut and a standard left-to-right algorithm (i.e., adding the first two numbers and then subtracting the third number) were demonstrated to participants and participants were asked if they approved of each approach. Bisanz et al. [9] argued that the evaluation of procedures task is a good measure of conceptual understanding as it permits children to demonstrate their understanding which they may have implemented during problem solving. However, in an earlier pilot study, we found that participants were very likely to approve of both the shortcut and the left-to-right algorithm for both inversion and associativity and thus a more stringent measure was needed. To gain more useful information about children's understanding of arithmetic concepts, the participants in Robinson and Dubé [13] were also asked to compare the two solution procedures for each problem type and decide which was better and why. Explicitly justifying a strategy suggests conceptual understanding because the ability to justify typically develops after the ability to assess a strategy's worth and even use the strategy during problem solving [14]. Robinson and Dubé [13] found that most of the participants (80% or more) approved of both the shortcut and the left-to-right procedure for both the inversion and associativity problems. The more stringent measure of choosing the better strategy was more sensitive as a clear majority of participants preferred the shortcut to the left-to-right algorithm for inversion problems (78%) but not for associativity problems (59%) with older students in Grades 3 and 4 more likely to prefer the associativity shortcut. Effects of the evaluation of procedures task on subsequent problem solving were not examined in that study.

The study by Robinson and Dubé [13] provided two conclusions regarding strategy instruction and attitudes about problem solving strategies. The first conclusion is that the children had distinctly positive or negative attitudes about the appropriateness of the shortcuts. For example, some participants commented on the cleverness of the shortcuts (e.g., "that's so easy, I wish I'd thought of doing it that way" while others strongly disapproved of the shortcuts "e.g., it's cheating not to do all the math"). This variability in attitudes across individuals suggests that some children may be open and flexible about learning new ways to problem solve while others may be rigid and inflexible. For example, across a series of studies, Torbeyns and colleagues [15–17] have shown that children are often resistant to using a more efficient arithmetic strategy, even when explicitly encouraged and/or instructed to use that strategy. Previous research has suggested that children's attitudes and beliefs about mathematics are critical to success in mathematics and to enrollment in advanced mathematics courses and therefore engaging children with mathematics is of critical importance [18]. During schooling, children begin to have strong attitudes and beliefs about mathematics [19]. Children who are intrinsically motivated [20], are mastery-oriented [21] or who have low levels of mathematics anxiety [22], are more likely to be successful in mathematics. Other factors relating to mathematics success include the role of peer pressure [23] and disengagement [24].

Although several studies have investigated children's attitudes and beliefs about mathematics, few studies have investigated children's attitudes about specific problem solving strategies. Ellis [25] and Verschaffel et al. [26] note that much of the research on the factors involved in children's strategy choices has focussed on the roles of speed and accuracy and has ignored other factors such as individual and sociocultural influences. The findings of Robinson and Dubé [13] suggest that children's attitudes towards the use of problem solving strategies that involve simplifying and reducing solution times are already entrenched by Grade 2 and that these attitudes may become even more firmly held by the end of the middle school years [27]. Current models of children's strategy choices emphasize the tendency for children to want to use the most efficient problem solving strategies [28, 29] and yet the findings of Robinson and Dubé [13] support Ellis' and Verschaffel et al.'s [26] proposal that other factors, in this case attitudes, may also impact strategy choices.

The second conclusion drawn from Robinson and Dubé [13] was that comparison of problem solving strategies yielded more information about children's understanding of arithmetic concepts than only asking them to evaluate strategies. Research on comparison of solution methods has been encouraging as it appears to be an effective learning tool [30–32]. In two studies, participants in Grades 7 and/or 8 were given the opportunity to compare different solution methods for solving algebraic equations [30, 31] and in Star and Rittle-Johnson [32], participants in Grades 5 and 6 compared different solution methods for computational estimation. In all of the studies, the opportunity to compare different methods led to greater increases in procedural and conceptual knowledge than simply being presented with different methods. None of the studies examined whether there were developmental changes in the effectiveness of comparison and no studies of the effects of comparison have been conducted with younger students. Extending the use of comparisons even further, Yakes and Star [33] found that teachers who participated in a workshop on how to use comparison as an instructional tool for teaching algebra changed their teaching practices. The teachers used comparison of different solution methods as a teaching tool and also began to recognize and emphasize the importance of procedural flexibility in their teaching.

Based on the findings of Robinson and Dubé [13] that there are marked individual differences in children's attitudes about the inversion and associativity shortcuts and that presenting solution methods concurrently improves comparison and is a useful learning technique for older children (e.g., [30, 31]), the first two goals of this study were to determine whether children's attitudes about the solution methods they were asked to evaluate would impact subsequent problem solving strategies and to examine whether presenting solution methods concurrently improves comparison and is an effective learning tool on inversion and associativity problems. The final two goals of the study were to examine whether attitudes and the impact of comparison would change across development and to assess the strength of the intervention task by investigating whether children would transfer their new knowledge about the shortcuts to transfer problems. When concepts such as inversion or associativity are effectively learned, then that knowledge should be applicable or transferable to new problem types [34]. Rittle-Johnson and Star [30, 31] found that comparison of solution methods promoted flexibility and Rittle-Johnson [35] proposed that explaining why a procedure works is an effective learning tool and can result in the ability to transfer knowledge to new situations. Children do not necessarily understand a concept that has been taught to them but the ability to generalize a problem-solving strategy based on conceptual knowledge is an indicator that learning of that concept has occurred [36].

2. Method

2.1. Participants. Twenty-four Grade 2 students (12 boys, 12 girls) (mean age = 7 years, 0 months), thirty-five Grade 3 students (14 boys, 21 girls) (mean age = 7 years, 11 months), and forty-three Grade 4 students (20 boys, 23 girls) (mean age = 8 years, 10 months) participated in the study. The age groups were selected to correspond with previous research [13] and to correspond to the time in which children are learning about addition and subtraction [18]. Participants were from a large Canadian city, were predominantly Caucasian, and from middle SES families. The study took place in the first half of the school year.

2.2. Design and Intervention. The same pretest-intervention-posttest design was used as in the studies by Rittle-Johnson and Star [30, 31] but the participants were tested individually throughout the study rather than being paired up for the intervention, and the posttest was divided into the first posttest with familiar problems and a second posttest with transfer problems to assess strength of learning from the intervention. Half the students per grade were randomly assigned to either the sequential condition ($n = 51$) or the concurrent condition ($n = 51$). The intervention was the evaluation of procedures task. For both inversion and associativity problems, two strategies were demonstrated. In the sequential group, for each problem type: (1) the first strategy was demonstrated and then participants were asked if they approved of the strategy; (2) the second strategy was demonstrated and then participants were asked if they approved of the second strategy; (3) participants were asked which of the two strategies they preferred. In the concurrent group, for each problem type: (1) both strategies were demonstrated consecutively; (2) participants were asked if they approved of both strategies at the same time; (3) participants were asked which of the two strategies they preferred. Problem type and strategy orders were counterbalanced across boys and girls as closely as possible within each grade. For the inversion problems, on one problem, participants were told how a fictitious child had solved the problem by using the inversion shortcut ("When X solved this problem, s/he said that the answer would be the first number because when you add and subtract by the same number, the answer is always the first number"). On the other problem, participants were told how a fictitious child had solved the problem using a left-to-right algorithmic approach ("When X solved this problem, she/he added the first two numbers together and then subtracted the third number from that answer"). For the associativity problems, on one problem, participants were told how a fictitious child had solved the problem by using the associativity shortcut ("When X solved this problem, she/he subtracted the third number from the second number and then took the answer and added it to the first number"). On the other problem, the same left-to-right algorithmic approach used on the inversion problem was used again.

2.3. Materials and Procedure. There were three sessions, which took place within a 7 day period with at least one day between each session. In the first session which was the pretest, participants solved 16 three-term addition and subtraction problems. Half the problems were inversion problems of the form $a + b - b$ and half were associativity problems of the form $a+b-c$. Half the problems of each type were small ($a, b, c < 10$) (e.g., $3+6-6$ and $3+6-4$) and half were large ($a < 10, b$ and c between 21 and 29, $b > c$) (e.g., $7+23-23$ and $7+23-21$). No more than two problems of each type or each size were presented consecutively. Problems were presented on a laptop screen using e-prime. Participants did not have the aid of paper and pencil. Solution latencies (measured from the time the problem appeared on the screen until the participant stated the answer and pressed the space bar), accuracy, and immediately retrospective verbal reports of problem solving strategy (i.e., "how did you solve that problem?") were collected for each problem. Participants who were unable to provide an answer within 30 seconds were given a "cut-off protocol" in which they were asked to report how they were trying to solve the problem before moving on to the next problem. Cut-off problems were coded as incorrect and no solution latencies were recorded.

In the second session which was the intervention and first posttest session, participants were randomly assigned to the concurrent or sequential conditions and completed the evaluation of procedures task and then solved the first posttest of a new set of 16 three-term addition and subtraction problems. The same measures and the same problem parameters were used as in the first session.

In the third session which was the second posttest session, participants solved 16 novel transfer problems. Half of the problems were inversion problems and the other half were associativity problems using the same parameters and measures as in the first and second sessions except that half of the inversion problems were of the form $b + a - b$ (e.g., 4 + 9 − 4) and half of the form $a - b + b$ (e.g., 7 − 23 + 23) and the associativity problems were of the form $b + a - c$ (e.g., 28 + 6 − 25).

3. Results

Data from boys and girls were collapsed together as no significant results involving gender were found. Tukey's Honestly Significant Difference test was used to examine post-hoc effects and the alpha level was .05 or less for all significant results. Analyses of verbal report data only are reported but accuracy, solution latency, and cutoff data matched expected patterns (higher accuracy, shorter solution latencies, and fewer cutoffs when shortcuts were used, see Table 1). Although differences between the concurrent and sequential conditions were expected, no differences were found (see Table 2) so the analyses reported below are all collapsed across condition. This lack of condition effect may have been a result of such a brief intervention or of the nature of the task. Both conditions included exposure to the same information and the same problems and the children in both conditions were asked to decide which strategy they preferred (the conceptually-based shortcut or the left-to-right strategy) yielding comparable data across conditions. This data allows the investigation of how children's attitudes towards different problem solving strategies impacts subsequent conceptually-based shortcut use.

3.1. Promotion of Conceptually-Based Shortcuts across Development. As can be seen in Table 3, some children were already using the inversion and associativity shortcuts in the pretest. Shortcut use between the pretest and the first posttest (familiar problems) was compared to determine if shortcut use on familiar problems increased after the evaluation of procedures task. Two separate 3 (Grade) × 2 (Size) × 2 (Session) analyses of variance were conducted on inversion and associativity shortcut use. Shortcut use increased from the pretest to the first posttest (43.6% versus 63.2% for inversion, 20.9% versus 35.9% for associativity), $F(1, 99) = 39.75$, $MSE = 929.93$, $\eta_p^2 = .29$ and $F(1, 99) = 17.43$, $MSE = 1231.66$, $\eta_p^2 = .15$ for inversion and associativity respectively. There was less shortcut use on small than large problems (50.7% versus 56.2% for inversion, 23.86% versus 32.86% for associativity), $F(1, 99) = 11.17$, $MSE = 259.68$, $\eta_p^2 = .10$ and $F(1, 99) = 15.67$, MSE = 496.78, $\eta_p^2 = .14$ for inversion and associativity respectively. For inversion, no grade differences were found (44.0%, 62.9%, and 53.5%, for Grades 2, 3, and 4) but for associativity (17.71%, 39.46%, and 27.91% for Grades 2, 3 and 4), there was more shortcut use by Grade 3 than Grade 2 students and Grade 4 students did not differ from Grade 2 or 3 students, $F(2, 99) = 3.92$, MSE = 882.88, $\eta_p^2 = .07$, and HSD = 17.7.

If the evaluation of procedures task was successful at promoting shortcut use, then participants should also use the shortcuts on the novel transfer problems in the second posttest. Shortcut use on typical problems before and after the evaluation of procedures task and shortcut use on transfer problems after the evaluation of procedures task were analyzed using two repeated measures ANOVAs. After the evaluation of procedures task, shortcuts were used less frequently on transfer problems in the second posttest than on typical problems in the first posttest (43.8% versus 65.0%, for inversion, 16.8% versus 37.6% for associativity) but were used just as frequently as shortcuts before the evaluation of procedures task (44.0% for inversion, 21.3% for associativity), $F(2, 202) = 25.68$, MSE = 588.35, $\eta_p^2 = .20$, HSD = 14.4, $F(2, 202) = 21.24$, MSE = 576.48, $\eta_p^2 = .17$, and HSD = 14.3 for inversion and associativity problems, respectively. This suggests that participants had greater difficulty applying the shortcuts to transfer problems than to typical problems after the evaluation of procedures task. However, shortcut use on the transfer problems after the intervention was the same as shortcut use on the typical problems before the intervention suggesting that the intervention may have promoted shortcut use on the transfer problems.

Shortcut use on the transfer problems in the second posttest was analyzed in greater detail to determine the effects of grade, problem size, and transfer type. For inversion problems, two types of transfer problems were possible, and a 3 (Grade) × 2 (Size) × 2 (Transfer type) ANOVA was conducted (see Figure 1). Inversion shortcut use was higher on large problems (32.7% versus 49.9% for small and large), $F(1, 99) = 34.32$, MSE = 828.65, $\eta_p^2 = .26$. There was a two-way interaction between transfer type and grade, $F(2, 99) = 5.22$, MSE = 1119.79, and $\eta_p^2 = .10$, with no grade differences on the first type of inversion transfer problem ($a - b + b$) but higher shortcut use by the Grade 4 than the Grade 2 students on the second type of transfer problem ($b+a-b$). There were no differences between transfer type in Grades 2 or 3 but in Grade 4, shortcut use was higher on the second type. This interaction was mediated by a three-way interaction between type, grade, and size, $F(2, 99) = 3.23$, MSE = 615.43, and $\eta_p^2 = .06$. There was a main effect of problem size with more shortcut use on large problems in all grades and both types of transfer problems, except for Grade 4 students who had no size difference on the first type of problem although the means were in the expected direction.

For associativity problems, a 3 (Grade) × 2 (Size) ANOVA was conducted on the transfer problems in the second posttest (see Figure 2). Associativity shortcut use was lower on small problems (12.4% versus 18.5% for small and large), $F(1, 99) = 5.89$, MSE = 303.04, and η_p^2 =.06, and there was a two-way interaction between grade and size, $F(2, 99) = 6.35$, MSE = 303.04, and $\eta_p^2 = .11$. On small problems, Grade 2 students used the associativity shortcut less frequently than the Grade 3 students, and on large problems the Grade 2 students used the shortcut less than both the Grade 3 and 4 students. There was no main effect of problem size in Grades 2 or 3, but Grade 4 participants used the shortcut more on large problems.

TABLE 1: Accuracy (%), solution latencies, and proportion of cutoffs (%) in the pretest, first posttest, and second posttest on inversion and associativity problems.

	Session 1	Session 2	Session 3
Accuracy		Inversion	
Shortcut	98.3 (2.1)	99.4 (1.7)	98.8 (2.1)
Algorithm	40.8 (2.2)	42.0 (3.0)	56.9 (2.6)
Solution latency			
Shortcut	5174 (293)	3216 (240)	4830 (298)
Algorithm	12407 (484)	114449 (646)	10346 (480)
Cutoffs			
Shortcut	1.4 (1.9)	.4 (1.6)	.9 (2.0)
Algorithm	37.0 (2.1)	36.8 (2.8)	17.2 (2.4)
Accuracy		Associativity	
Shortcut	65.0 (3.4)	76.2 (2.3)	65.0 (3.4)
Algorithm	48.8 (1.6)	47.2 (1.8)	48.8 (1.6)
Solution Latency			
Shortcut	11927 (524)	9389 (361)	10479 (585)
Algorithm	13396 (347)	12358 (373)	13359 (327)
Cutoffs			
Shortcut	16.1 (2.8)	9.1 (2.1)	10.2 (3.2)
Algorithm	33.3 (1.5)	36.3 (1.7)	28.8 (1.5)

Note. Standard errors are in parentheses.

TABLE 2: Percentage shortcut use in the pretest, first posttest (familiar problems), and second posttest (transfer problems) for the sequential and concurrent groups in each grade.

		Session					
		Pretest	1st posttest	2nd posttest	Pretest	1st posttest	2nd posttest
Grade 2	n		Inversion			Associativity	
Sequential	13	42.3 (11.1)	51.0 (11.1)	42.3 (8.6)	15.4 (8.8)	22.1 (11.1)	6.7 (4.8)
Concurrent	11	31.8 (12.0)	50.0 (12.1)	29.5 (7.3)	11.4 (8.8)	21.6 (12.1)	5.6 (3.9)
Grade 3							
Sequential	16	57.0 (10.0)	75.8 (10.0)	53.9 (10.1)	35.2 (7.2)	48.4 (10.0)	29.7 (10.0)
Concurrent	19	51.3 (9.1)	68.4 (9.2)	40.8 (7.5)	30.9 (6.7)	44.1 (9.2)	12.5 (4.8)
Grade 4							
Sequential	23	37.0 (8.3)	70.1 (8.3)	48.9 (6.3)	18.5 (6.1)	41.3 (8.3)	21.7 (5.4)
Concurrent	20	42.5 (8.9)	64.4 (9.0)	41. (7.8)	13.8 (6.5)	37.5 (8.9)	17.5 (5.5)

Note. Standard errors are in parentheses.

3.2. The Effects of Attitudes about Conceptually-Based Shortcuts across Development. In the evaluation of procedures task, participants were asked which they preferred: the shortcut or the left-to-right algorithm for both inversion and associativity problems. For inversion problems, participants were more likely to prefer the shortcut than the algorithm (71.8% versus 28.2%), $\chi^2(1, N = 103) = 19.66$, and that preference was similar across grade (58.3%, 77.1%, and 76.7% for Grades 2, 3, and 4). For associativity problems, participants, however, were not more likely to prefer the shortcut (58.3% versus 41.7%) but older children were more likely to prefer the shortcut (29.2%, 62.9%, and 72.1% for Grades 2, 3, and 4), $\chi^2(2, N = 103) = 12.08$. Thus, the success of the evaluation of procedures task may vary depending on whether participants "bought in" to the shortcuts.

To determine whether increases in shortcut use between sessions were attributable to participants "buying in" to the training provided by the evaluation of procedures task or whether they were attributable to practice or exposure effects, changes in inversion and associativity shortcut use within the pretest and the first posttest were compared to changes in shortcut use between the pretest and the first posttest using two 4 (1st half of pretest, 2nd half of pretest, 1st half of first posttest, 2nd half of first posttest) × 2 (Preference: shortcut, algorithm) ANOVAs (see Figure 3).

For inversion, shortcut use did not change within the pretest of the first posttest (34.6% versus 42.7%, 56.6% versus 58.8% for the 1st and 2nd half of the prestest and first posttest, resp.) but did increase between the 2nd half of the pretest and the first half of the first posttest, $F(3, 300)$

TABLE 3: Percentage shortcut use in the pretest and first posttest on small and large problems in each grade.

	Session	
	Pretest	First posttest
Grade 2	Inversion	
Small	37.5 (7.8)	49.0 (8.7)
Large	37.5 (8.7)	52.1 (8.2)
Grade 3		
Small	51.4 (6.4)	69.3 (7.2)
Large	56.4 (7.3)	74.3 (6.8)
Grade 4		
Small	34.3 (5.9)	62.8 (6.5)
Large	44.8 (6.5)	72.1 (6.1)
Grade 2	Associativity	
Small	11.5 (5.9)	18.8 (8.1)
Large	15.6 (7.0)	25.0 (9.0)
Grade 3		
Small	30.7 (4.9)	42.1 (6.7)
Large	35.0 (5.8)	50.0 (7.4)
Grade 4		
Small	8.7 (4.4)	31.4 (6.1)
Large	23.8 (6.7)	47.7 (6.7)

Note. Standard errors are in parentheses.

= 20.8, MSE = 516.29, η_p^2 = .17, HSD = 13.3. Participants who preferred the inversion shortcut used the shortcut more frequently than participants who preferred the algorithm (62.2% versus 34.2%, resp.), $F(1, 100)$ = 13.2, MSE = 4826.17, and η_{p2} = .11.

For associativity, shortcut use did not change within the pretest of first posttest (17.3% versus 23.9%, 32.9% versus 36.8% for the 1st and 2nd half of the pretest and first posttest, resp.) nor did it change between the 2nd half of the pretest and 1st half of the first posttest, $F(3, 300)$ = 14.552, MSE = 526.11, η_p^2 = .13, and HSD = 12.1. Participants who preferred the associativity shortcut used the shortcut more frequently than participants who preferred the algorithm (37.6% versus 17.9%, resp.), $F(1, 100)$ = 11.38, MSE = 3387.69, and η_p^2 = .10. There was a two-way interaction between session and preference, $F(3, 300)$ = 9.38, MSE = 526.11, η_p^2 = .09, and HSD = 14.2. For participants who preferred the algorithm, shortcut use did not change within the pretest or the first posttest nor did it change between the two. For participants who preferred associativity, shortcut use did not change within the pretest or the first posttest but did increase between the 2nd half of the pretest and the 1st half of the first posttest. Furthermore, the difference in shortcut use between participants who preferred the associativity shortcut and participants who preferred the algorithm was not significant in the pretest but was significant in the first posttest.

To determine if participants "buying in" to the training affected shortcut use on transfer problems, two independent sample t-tests were conducted comparing shortcut use in Session 3 between participants who preferred the shortcut and participants who preferred the algorithm. For inversion

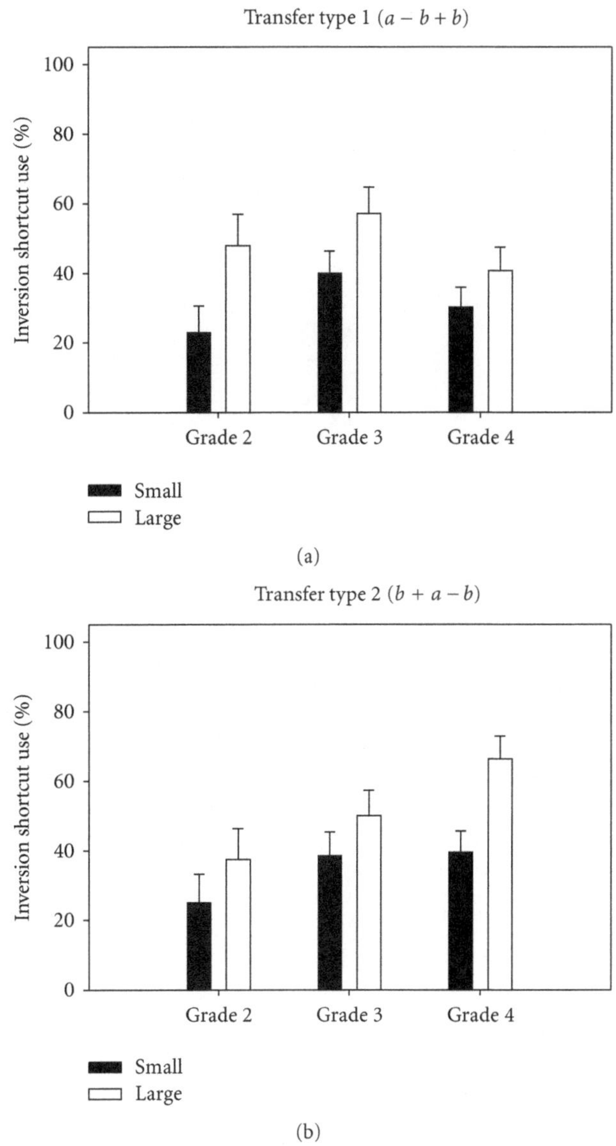

FIGURE 1: Inversion shortcut use on transfer problems in the second posttest for each grade and problem size Type 1 (a) problems ($a - b + b$) and Type 2 (b) problems ($b + a - b$). Error bars are SE.

problems, participants who preferred the shortcut used shortcuts more frequently (M = 48.0%, SE = 3.8%) than participants who preferred the algorithm (M = 32.6%, SE = 5.8%), $t(100) = -2.15$. For associativity problems, participants who preferred the shortcut used the shortcut just as frequently (M = 20.2%, SE =3.6%) as participants who preferred the algorithm (M = 11.9%, SE = 3.6%), $t(100) = -1.58$, $P = .17$.

4. Discussion

The brief evaluation of procedures task appears to have been successful in promoting conceptually-based shortcut use and decreasing the use of the less efficient left-to-right problem solving algorithm in many children in Grades 2,

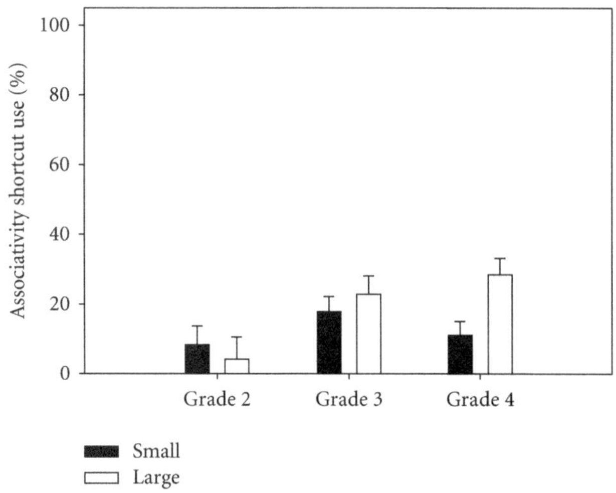

FIGURE 2: Associativity shortcut use on transfer problems in the second posttest for each grade and problem size. Error bars are SE.

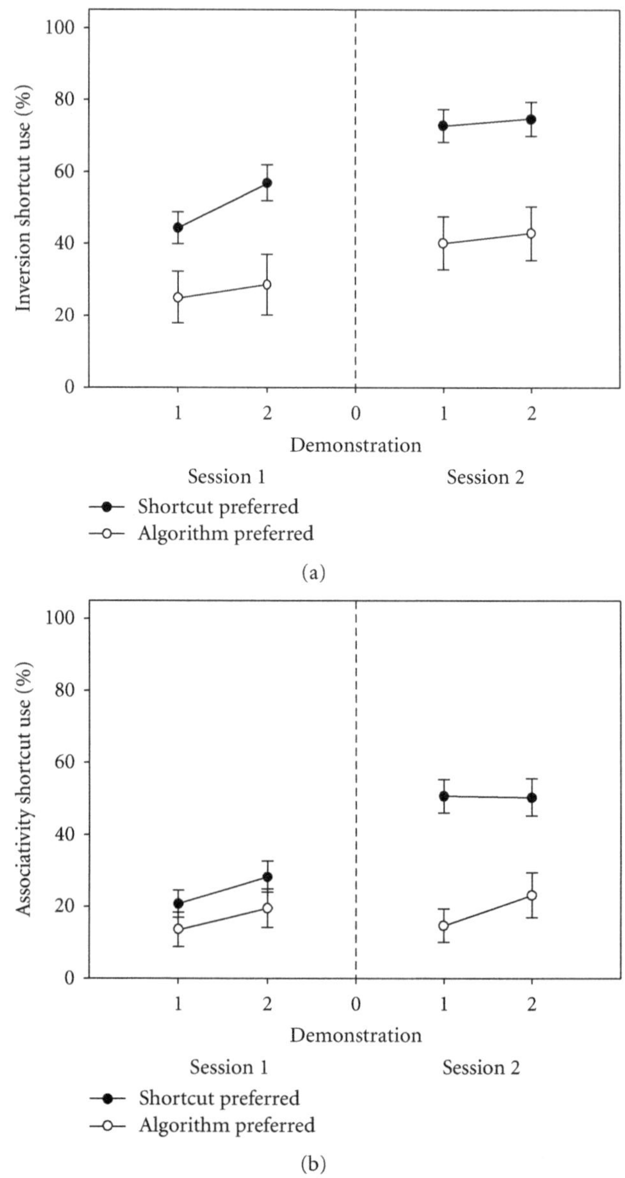

FIGURE 3: Shortcut use in 1st and 2nd half of the pretest and the first posttest on inversion (a) and associativity (b) problems by preference. Error bars are SE.

3, and 4. Children who use a conceptually-based shortcut are implementing an efficient problem solving strategy or procedure that is dependent on the inverse or associate relation between addition and subtraction, that is, they are using a procedure that is based on an arithmetic concept. The successful promotion of shortcuts that arise from arithmetic concepts is a finding consistent with a recent study with slightly older children showing that the task promoted more conceptually-based shortcut use in a condition similar to the present study's concurrent condition than in a control condition [37]. To learn and implement new problem solving strategies such as the inversion and associativity shortcuts is integral to increasing mathematical knowledge [8] as children with stronger conceptual knowledge of arithmetic will be able to represent problems in arithmetic and algebra more accurately [14, 38]. Children are expected to understand and discover the inversion and associativity concepts and shortcuts on their own [8] and few studies have attempted to teach children about the inverse relationship between addition and subtraction [11] and none have been conducted on teaching children about the associative relationship between addition and subtraction. The results of the current study support both the ability of many children in Grades 2, 3, and 4 to spontaneously discover and apply conceptually-based shortcuts during problem solving and the capacity of children to learn how to use these shortcuts immediately after a brief intervention where children are given demonstration of the shortcuts. Interestingly, children's attitudes towards the shortcuts were much more critical for children adopting a shortcut during subsequent problem solving. In contrast, being in the concurrent or sequential condition had little impact [30–32].

The lack of grade differences in spontaneous inversion shortcut use (see also [3]), the higher use of the inversion shortcut for all students after the evaluation of procedures task, and the more frequent use of the inversion shortcut than the associativity shortcut all suggest that the inversion shortcut is easier to discover, learn, and apply than the associativity shortcut. The associativity shortcut, on the other hand, was more likely to be used by the Grade 3 than the Grade 2 and 4 students. The shortcut requires calculation and therefore the advantage of using the shortcut may not be clear to Grade 2 students struggling with calculation, whilst the Grade 4 students may be good enough calculators that the shortcut does not seem superior. Demonstrating the conceptually-based shortcuts may be most suitable for Grade 3 students who have just enough calculation skills to be able to cope with the shortcut but not enough that the shortcut and the algorithm seem equally efficient. When typical solution methods are too difficult or inefficient, students are more likely to use alternative methods [39], which is consistent with the finding in the current study that students in all grades had higher use of shortcuts on problems with larger numbers.

When children have good conceptual knowledge of inversion and associativity, they should be able to appropriately transfer the conceptually-based shortcuts to solve novel problems [1]. Our findings suggest that the evaluation of procedures task promoted the use of conceptually-based shortcuts on similar problems and that students were also able to apply the shortcuts to transfer problems. Consistent with the findings of Siegler and Stern [12], inversion shortcut use was lower on transfer problems than in the previous session with typical inversion problems, and the pattern was similar for associativity shortcut use. However, shortcut use on the transfer problems was similar to that of spontaneous shortcut use in the first session. It is possible that, without the intervention, use of the shortcuts on the transfer problems might have been even lower and therefore future studies that investigate spontaneous use of the shortcuts on transfer problems before and after an intervention are needed. Children in all grades were able to spontaneously apply their knowledge of the shortcuts to the novel problems in the first session indicating a strong schema or strong understanding of inversion and associativity [40]. After the very brief intervention, shortcut use may not have transferred because children had learned to use the shortcut rather than understanding the concept behind the shortcut.

Contrary to expectations, the presentation format for the evaluation of procedures task, either sequential or concurrent, made little difference to the promotion of conceptually-based shortcuts. Rittle-Johnson and Star's [30–32] studies differed from the present task in that our task was briefer, the problems and solution procedures in our task were simpler, and our participants were not required to provide as much information about their mathematical reasoning. Future work could use an intervention containing more problems and include problems that are similar in structure but to which the shortcuts do not apply—this could improve the effectiveness of the instruction by showing children the limitations of the shortcuts. Our results indicate that providing multiple problem solving approaches was effective in promoting shortcut use and the presentation of the approaches and the opportunity for comparison was not critical as it was in the Rittle-Johnson and Star studies. However, Rittle-Johnson, Star, and Durkin [41] found that comparison of solution strategies was not always effective. Based on children's shortcut use before and after the evaluation of procedures task, we propose that the evaluation task used in the present study provides a quick and effective instructional tool that can be implemented in the classroom to promote children's understanding of the relations between addition and subtraction.

Children's attitudes about the demonstrated shortcuts, compared to a left-to-right algorithm on inversion and associativity problems, had a clear effect on subsequent problem solving procedures. Inversion and associativity shortcut use was higher for participants who preferred the shortcut, with associativity shortcut use significantly increasing after the demonstration for participants who preferred the shortcut. On transfer problems, preferring the inversion shortcut also led to higher shortcut use and preferring the associativity shortcut did not. This latter finding provides further evidence that the associativity shortcut is more difficult for students perhaps because it can overtax cognitive resources. The associativity transfer problems require students to pay attention to all three numbers and notice that the third number can be subtracted from the first number and then to subsequently perform that subtraction and then add the middle number while keeping track that all of the numbers have been added or subtracted. However, associativity shortcut use was similar on the transfer problems as it was in the pretest so the intervention may still have had a beneficial effect.

As most intervention studies involve providing students with information or instruction without assessing children's attitudes or beliefs about that information or instruction, the finding that children's views of problem solving procedures impact their subsequent procedure or strategy choices also needs to be further investigated and current theories of strategy choice need to include children's attitudes as a factor in strategy choice [27]. The current study used a brief intervention task and children had the opportunity to only provide brief information about their strategy preferences. As Verschaffel et al. [26] propose, more extensive interviews with children to gain deeper insight into their strategy choices and the influences on their strategy choices are needed. However, this is the first study to examine the consequences of children being more or less receptive to conceptually-based shortcuts and the consequences, particularly for the associativity shortcut, were marked. In areas outside of mathematics, research has shown that children's attitudes significantly contribute to their actions [5]. The present study indicates that children's attitudes towards mathematics, even simple preferences between two strategies, can be the basis for action during problem solving.

Researchers are increasingly focussing attention on how attitudes impact children's mathematics performance, decisions to take advanced mathematics courses, and career choices (e.g., [24]). However, there is also a need to investigate how attitudes impact smaller components of mathematics learning such as strategy choice. Conceptually-based shortcut use has important advantages. First, using shortcuts frees up cognitive resources [42] that can then be used to deal with more complex problems such as algebra problems [38]. Second, using shortcuts may make children more likely to pay attention to problem characteristics to guide strategy choices [39, 42] rather than being "mindless" problem solvers who are rigid rather than flexible [43]. Further research on why some children have more positive attitudes towards accepting strategies that are highly efficient but are novel to their current strategy repertoire of algorithmic approaches may help explain some of the large individual differences found in children's procedural and conceptual knowledge of arithmetic.

Acknowledgment

This paper was supported in part by an NSERC discovery grant. Thanks to Jen Gibson, John Brand, and Anna Maslany for assistance with the collection and coding of the data. Many thanks to the children, teachers, and principals from the participating schools.

References

[1] National Mathematics Advisory Panel, *Foundations for Success: The Final Report of the National Mathematics Advisory Panel*, U.S. Department of Education, Washington, DC, USA, 2008.

[2] J. Bisanz, "The development of mathematical cognition: arithmetic," *Journal of Experimental Child Psychology*, vol. 74, no. 3, pp. 153–156, 1999.

[3] C. K. Gilmore and M. Papadatou-Pastou, "Patterns of individual differences in conceptual understanding and arithmetical skill: a meta-analysis," *Mathematical Thinking and Learning*, vol. 11, no. 1-2, pp. 25–40, 2009.

[4] J. S. Klein and J. Bisanz, "Preschoolers doing arithmetic: the concepts are willing but the working memory is weak," *Canadian Journal of Experimental Psychology*, vol. 54, no. 2, pp. 105–116, 2000.

[5] K. Bartsch and H. Wellman, "Young children's attribution of action to beliefs and desires," *Child Development*, vol. 60, no. 4, pp. 946–964, 1989.

[6] J. Kilpatrick, J. Swafford, and B. Findell, *Adding it up: Helping Children Learn Mathematics*, National Academy Press, Washington, DC, USA, 2001.

[7] J. Bisanz and J. LeFevre, "Strategic and nonstrategic processing in the development of mathematical cognition," in *Children's Strategies: Contemporary Views of Cognitive Development*, D. F. Bjorklund, Ed., pp. 213–244, Erlbaum, Hillsdale,, NJ, USA, 1990.

[8] M. Schneider and E. Stern, "The inverse relation of addition and subtraction: a knowledge integration perspective," *Mathematical Thinking and Learning*, vol. 11, no. 1-2, pp. 92–101, 2009.

[9] J. Bisanz, R. P. D. Watchorn, C. Piatt, and J. Sherman, "On "understanding" children's developing use of inversion," *Mathematical Thinking and Learning*, vol. 11, no. 1-2, pp. 10–24, 2009.

[10] M.-L. Lai, A. J. Baroody, and A. R. Johnson, "Fostering Taiwanese preschoolers' understanding of the addition-subtraction inverse principle," *Cognitive Development*, vol. 23, no. 1, pp. 216–235, 2008.

[11] T. Nunes, P. Bryant, D. Hallett, D. Bell, and D. Evans, "Teaching children about the inverse relation between addition and subtraction," *Mathematical Thinking and Learning*, vol. 11, no. 1-2, pp. 61–78, 2009.

[12] R. S. Siegler and E. Stern, "Conscious and unconscious strategy discoveries: a microgenetic analysis," *Journal of Experimental Psychology*, vol. 127, no. 4, pp. 377–397, 1998.

[13] K. M. Robinson and A. K. Dubé, "Children's understanding of addition and subtraction concepts," *Journal of Experimental Child Psychology*, vol. 103, no. 4, pp. 532–545, 2009.

[14] R. W. Prather and M. W. Alibali, "The development of arithmetic principle knowledge: how do we know what learners know?" *Developmental Review*, vol. 29, no. 4, pp. 221–248, 2009.

[15] B. De Smedt, J. Torbeyns, N. Stassens, P. Ghesquière, and L. Verschaffel, "Frequency, efficiency and flexibility of indirect addition in two learning environments," *Learning and Instruction*, vol. 20, no. 3, pp. 205–215, 2010.

[16] J. Torbeyns, B. De Smedt, P. Ghesquière, and L. Verschaffel, "Acquisition and use of shortcut strategies by traditionally schooled children," *Educational Studies in Mathematics*, vol. 71, no. 1, pp. 1–17, 2009.

[17] J. Torbeyns, B. De Smedt, P. Ghesquière, and L. Verschaffel, "Solving subtractions adaptively by means of indirect addition: influence of task, subject, and instructional factors," *Mediterrannean Journal for Research in Mathematics Education*, vol. 8, no. 2, pp. 1–30, 2009.

[18] National Council of Teachers of Mathematics, *Principles and Standards for School Mathematics*, NCTM, Reston, Va, USA, 2000.

[19] D. B. McLeod, "Connecting research to teaching," *Mathematics Teacher*, vol. 86, pp. 761–763, 1993.

[20] M. R. Lepper, H. J. Corpus, and S. S. Iyengar, "Intrinsic and extrinsic motivational orientations in the classroom: age differences and academic correlates," *Journal of Educational Psychology*, vol. 97, no. 2, pp. 184–196, 2005.

[21] C. A. Wolters, "Advancing achievement goal theory: using goal structures and goal orientations to predict students' motivation, cognition, and achievement," *Journal of Educational Psychology*, vol. 96, no. 2, pp. 236–250, 2004.

[22] M. H. Ashcraft, J. A. Krause, and D. R. Hopko, "Is math anxiety a mathematical learning disability?" in *Why is Math so Hard for Some Children? The Nature and Origins of Mathematical Learning Difficulties and Disabilities*, D. B. Berch and M. M. M. Mazzocco, Eds., pp. 329–248, Paul H. Brookes, Baltimore, Md, USA, 2007.

[23] National Research Council, *Knowing and Learning Mathematics for Teaching: Proceedings of a Workshop*, National Academy Press, Washington, DC, USA, 2001.

[24] A. J. Martin, J. Anderson, J. Bobis, R. Vellar, and J. Way, "Switching on and switching off in mathematics: an ecological study of future intent and disengagement among middle school students," *Journal of Educational Psychology*, vol. 104, no. 1, pp. 1–18, 2012.

[25] S. Ellis, "Strategy choice in sociocultural context," *Developmental Review*, vol. 17, no. 4, pp. 490–524, 1997.

[26] L. Verschaffel, K. Luwel, J. Torbeyns, and W. Van Dooren, "Conceptualizing, investigating, and enhancing adaptive expertise in elementary mathematics education," *European Journal of Psychology of Education*, vol. 24, no. 3, pp. 335–359, 2009.

[27] K. M. Robinson and J. LeFevre, "The inverse relation between multiplication and division: concepts, procedures, and a cognitive framework," *Educational Studies in Mathematics*, vol. 79, no. 3, pp. 409–428, 2012.

[28] A. J. Baroody, S. H. Tiilikainen, and Y.-C Tai, "The application and development of an additional goal sketch," *Cognition and Instruction*, vol. 24, no. 1, pp. 123–170, 2008.

[29] R. S. Siegler and R. Araya, "A computational model of conscious and unconscious strategy discovery," in *Advances in Child Development and Behavior*, R. V. Kail, Ed., vol. 33, pp. 1–42, Elsevier, New York, NY, USA, 2005.

[30] B. Rittle-Johnson and J. R. Star, "Does comparing solution methods facilitate conceptual and procedural knowledge? An experimental study on learning to solve equations," *Journal of Educational Psychology*, vol. 99, no. 3, pp. 561–574, 2007.

[31] B. Rittle-Johnson and J. R. Star, "Compared with what? The effects of different comparisons on conceptual knowledge and procedural flexibility for equation solving," *Journal of Educational Psychology*, vol. 101, no. 3, pp. 529–544, 2009.

[32] J. R. Star and B. Rittle-Johnson, "It pays to compare: an experimental study on computational estimation," *Journal of Experimental Child Psychology*, vol. 102, no. 4, pp. 408–426, 2009.

[33] C. Yakes and J. R. Star, "Using comparison to develop flexibility for teaching algebra," *Journal of Mathematics Teacher Education*, vol. 14, no. 3, pp. 175–191, 2011.

[34] D. C. Geary, *Children's Mathematical Development: Research and Practical Implications*, American Psychological Association., Washington, DC, USA, 1994.

[35] B. Rittle-Johnson, "Promoting transfer: effects of self-explanation and direct instruction," *Child Development*, vol. 77, no. 1, pp. 1–15, 2006.

[36] T. P. Carpenter, "Conceptual knowledge as a foundation for procedural knowledge: implications from research on the initial learning of arithmetic," in *Conceptual and Procedural Knowledge: The Case of Mathematics*, J. Hiebert, Ed., pp. 113–132, Erlbaum, Hillsdale,, NJ, USA, 1986.

[37] K. M. Robinson and A. K. Dubé, "Children's additive concepts: promoting understanding and the role ofinhibition," *Learning and Individual Differences*. In press.

[38] T. Nunes, P. Bryant, D. Burman et al., "Deaf children's understanding of inverse relationships," in *Deaf Cognition: Foundations and Outcomes*, M. Marschark and P. C. Hauser, Eds., pp. 201–225, Oxford University Press, New York, NY, USA, 2008.

[39] K. J. Newton, J. R. Star, and K. Lynch, "Understanding the development of flexibility in struggling algebra students," *Mathematical Thinking and Learning*, vol. 12, no. 4, pp. 282–305, 2010.

[40] A. J. Baroody, "The development of adaptive expertise and flexibility: the integration of conceptual and procedural knowledge," in *The Development of Arithmetic Concepts and Skills: Constructing Adaptive Expertise*, A. J. Baroody and A. Dowker, Eds., pp. 1–33, Erlbaum, Mahwah, NJ, USA, 2003.

[41] B. Rittle-Johnson, J. R. Star, and K. Durkin, "The importance of prior knowledge when comparing examples: influences on conceptual and procedural knowledge of equation solving," *Journal of Educational Psychology*, vol. 101, no. 4, pp. 836–852, 2009.

[42] D. J. Mabbott and J. Bisanz, "Developmental change and individual differences in children's multiplication," *Child Development*, vol. 74, no. 4, pp. 1091–1107, 2003.

[43] N. M. McNeil, B. Rittle-Johnson, S. Hattikudur, and L. A. Petersen, "Continuity in representation between children and adults: arithmetic knowledge hinders undergraduates' algebraic problem solving," *Journal of Cognition and Development*, vol. 11, no. 4, pp. 437–457, 2010.

Observed Human Actions, and Not Mechanical Actions, Induce Searching Errors in Infants

Yusuke Moriguchi,[1,2] Reiko Matsunaka,[3] Shoji Itakura,[4] and Kazuo Hiraki[5]

[1] *Department of School Education, Joetsu University of Education, Joetsu 943-8512, Japan*
[2] *Japan Science and Technology Agency, Precursory Research for Embryonic Science and Technology, Tokyo 102-0076, Japan*
[3] *Department of General Systems Studies, Graduate School of Arts and Sciences, The University of Tokyo, Tokyo 153-8902, Japan*
[4] *Department of Psychology, Graduate School of Letters, Kyoto University, Kyoto, Japan*
[5] *The Interfaculty Initiative in Information Studies, The University of Tokyo, Tokyo 113-0033, Japan*

Correspondence should be addressed to Yusuke Moriguchi, moriguchi@juen.ac.jp

Academic Editor: Masha Gartstein

Recent neurophysiological studies have shown that several human brain regions involved in executing actions are activated by merely observing such actions via a human, and not by a mechanical hand. At a behavioral level, observing a human's movements, but not those of a robot, significantly interferes with ongoing executed movements. However, it is unclear whether the biological tuning in the observation/execution matching system are functional during infancy. The present study examines whether a human's actions, and not a mechanical action, influence infants' execution of the same actions due to the observation/execution matching system. Twelve-month-old infants were given a searching task. In the tasks, infants observed an object hidden at location A, after which either a human hand (human condition) or a mechanical one (mechanical condition) searched the object correctly. Next, the object was hidden at location B and infants were allowed to search the object. We examined whether infants searched the object at location B correctly. The results revealed that infants in the human condition were more likely to search location A than those in the mechanical condition. Moreover, the results suggested that infants' searching behaviors were affected by their observations of the same actions by a human, but not a mechanical hand. Thus, it may be concluded that the observation/execution matching system may be biologically tuned during infancy.

1. Introduction

It has been proposed that actions are intrinsically linked to perception, and that imagining, observing, or in any way representing an action, excites the motor programs used to execute such actions. This proposal is originally derived from James' ideomotor theory [1] and recently developed by Prinz's common coding framework [2]. According to this framework, the representation of a perceived action involves simulative production of that action on the part of the observer. This covert motor activation results in the observation of an action facilitating its execution. Neurophysiological studies have supported the common coding framework by showing that several brain regions (e.g., the primary motor cortex) involved in executing actions are activated by the mere observation of such actions, through what is known as the mirror neuron in animals [3, 4] and the mirror neuron system in human [5, 6]. Importantly, the mirror neuron system can respond only to biological actions [7]. On the behavioral level, the biological tuning leads to the fact that observing a human's arm movements, but not those of a robot, significantly interferes with ongoing executed movements [8, 9].

Given this evidence, it has been proposed that we should understand another person's actions through matching between observed actions and internal motor repertories. Biological tuning has been interpreted as suggesting that non-biological actions are not part of behavioral repertories and therefore we do not understand those actions through matching processes [7, 10]. In other words, biological tuning may be one important property in the observation/execution matching system.

Developmental literature has reported that the observation/execution matching system can be functional during the initial years of life. For example, Shimada and Hiraki [11] showed that the neuroimaging data of the primary motor cortex among six-month-old infants was activated when observing another person's actions. Falck-Ytter et al. [12] reported that 12-month-old infants produced a proactive goal-directed movement during the observation of another person's actions and suggested that this reflected that the infants were able to map observed actions onto their internal motor representations. Taken together, the developmental research suggests that during the initial years of life infants, can understand another person's actions through the observation/execution matching system.

However, whether the observation/execution system in infants is biologically tuned is still unclear. This is in spite of the fact that biological tuning is a key aspect of the observation/matching system. There is some evidence that young children's observation/execution matching systems may be biologically tuned, in which observing a human's actions, but not a mechanical action, affected the children's execution of the same actions [13, 14]. Moreover, in an infant study, Kanakogi and Itakura [15] reported that infants' motor skills (grasping skills) were correlated with their ability to predict another person's goal of the same actions. Importantly, the infants were able to predict the goal-directed actions by a human hand, but not by a mechanical hand. The results suggest that the observation/execution matching system may be biologically tuned during the initial years of life. Nevertheless, the correlational data was not sufficient to draw a conclusion that the system might be biologically tuned. Rather, as in behavioral studies among adults [9], the functional dependency between the observation and execution of the same actions should be addressed for infants. If the infants' matching systems are biologically tuned, it may follow that observing a human's actions, but not mechanical actions, may interfere with the infants' execution actions.

Recently, the possibility that the infants' observation/execution matching system might be biologically tuned was reported from an A-not-B task [16, 17]. This task was first developed by Piaget [18], and the phenomenon was replicated and discussed by many researchers [19–21]. In the searching task, infants correctly searched an object they see hidden in one location (location A) and retrieved the object, after which they were allowed to search for the object hidden in the other location (location B). In the A-not-B task situation, infants aged 8 to 12 months continued to search in location A and were unable to retrieve the object in location B correctly. There were several explanations regarding why infants committed errors in the task, but many researchers suggest that reaching experiences in location A would cause the A-not-B errors [22–24].

Importantly, the "real" reaching behaviors were not necessarily for the occurrence of the A-not-B errors. Longo and Bertenthal [17] reported that the mere observation of an experimenter's reaching out toward location A caused A-not-B like errors in infants. The researchers indicated that infants simulated the experimenter's searching behaviors at location A while observing, which caused the infants' reaching out toward location A in the B trials. Moreover, Boyer et al. [16] showed that infants were unlikely to commit the A-not-B errors after the observation of the actions performed by a mechanical devise, and that the familiarity with the devise may increase the likelihood for perseverative errors. Boyer et al. suggested that infants were less likely to commit the A-not-B errors when observing the actions by a mechanical devise than by human agents. However, the researchers have not directly compared the mechanical condition with the human condition. That is, there were no human conditions used in the previous study. To argue for biological tuning, a direct comparison between the human condition and the mechanical condition is needed. In addition, there were no control conditions in the previous study. Without a control condition, it was unclear whether infants' searching errors were due to the infants simply failing to search for objects or that the observation in the A trials affected the infants' performances in the B trials. The present study directly examined whether observations of a human's actions, and not a mechanical action, induced infants' searching errors.

In the present study, infants aged approximately 12 months observed either a human (human condition) or a mechanical hand (mechanical condition) searching an object at location A, after which they were allowed to search the object at location B. Infants were given four consecutive A trials, followed by four consecutive B trials. In addition to the two experimental conditions, a control condition was added. The control condition was the same as the human condition except for the A trials. In the A trials of the control condition, there was one cup instead of two cups used in the human condition. For each condition, there were two experimenters. The first experimenter hid the object and the second experimenter retrieved the object using her hand or a mechanical hand (Figure 1).

2. Materials and Method

2.1. Ethics Statement. Participants were recruited from nursery schools in Tokyo and Kyoto. Written informed consent was obtained from the parents and teachers of children prior to their involvement in the study. The study was conducted in accordance with the principles of the Declaration of Helsinki and the study design was approved by the ethics review board at the University of Tokyo.

2.2. Participants. Forty-two twelve-month-old infants (mean = 12.1, SD = 0.4; twenty-four boys and eighteen girls) participated in the study. Of these, seven infants were not included in the final data because of a failure to observe the demonstration (four), fussiness (one), and reaching out toward both locations simultaneously (two). The remainder of the infants were randomly assigned to three conditions: a human condition ($N = 12$, five girls), a mechanical condition ($N = 11$, six girls), and a control condition ($N = 12$, four girls). There were no significant differences in age (in weeks) between conditions. Parents provided written informed consent and were informed verbally of the purpose of the study.

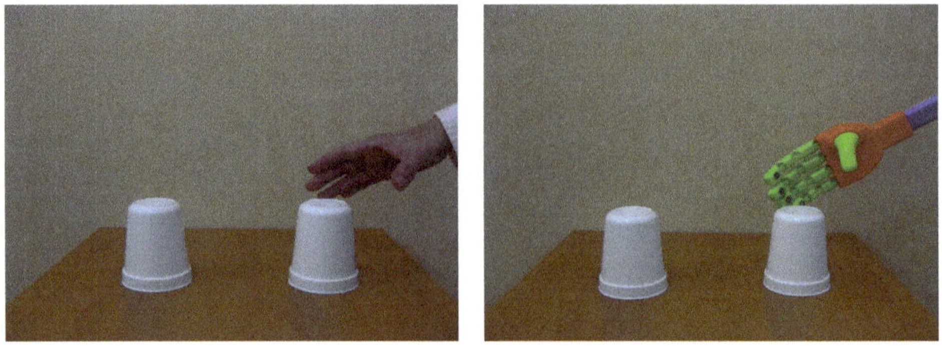

(a) (b)

Figure 1: Infants observed either (a) a human or (b) a mechanical hand searching a toy.

2.3. Stimuli and Procedure. The experimental apparatus consisted of a tray with two cups placed on it. The cups were placed 10.0 cm apart.

Infants were seated on their mother's lap in front of a table and allowed to play with a toy (a cartoon character) for several seconds. Three warm-up trials were administered by an experimenter using procedures by Smith et al. [23] and Longo and Bertenthal [17]. On the first warm-up trial, the toy was placed on top of a single cup, after which infants were allowed to take the toy. During the second trial, the toy was placed in the cup but left uncovered and infants were required to get the toy. For the final trial, the toy was completely inside the cup, and infants were allowed to search for the toy.

The experimental trials used a two-cup apparatus and comprised four A trials and four B trials. Infants were first given four consecutive A trials, followed by four consecutive B trials. There were two experimenters in the experimental trials. In the A trials of the human condition, the first experimenter showed the toy to the infants and the second experimenter hid it in one of the cups and waited for five seconds. Thereafter, the tray and cups were presented to the second experimenter. The second experimenter successfully searched for the toy. Infants observed the second experimenter's searching behavior (Figure 1(a)). The A-location of the toy (right or left) was counterbalanced across infants. In order to exclude the possibility that infants failed to observe the second experimenter's behaviors, in both trials, the toy was waved in the air and the infants' name was called to attract their attention. In the B trials, infants were presented with the tray with cups by the first experimenter in a similar manner as done in the A trials and they were allowed to search for the toy.

The mechanical condition was presented exactly in the same manner as the human condition, except for in the A trials. In these trials, infants observed a mechanical hand that searched for the toy (Figure 1(b)). The mechanical hand was operated by the second experimenter behind a screen, and infants were unaware of the experimenter's presence.

The control condition was the same as the human condition, except in the A trials. In the A trials of the control condition, there was one cup instead of two in the human condition. The first experimenter showed the toy to the infants and the second experimenter hid it inside the cup and presented both the tray and cup. Infants observed the second experimenter's searching behavior.

Infants received a score of 1 when they successfully searched for the toy in each of the B trials (0–4). If infants did not show any searching behaviors fifteen seconds after the tray was presented, the trials were excluded from the data. In total, four trials from the human condition, seven trials from the mechanical condition, and six trials from the control condition were excluded from further analyses.

3. Results

Infants were given a score of 1 if they successfully searched the toy in each of the B trials (0–4). The mean error rates out of the trials where children produced searching behaviors were calculated in each condition. If infants produced searching behaviors on 4 trials and failed to search the toy on 2 trials, the error rate of the infants was 0.5. The results are presented in Figure 2. We assume that the control condition would evaluate "pure" infants' searching abilities. Infants in the control condition observed the searching behaviors by the second experimenter in the A trials; however, the experimenter's behaviors did not provide any biases with infants' behaviors in the B trials because there was only one cup in the A trials of the control condition. In the control condition, infants were able to search the toy rather easily (mean error rate = 15.5%). On the other hand, infants' behaviors in the human control condition were strongly affected by observing the second experimenter's behaviors. They performed only 50.0% of the B trials correctly, which was consistent with previous results that observing another person's behaviors could induce A-not-B like errors. Finally, interestingly, infants' performances in the mechanical condition were similar to those in the control condition. Infants in the mechanical condition had an error rate of 20.5% in the B trials.

The mean error rates was analyzed using a one-way ANOVA, and we observed a significant main effect of condition, $F(2, 32) = 4.126$, $P < .02$. The post hoc analyses using

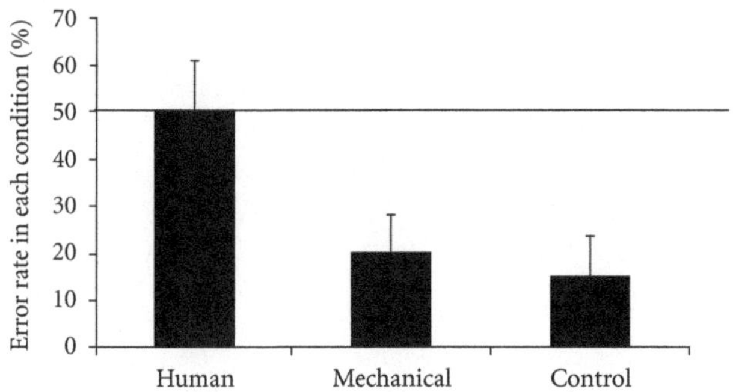

FIGURE 2: The mean error rates in the B trials in each condition. The bar indicates the standard error.

Tukey's HSD revealed that infants in the human condition performed the B trials significantly worse than those in the control conditions ($P < .05$). There were marginal differences between the human condition and the mechanical condition ($P < .09$), but no significant differences between the mechanical condition and the control condition.

Further, we also examined whether the error rates of infants in each condition were significantly different from what would have been expected to occur by chance. The chance level for each trial was 50%; therefore, the score expected by chance was 2 in the B trials. A one-sample t-test revealed that infants in the human condition performed at chance level in the B trials, $t(12) = 0.000$, $P > .99$, whereas the infants in the mechanical and control conditions correctly searched the toy in the B trials below chance level, $t(11) = 3.633$, $P < .001$ and $t(12) = 4.080$, $P < .001$, respectively.

Finally, we examined whether there were some learning effects in the B trials. We divided the four B trials into the first two and second two trials and compared the performances. The results revealed no significant differences between conditions ($P > .10$).

4. Discussion

The present study examined whether observing another person's actions, and not a mechanical action, interfered in infants' execution of the same actions using the A-not-B task. Previous studies showed that infants were likely to commit perseverative errors after the observation of a human's actions, but observation of the mechanical actions may not induce these errors [16, 17]. However, there were no direct comparisons between them. The results revealed that 12-month-old infants committed searching errors after observing a human's actions, but not mechanical actions. That is, after infants observed another person searching for an object at location A, infants tended to search it at location A, even though the object was at location B. On the other hand, infants successfully retrieved the object after observing a mechanical hand searching the object at location B. The results suggested that infants' observation/execution matching systems might be biologically tuned during the initial years of life.

One can argue that infants pay more attention to the human's actions, but not to the mechanical hand's actions in the A trials, which might explain the different results between the conditions. However, in this experiment, we carefully monitored an infant's gazing behavior during the A trials and excluded the trials where the infants did not observe the demonstration in both conditions from the final analyses. At least at the observable level, it is unlikely that infants paid more attention to the human's actions but not to those of the mechanical hand in the A trials.

The results in the present study are generally consistent with the evidence regarding the observation/execution matching system during infancy. On the behavioral level, Sommerville et al. [25] revealed that the action experience among three-month-old infants facilitated their perception of another person's actions. Falck-Ytter et al. [12] reported that 12-month-old infants produced a proactive goal-directed movement during the observation of another person's actions. At the neural level, the mirror neuron system might be functional during the initial years of life. Shimada and Hiraki [11] showed that six-month-old infants activated the primary motor cortex when observing another person's actions. Southgate et al. [26] recorded nine-month-old infants' electroencephalographs (EEGs) during their reaching and observation of the actions and found that the motor activities during observation was also similar during execution.

The critical property of the observation/execution matching system may be biological tuning. In this regard, there was little evidence during infancy. At the perceptual level, Woodward [27] showed that six-month-old infants attributed the goal to a human's actions, but not a mechanical hand's actions. Kanakogi and Itakura [15] reported that six-month-old infants were able to predict goal-directed actions by a human hand, but not by a mechanical hand. The infants' ability to predict another person's goal is correlated with their ability to perform the same actions. Moreover, Longo and Bertenthal [17] showed that infants' searching behaviors were strongly affected by their observation of the same actions by another person. Boyer et al. [16] reported that infants were unlikely to commit the errors after observation of mechanical actions. The present study directly compared the effects of human actions with those of mechanical ones and found that infants committed the errors after the observation of human actions, but not mechanical actions. Taken together, the results indicate that the observation/execution system may be biologically tuned during infancy.

Acknowledgments

The authors would like to thank parent and infants who participated in this study. The research was supported by Grants from Japan Society for the Promotion of Sciences for the first, third, and forth authors.

References

[1] W. James, *Principles of Psychology*, Holt, New York, NY, USA, 1890.

[2] W. Prinz, "A common coding approach to perception and action," in *Relationships Between Perception and Action*, O. Neumann and W. Prinz, Eds., pp. 167–201, Springer, Heidelberg, Germany, 1990.
[3] V. Gallese, L. Fadiga, L. Fogassi, and G. Rizzolatti, "Action recognition in the premotor cortex," *Brain*, vol. 119, no. 2, pp. 593–609, 1996.
[4] G. Rizzolatti, L. Fadiga, V. Gallese, and L. Fogassi, "Premotor cortex and the recognition of motor actions," *Cognitive Brain Research*, vol. 3, no. 2, pp. 131–141, 1996.
[5] G. Buccino, F. Binkofski, G. R. Fink et al., "Action observation activates premotor and parietal areas in a somatotopic manner: an fMRI study," *European Journal of Neuroscience*, vol. 13, no. 2, pp. 400–404, 2001.
[6] J. Decety, J. Grèzes, N. Costes et al., "Brain activity during observation of actions. Influence of action content and subject's strategy," *Brain*, vol. 120, no. 10, pp. 1763–1777, 1997.
[7] Y. F. Tai, C. Scherfler, D. J. Brooks, N. Sawamoto, and U. Castiello, "The human premotor cortex Is 'mirror' only for biological actions," *Current Biology*, vol. 14, no. 2, pp. 117–120, 2004.
[8] C. Press, G. Bird, R. Flach, and C. Heyes, "Robotic movement elicits automatic imitation," *Cognitive Brain Research*, vol. 25, no. 3, pp. 632–640, 2005.
[9] J. M. Kilner, Y. Paulignan, and S. J. Blakemore, "An interference effect of observed biological movement on action," *Current Biology*, vol. 13, no. 6, pp. 522–525, 2003.
[10] G. Rizzolatti, L. Fogassi, and V. Gallese, "Neurophysiological mechanisms underlying the understanding and imitation of action," *Nature Reviews Neuroscience*, vol. 2, no. 9, pp. 661–670, 2001.
[11] S. Shimada and K. Hiraki, "Infant's brain responses to live and televised action," *NeuroImage*, vol. 32, no. 2, pp. 930–939, 2006.
[12] T. Falck-Ytter, G. Gredebäck, and C. von Hofsten, "Infants predict other people's action goals," *Nature Neuroscience*, vol. 9, no. 7, pp. 878–879, 2006.
[13] Y. Moriguchi, T. Kanda, H. Ishiguro, and S. Itakura, "Children perseverate to a human's actions but not to a robot's actions," *Developmental Science*, vol. 13, no. 1, pp. 62–68, 2010.
[14] A. N. Meltzoff, "Understanding the intentions of others: re-enactment of intended acts by 18-month-old children," *Developmental Psychology*, vol. 31, no. 5, pp. 838–850, 1995.
[15] Y. Kanakogi and S. Itakura, "Developmental correspondence between action prediction and motor ability in early infancy," *Nature Communications*, vol. 2, no. 1, article 341, 2011.
[16] T. W. Boyer, J. Samantha Pan, and B. I. Bertenthal, "Infants' understanding of actions performed by mechanical devices," *Cognition*, vol. 121, no. 1, pp. 1–11, 2011.
[17] M. R. Longo and B. I. Bertenthal, "Common coding of observation and execution of action in 9-month-old infants," *Infancy*, vol. 10, no. 1, pp. 43–59, 2006.
[18] J. Piaget, *The Construction of Reality in the Child*, Basic Books, New York, NY, USA, 1954.
[19] Y. Munakata, J. L. McClelland, M. H. Johnson, and R. S. Siegler, "Rethinking infant knowledge: toward an adaptive process account of successes and failures in object permanence tasks," *Psychological Review*, vol. 104, no. 4, pp. 686–713, 1997.
[20] H. M. Wellman, D. Cross, and K. Bartsch, "Infant search and object permanence: a meta-analysis of the A-not-B error," *Monographs of the Society for Research in Child Development*, vol. 51, no. 3, pp. 1–67, 1986.
[21] E. Thelen, G. Schöner, C. Scheier, and L. B. Smith, "The dynamics of embodiment: a field theory of infant perseverative reaching," *Behavioral and Brain Sciences*, vol. 24, no. 1, pp. 1–34, 2001.
[22] S. Marcovitch and P. D. Zelazo, "A hierarchical competing systems model of the emergence and early development of executive function," *Developmental Science*, vol. 12, no. 1, pp. 1–25, 2009.
[23] L. B. Smith, E. Thelen, R. Titzer, and D. McLin, "Knowing in the context of acting: the task dynamics of the A-not-B error," *Psychological Review*, vol. 106, no. 2, pp. 235–260, 1999.
[24] A. Diamond, "Neuropsychological insights into the meaning of object concept development," in *The Epigenesis of Mind: Essays on Biology and Cognition*, S. Carey and R. Gelman, Eds., pp. 67–110, Lawrence Erlbaum Associates, Hillsdale, NJ, USA, 1991.
[25] J. A. Sommerville, A. L. Woodward, and A. Needham, "Action experience alters 3-month-old infants' perception of others' actions," *Cognition*, vol. 96, no. 1, pp. B1–B11, 2005.
[26] V. Southgate, M. H. Johnson, T. Osborne, and G. Csibra, "Predictive motor activation during action observation in human infants," *Biology Letters*, vol. 5, no. 6, pp. 769–772, 2009.
[27] A. L. Woodward, "Infants selectively encode the goal object of an actor's reach," *Cognition*, vol. 69, no. 1, pp. 1–34, 1998.

19

What Makes an Act a Pretense One? Young Children's Pretend-Real Judgments and Explanations

Lili Ma[1] **and Angeline S. Lillard**[2]

[1] *Department of Psychology, Ryerson University, 350 Victoria Street, Toronto, ON, Canada M5B 2K3*
[2] *Department of Psychology, University of Virginia, P.O. Box 400400, Charlottesville, VA 22904-4400, USA*

Correspondence should be addressed to Lili Ma; lilima@psych.ryerson.ca

Academic Editor: Tricia Striano

The present study examined what makes an act a pretense one for adults and preschoolers. Participants watched pretense versus real acts, judged whether each act was pretend or real, and justified their judgment by citing the cues they used. These reported cues are presumed to reflect viewers' conception of what makes an act a pretense one. The results suggested that like adults, 5-year-olds represented pretense behavior in the form of contrasts between pretense and its real counterpart. However, children placed greater weight on deviant content than on behavioral cues, whereas adults used behavioral cues, especially movement, when content information was not available. These results are discussed in terms of how children's intuitive theories of pretense might differ from those of adults.

1. Introduction

Pretense is one of the earliest symbolic activities of young humans. In pretending, a child projects a mental representation onto reality, in a spirit of fun; the projection is done intentionally and with full awareness, and is often (but not always) accompanied by activities [1]. For example, a boy might take a stick and project onto it his mental representation of a horse, proceeding to "gallop" around with the stick. Children begin to engage in pretend play at around 12 months, and their pretense activities become more elaborate as they move into the central pretend play years of 3 to 5 [2–5]. Adults also engage in various forms of make believe, from pretending a spoon is an airplane in front of their young children to acting on a stage [6, 7]. Given the prevalence of pretense throughout the lifespan, an intriguing question is how people, especially young children, make pretense interpretations. Pretense involves distortions of the real world. If a young child reads a pretense event literally, his or her developing representations of the real world might get confused [8]. Thus, it is vital that young children interpret pretense in its nonliteral mode and distinguish it from what is real. The goal of this research is to examine how well children, as compared to adults, discriminate certain pretense and real acts and on what basis they think they make their judgments. The findings have the potential to provide insight into how young children's intuitive theories of pretense might differ from those of adults.

Pretense acts differ from real ones in both underlying intentions and external manifestations. Children from ages 3 to 5 are developing an understanding of the former difference, namely, the underlying intentions that are essential in defining pretense versus real behavior (e.g., [9–11]). We focus on the latter difference here: what aspects of external manifestations distinguish pretense acts from real ones, and which of these do adults and children pick up on?

There are at least two ways in which one might use external cues to discriminate pretense and real acts. The first possibility is that the pretenders signal pretending to others verbally. For instance, pretenders might use flagging words like "pretend," "fake," or "not real" when commenting on their own pretense actions. However, such cues are rare: pretending adults seldom explicitly tell young children that they are pretending [12]. The second possibility is that one might decipher pretense based on deviant content and behavioral signs, such as absence of necessary materials or outcomes and modifications in the actions of the pretender. This second way might be the most pertinent for very young children's pretense interpretations: deviant content and behavioral signs are the most salient cues to pretense that can be directly observed and easily contrasted with what children already know is real.

In terms of deviant content, pretense acts can differ from real ones in that the necessary materials and outcomes of familiar activities are often absent [4]. In pretense, some necessary materials (were the act real) might manifestly not exist—they might be represented by substitute objects, or might be purely imaginary. For example, when one is pretending to eat, the eating behavior is often performed in the absence of real food. In addition, pretense acts often do not result in the usual outcomes of the activities performed for real [4, 10]. For instance, when one is pretending to write, it is very likely that there would be no ink traces left on the paper.

Pretense acts can also differ from real ones in terms of the behavioral modifications of the pretender, including aspects of movement and paralinguistic features. As an example of a variation in movements that has been observed in pretense, people move faster when pantomiming pouring into and drinking from a "glass" than they do when executing the same actions with a real bottle and a real glass [13]. In addition, in pretense, movements are often truncated, exaggerated, or oddly timed [12, 14, 15]. With regard to paralinguistic features, both adults and children make sound effects when pretending. For instance, when children are pretending about cars, they sometimes make "vroom vroom" sounds [6, 16]; when adults are pretending to drink imaginary juice, they often make nonverbal noises that mimic sounds made during the course of real drinking [12]. Changes in voice might also accompany pretense acts, such as mothers talking more loudly and using a more variable pitch when pretending [15].

Thus, pretense activities can involve both deviant content and specific behavioral signs. At issue here is whether these external cues are salient markers of pretense for children. Deviant content, in particular, might readily bring to mind that an act contrasts with the real and thus might lead to a pretense interpretation. For example, upon seeing that there is no real juice in an empty glass, a child might immediately realize that a person who is "drinking" from that glass is pretending. Because pretense is clearly occurring when content is obviously not there, in the present study we did not examine the use of this cue (but see controls in Study 2). However, there are pretense situations in which content information is either absent or insufficient, and it was the cues used in such cases that were of interest here. For instance, a person might pretend to eat but observers might not be able to see whether actual food is involved, or a person might hold a real apple but pretend to bite it in such a way that observers could not see if an actual bite were taken. In such circumstances, children must rely on other cues to tell pretense from real events.

Previous research has shown that pretenders emit non-verbal behavioral cues [12] and observers use such cues to detect pretense. In Richert and Lillard's work [17], adults and children (ages 3 to 10) watched short video clips of mothers engaging in pretense and real snacks and judged whether each event was pretend or real. The clips were selected based on the presence of different behavioral cues that previous research had shown varied with pretense [12], such as mothers looking longer at the child, moving faster, holding their hands at the mouth longer while "eating," and producing pretend sound effects. Content information (e.g., presence or absence of food) was blocked from view by video-editing a small black rectangle over the place where that content would be. In addition, the word "pretend" was not used in the clips. Although there was improvement with age, even the youngest participants made correct judgments most of the time in response to clips containing more marked variation in certain cues, such as the extent to which mothers looked at the child and how rapidly mothers moved. However, in that study it is unclear which cues viewers used to make their judgments, because participants were not asked for the basis of their judgments. When making a pretense interpretation, the viewers could have picked up a different cue in each clip than what the experimenters selected in the stimuli.

The present work addressed this by having adults and preschoolers state what cue they believe they used in making a pretend-real judgment about an action they watched on a film. In this way, it both replicated the prior study by looking at the proficiency at judging real versus pretense acts, and it examined viewers' conception of what makes an act a pretense one. Five-year-olds were tested because they are well-practiced pretenders, nearing the end of the "high season" of pretend play, but they are still developing their ability to judge pretense; not until the age of 7 are children as proficient at judging pretense as adults are [17]. As in Richert and Lillard's work [17], participants watched short video clips of pretense and real acts in which content cues were blocked and judged whether each act was pretend or real ("judgment of the act"); new in this study, they also indicated the cues they believed they had used for that judgment ("reported cues"). We reasoned that the association between the pretend-real judgment and reported cues would reveal viewers' conception of what makes an act a pretense one. First, when asked to explain their pretend-real judgment, we expected that viewers would only report cues that they believe are characteristic of pretense or real behavior. Second, we speculated that viewers might even go so far as to report making their judgments on the basis of cues that were not actually perceptible in the video clips. In such cases, their theories of what should allow them to identify pretense event would actually trump reality, similar to misrecalling sentences or scenes based on typical real-world representations rather than what was actually perceived [18].

To examine what cues viewers are likely to rely on to make pretense or real interpretations, the association between the two categorical variables—judgment of the act and reported cues—was examined by correspondence analysis. Correspondence analysis is an exploratory technique related to principle components analysis. It displays two or more categorical variables in a property space that plots their association in two or more dimensions. The degree of association between two data points can be displayed as the distance between them on the plot [19, 20]. We discuss this method further below.

2. Study 1

2.1. Method

2.1.1. Participants. Adult participants were 55 college students (M = 19.5 years; 28 females). They were recruited from a public university in a small city and received experiment credit for their participation. Child participants were 44 children around 5 years of age (M = 63.3 months, range = 54.0–71.2 months; 25 girls). All children were normally developing and had normal vision. Five additional children were excluded due to unwillingness to participate. Children were recruited through a participant database maintained by a research laboratory at a public university or from local preschools (about half from each source). They were predominately from white, middle-class families.

2.1.2. Materials. Twenty video clips of mother-child interactions (M = 20.1 seconds, SD = 0.36 seconds) were shown to participants. These clips were refined adaptations of those used by Richert and Lillard [17, Experiment 2], who had taken the clips from a study of mother-child interactions [12]. In each clip, a mother engaged in snacking behaviors that were either pretend or real. Half of the clips showed pretense snacking behaviors, and half showed real snacking behaviors.

Each clip had three pertinent characteristics. First, each clip contained at least two instances of complete snacking behaviors (among them eating, drinking, or pouring) that were either pretend or real. Second, the words "pretend" and "real" were not used in any of the clips. Third, effort was made to eliminate obvious signs about the content through video editing using *Final Cut Pro*: visual signs of content (e.g., the presence or absence of food or drink in the container) were blocked by video-editing a black rectangle over the content, and auditory signs of real content (e.g., the sounds of consuming the food or drink) were removed.

Four adults previewed all the video clips. They were asked to indicate whether they could hear or see any content cues in each clip (e.g., Cheerios being munched, or lack of juice in the cup), without making any pretend-real judgment. All viewers ascertained that one could not see or hear any direct perceptual information indicating the presence or absence of content in the clips.

2.1.3. Procedure. The adult participants viewed the 20 clips in a quiet room. The clips were randomly arranged in two orders. Half of the participants viewed the clips in one order, and half of them viewed the clips in the other order. After viewing each clip, participants judged the veracity of the mother's behavior on a 4-point scale: "real," "probably real," "probably pretend," and "pretend." They also wrote down why they made that judgment ("Please write down the reasons or the cues you have used for your judgment.").

The child participants were tested individually in a laboratory or in a quiet room at their preschools. The procedure was similar to that with the adults, except for the following changes. After each clip, one experimenter asked the child to judge whether the act was pretend or real, by presenting the 4-point scale verbally. Then the child was asked to justify his or her judgment (e.g., "How could you tell that she was really eating/pretending to eat?"). On the response form, a second experimenter noted children's verbal responses and body language if there was any (e.g., child mimicking the mother's exaggerated lip smacking behavior when explaining a pretend judgment). The average number of clips watched was 15 (out of 20; SD = 4.84). This had no significant impact on the correspondence analysis.

2.1.4. Data Coding

Judgment. The total number of judgments made by adults was 1100 and by children was 657. The majority of the children (70%) judged every clip as either pretend or real, without including any "probably real" or "probably pretend" responses in their reports. Because of this tendency, and for ease of comparison, data were adjusted so the "probably" judgments were assigned to the definite category. Then each judgment was coded as either correct (PP, a pretense act judged as pretend, or RR, a real act judged as real) or incorrect (PR, a pretense act judged as real, or RP, a real act judged as pretend).

Reported Cues. After excluding unrecognizable reports and "not sure" or "do not know" responses (adults: 72; children: 100), there were 1044 valid reports from adults and 557 from children, and most of these reported cues (adults: 85.7%; children: 90.2%) were coded into four categories: *movement*, *content*, *sound or noise*, and *general impression*, each with two bipolar subcategories indicating either "appropriate" or "variant" features of the observed behavior (e.g., *aContent* or *vContent*; see Table 1). For example, "Her chin moved in a way indicating that she was really chewing," "it seemed that there's juice in the cup," "crunching sounds (some participants claimed to use sounds even though they had been edited out, as confirmed by pre-testing)," and "it looked real" were considered appropriate features, meaning consistent with the real behavior. In contrast, "she held her fingers at her mouth for too long and she did not swallow at all," "the cup seemed empty," "couldn't hear any chewing sounds," and "it's just fake" were considered variant or deviant features as compared to those of real behavior.

The remaining reported cues of the adult participants (14.3%) included references to appropriate or variant features of the mother's coordination of movements (e.g., "talking when should be chewing"), interaction with the child (e.g., "fake interactions with baby"), emotional expressions (e.g., "fake smiles"), and voice (e.g., "she spoke in a much higher pitch"). The remaining reported cues of the children (9.8%) included references to the mother's desires (e.g., "she's hungry and she wanted to be strong") or intent (e.g., "she wanted to trick the child") (*other*, see Table 1).

Occasionally a participant noted two different cues for a judgment of a single act. Such instances were coded as two separate observations. Each observation consisted of one

TABLE 1: Categories of reported cues.

Category	Subcategory	Examples	Variable name
Movement	Appropriate	She was really swallowing; the way her chin moved indicated real chewing	aMovement
	Variant	Exaggerated or too fast movement	vMovement
Content	Present	Food in the bowl; cup has weight	aContent
	Absent	There's no real food; cup has no weight	vContent
Sound/noise	Appropriate	Snack-related sounds	aSound
	Variant	Pretend or exaggerated sound effects	vSound
General impression	Appropriate	It looked real or convincing	aGeneral
	Variant	It looked pretend or fake; overacting	vGeneral
Other	—	Adult: facial expressions, voice, interaction with the child, and coordination of movements Child: desires and intent	—

judgment and the corresponding reported cue. For example, if the participant judged a pretense act as pretend and cited both "fake chewing sounds" and "too fast movements," two observations were coded out of this instance: PP with variations in sound/noise (*vSound*) and PP with variations in movement (*vMovement*).

2.1.5. Reliability. Two trained research assistants coded the reported cues from the response forms; both were blind to the underlying hypotheses. One assistant coded the adult sample, and the other assistant coded the child sample. A third coder coded 40% of the adult sample and 50% of the child sample, and she agreed with the first two coders 89% and 96% of the time (Cohen's kappa = .84 and .95, resp.). Disagreements were resolved by discussion. All three coders were blind to the pretend-real judgment of the participants when they coded the reported cues.

2.2. Results and Discussion

2.2.1. Proficiency at Identifying Pretense versus Real Acts. Preliminary analyses revealed no gender effect on the main variables, so gender was not included in the main analyses. All reported P values are 2-tailed. Proportions of correct judgments of pretense versus real acts were averaged across participants in each age group, and the means and standard deviations are presented in Table 2. Adult participants exhibited a high degree of proficiency. Overall, they correctly judged the clips at an above-chance level (88% correct), $t(54) = 26.45$, $P < .001$, which is comparable to the performance of the adults (80% correct) in Richert and Lillard's work [17, Experiment 2]. More specifically, they correctly identified the pretense acts 90% of the time and the real acts 87% of the time, both at above-chance levels, $t(54) = 22.56$, $P < .001$, and $t(54) = 21.14$, $P < .001$, respectively (one-sample t tests).

TABLE 2: Mean proportion of correct judgments.

	N	Pretense acts		Real acts		Overall	
		M	SD	M	SD	M	SD
Study 1							
Adults	55	$.90^{**}$	.130	$.87^{**}$	.130	$.88^{**}$	.107
Children	44	$.74^{**}$	.229	.46	.340	$.61^{**}$	.160
Study 2							
Children	39	$.83^{**}$	.186	.53	.332	$.68^{**}$	.147

$^{**}P < .001$ as compared to chance (.50).

Children's overall proficiency (61% correct) was significantly above chance, $t(43) = 4.50$, $P < .001$, which is comparable to that of the preschoolers (57% correct) in Richert and Lillard's work [17, Experiment 2]. Children correctly identified the pretense acts at an above-chance level (74% correct), $t(43) = 6.97$, $P < .001$. For the real acts, their performance was at chance (46% correct), $t(43) = -0.74$, $P = .465$. This high error rate is discussed later.

Participants' proficiency was further analyzed using a mixed-design analysis of variance, with clip type (pretense versus real acts) as the within-subjects factor and age (children versus adults) as the between-subjects factor. The results indicated a significant main effect of clip type, $F(1,97) = 18.48$, $P < .001$, $\eta_p^2 = .160$. In general participants were more proficient at judging the pretense acts (83% correct) than the real ones (69% correct). The main effect of age was also significant $F(1,97) = 117.64$, $P < .001$, $\eta_p^2 = .548$, in that adults were more competent than children. The interaction between clip type and age was also significant, $F(1,97) = 13.11$, $P < .001$, $\eta_p^2 = .119$. Paired-samples t tests indicated that adults were equally competent in judging both pretense and real acts, $t(54) = 1.21$, $P = .232$, whereas children were more proficient at judging the pretense acts than the real ones, $t(43) = 3.73$, $P = .001$.

2.2.2. Association between Pretend-Real Judgment and Reported Cues. Correspondence analysis was applied to explore the association between pretend/real judgment and reported cues. This method can represent the association between two or more categorical variables in terms of the distances between the data points on a plot [19, 20]. In a two-way correspondence analysis, a cross-tabulation table of frequencies is first standardized, so that the relative frequencies across all cells sum to 1.0. The entries in the table of relative frequencies are represented in the form of distances between individual data points of the rows and columns in a low-dimensional space. During this computation, the overall inertia or chi-square for the two-way table is decomposed, where inertia equals the overall

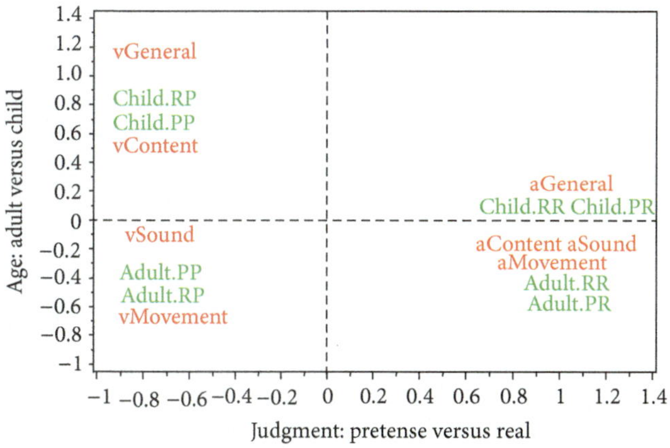

FIGURE 1: Association between judgment and reported cues—adults versus children in Study 1. Judgments identified with "child" were made by children; judgments identified with "adult" were made by adults.

chi-square divided by the total number of observations. On the plot, the distances between the data points represented by the coordinates are weighted (i.e., chi-square) distances between the relative frequencies, which indicate the strength of the association between the data points of the categorical variables (see [19, 20], for detailed introduction).

Table 3 shows the frequency of each type of the reported cues, by judgment type and age group. In order to provide a direct comparison between adults and children, data from both age groups were collapsed to carry out a single correspondence analysis, with focus on the four bipolar categories of justifications that represented most of the responses of both ages (e.g., *movement*, *content*, *sound or noise*, and *general impression*). Age (*child* versus *adult*) and judgment type (e.g., PP) were combined as a single, interactive variable (e.g., *child*.PP and *adult*.PP). The resulting two-way table was then analyzed, with age-judgment combinations as the rows and reported cues as the columns.

The analysis included 1397 observations (895 adult observations). The results indicated that the first two dimensions could explain 86.9% of the total inertia (i.e., chi-square) for the association between the participants' pretend-real judgment and the reasons they claimed. Most of the association was in fact attributable to the first dimension, accounting for 69.8% of the total inertia. A two-dimensional solution therefore has a satisfactory fit to the data and can give an excellent summary of the association between the variables.

Figure 1 shows the association between the participants' judgments and reported cues on those two dimensions. The first dimension, a clear left-right dimension of pretend versus real judgment, shows that cues considered "appropriate" to the activity were closely associated with real judgments, whereas cues believed to be deviant were closely associated with pretend judgments. Normal movements, "expected" normal sounds when consuming the food or drink, and "inferred" existence of content were the most pertinent. On the other hand, an act was judged as pretend when the participant *believed* that it was accompanied with deviant signs (e.g., "inferred" absence of content, deviant sound effects, or nonstandard movements). Thus, as might be expected, in general both adults and children judged pretense acts by their deviance from their real counterparts.

The second dimension accounts for 17.1% of the total inertia and displays the age difference. Adults were more likely to cite nonstandard features of movements when justifying their pretense interpretations. In contrast, children tended to justify their pretense interpretations by referring to absence of real content. This is despite the fact that we eliminated content cues by blocking visual information and removing auditory clues like chewing sounds. This is the case for both children's correct detection of pretense (PP) and their false identification of real acts as pretense (RP).

An interesting finding of Study 1 is children's frequent false identification of real acts as pretense (about half the time), seeming to reflect a "pretense bias." In the current stimuli, cues about the necessary content (e.g., food or juice) were blocked. One might worry that this video blocking might have confused children and led to this "pretense bias." This seems unlikely for two reasons. First, pretense clips were edited in the same way, with a black rectangle placed over where the content would be. Second, we know from other research that children can clearly read what is going on behind visual blocks on video—it is the basis for a wealth of research on infant cognition (e.g., [21, 22]). Thus, we speculate that in this study children read the person to be eating (or pretend eating) even when content cues were not visible due to the block.

One possible explanation for the "pretense bias" is that children judge everything they see on television as pretense. Previous research has suggested that before the age of 5 children view what is on television as truly real—when the screen shows an ocean, water will come out if one turns the TV set over [23]. But between the ages of 5 and 12, although they judge actors on television to be "real" people (e.g., Mr. and Mrs. Cosby really are married), they see the acting as "pretend" [24]. It is possible that some children in the current study viewed the mothers in the video clips as acting and thus judged all their behaviors to be "pretend" simply because they were on television. To test this, in Study 2 real content was shown for some clips. If all video material is pretend at this age, then even when real content is available, children should judge the acts as pretense.

A more interesting possibility is that the "pretense bias" reveals something about the basis by which children make pretend judgments. Content cues were blocked in the current stimuli, and in this situation adults easily moved to using behavioral cues, particularly how people moved. For example, on the real clips they used cues to reality such as well-timed or nonexaggerated movement. Five-year-olds, however, did not benefit from such behavioral cues. When content cues were not available, on the real clips, half the time they guessed that the mothers were pretending to eat, and, half the time, they guessed them to be really eating. Why were children not also thrown to guessing by the pretense clips? Perhaps it is because behavioral cues to pretense are marked—when judging the pretense clips, children could and did sometimes use pretender (behavioral) cues. In the real

TABLE 3: Frequencies of reported cues (number of total observations in parentheses).

	Judgment	Reported cues							
		aMovement	aContent	aSound	aGeneral	vMovement	vContent	vSound	vGeneral
Study 1: adults (895)	PP	0	3	0	0	261	86	92	7
	PR	17	7	3	3	2	0	0	0
	RP	1	0	0	0	28	9	5	1
	RR	282	39	26	14	5	1	2	1
Study 1: children (502)	PP	0	0	0	1	37	102	41	31
	PR	16	21	10	13	0	0	0	0
	RP	0	0	0	1	22	77	20	19
	RR	37	24	9	18	1	1	0	1
Study 2: children (617)	PP	1	0	1	0	68	105	73	25
	PR	20	13	8	7	0	0	0	0
	RP	2	0	1	0	19	64	32	10
	RR	95	42	15	16	0	0	0	0

PP: a pretense act judged as pretend; PR: a pretense act judged as real; RP: a real act judged as pretend; RR: a real act judged as real.

clips, however, behavioral cues to reality were not salient to children; lacking access to content cues, they (unlike adults) had to guess. Study 1 strongly suggests this possibility, and Study 2 was undertaken to test it.

One concern that must be addressed is whether our procedure obscured children's ability by asking children to quantify their confidence in their judgment. Past research has suggested that 3- to 5-year-olds show little comprehension of the differences between adverbs that denote different degrees of likelihood of judgment, such as *possibly*, *probably*, and *definitely* [25]. In a related vein, preschoolers have difficulty with multiple possibilities when asked to predict the outcome of undetermined events [26]. Perhaps children in the current study had difficulty processing or considering four possible judgments at the same time, so in Study 2 we simply asked for pretend versus real judgments.

3. Study 2

3.1. Method

3.1.1. Participants. The final sample included 39 children around 5 years of age ($M = 64.9$ months, range = 56.9–73.4 months; 20 girls). All children were normally developing and had normal vision. Four additional children were excluded due to unwillingness to participate. Children were recruited through a participant database maintained at a public university and predominantly from white, middle-class families.

3.1.2. Materials. The stimuli were 20 video clips, including 16 test clips randomly selected from the ones used in Study 1 (8 pretense acts and 8 real acts) and four control clips. Two control clips showed obvious real snacking behaviors, with the content cues visible, so viewers could see the real food or drink. The other two control clips showed obvious pretense acts: in addition to salient behavioral signs, the viewers could clearly see that all the containers were empty.

3.1.3. Procedure. Each child was tested individually in a laboratory room. The experimenter showed the child the 20 video clips, one at a time. At the end of each clip, the child was asked to judge whether the act was pretend or real (e.g., "was she really eating or was she just pretending?") and to justify that judgment (e.g., "how could you tell that she was really eating/pretending to eat?"). A video camera recorded the child's responses. All children watched all four control clips. The average number of test clips watched was 15 (out of 16; SD = 2.08).

3.1.4. Coding and Reliability. Children's reported cues were transcribed from videotapes. Two trained research assistants coded the reported cues from the transcripts into the same categories as those in Study 1, and on another occasion they coded children's pretend-real judgments from the videotapes. The coders were blind to the pretend-real judgments of the children when they coded the reported cues. Intercoder reliability based on 40% of the sample was very good. The coders agreed 99% of the time on pretend-real judgment (Cohen's kappa = .98) and 90% of the time on reported cues (Cohen's kappa = .88). Disagreements were resolved by discussion.

3.2. Results and Discussion. To preview, the 5-year-olds in this study had no difficulty identifying the control clips (about 90% correct). Their performance in judging the test clips exhibited patterns similar to those of the 5-year-olds in Study 1. Child data from both studies were collapsed to carry out a single correspondence analysis, which indicated similar results across studies.

3.2.1. Proficiency at Identifying Pretense versus Real Acts. Children correctly detected the "pretend" control clips 86% of the time, and for 84% of the correctly identified clips they referred to the absence of real content to justify their judgments. Moreover, children correctly identified the "real" control clips 94% of the time, and they referred to the presence of real food or drink when explaining their judgments (88%). An examination of individual performance patterns suggests that this proficiency is characteristic of most children: 90% of the children (35/39) correctly identified at least 3 of the 4 control clips, with 74% of the children (29/39) correctly identifying all four clips. In other words, 5-year-olds had no difficulty identifying acts displayed on television when it was abundantly clear whether an act was pretend or real. Therefore, the "pretense bias" in Study 1 was not due to children's difficulty in recognizing that events in videos are sometimes "real."

Children's performance in judging the test clips exhibited patterns similar to those of the 5-year-olds in Study 1 (see Table 2). Their overall proficiency (68% correct) was significantly above chance, $t(38) = 7.28$, $P < .001$. More specifically, they correctly identified the pretense acts at an above-chance level (83% correct), $t(38) = 11.19$, $P < .001$. For the real acts, their performance (53% correct) did not differ significantly from chance, $t(38) = 0.50$, $P = .619$. Additional analyses revealed that children outperformed the 5-year-olds in Study 1 (74% correct) in judging the pretense acts, $t(81) = 2.18$, $P = .032$. Their performance in judging the real acts was comparable to that of the 5-year-olds in Study 1 (46% correct), $t(34) = 0.87$, $P = .387$.

Thus, reducing the number of judgment choices to two did not significantly reduce children's errors in judging the real acts, suggesting that children's "pretense bias" in Study 1 was not due to difficulty with the 4-point judgment scale. Instead, it seems that false identification of the real acts stemmed from children relying heavily on content to the exclusion of behavioral cues. When content cues were not available, children guessed (50-50) as to whether the real content was behind the video block and made their pretend-real judgment accordingly.

3.2.2. Association between Pretend-Real Judgment and Reported Cues. Table 3 shows the frequency of each type of justifications cited by the children. A correspondence analysis was carried out with the collapsed data of the children from both studies, using the same four bipolar categories of justifications as in Study 1 (i.e., *movement*, *content*, *sound or noise*, and *general impression*). Study (1 versus 2) and judgment type (e.g., PP) were combined as a single variable (e.g., 1.PP and 2.PP), and the resulting two-way table was then analyzed, with study-judgment combinations as the rows and reported cues as the columns.

The analysis included 1119 observations (617 from Study 2). The results indicated that the first dimension could explain 91.2% of the total inertia for the association between children's judgment of the acts and the reasons they claimed. The second dimension only accounted for 5.0% of the total inertia. Thus, a one-dimensional solution has a sufficient fit to the data.

As Figure 2 shows, the first dimension is a clear left-right dimension of pretend versus real judgment, for children from both studies. Along this dimension, cues considered "appropriate" to the activity were closely associated with real

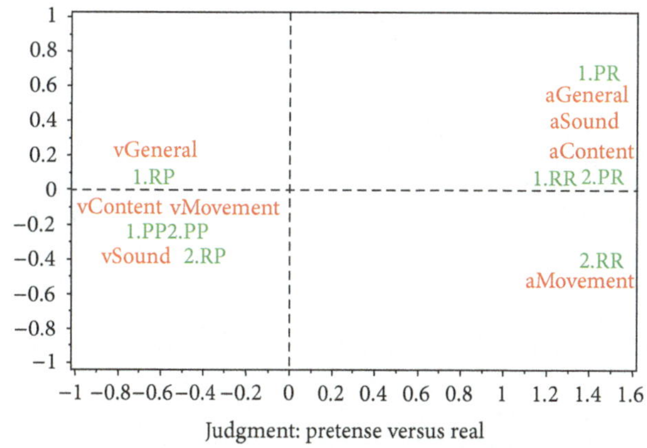

Figure 2: Association between judgment and reported cues—children in Studies 1 versus 2. Judgments identified with "1" were made by children in Study 1; judgments identified with "2" were made by children in Study 2.

judgments whereas cues believed to be deviant were closely associated with pretend judgments. Importantly, across both studies, children tended to justify their pretend judgments by referring to absence of real content, despite the fact that we had removed content cues from the test video clips.

4. General Discussion

The present work provides evidence of what cues children and adults find most pertinent to judging an act as pretend or real. In this research, 5-year-olds and adults viewed pretense versus real acts, judged whether each act was pretend or real, and justified their judgment by naming the cues on which they based their judgments. The claimed cues suggested what elements of pretense acts are the most pertinent in the viewers' conception of what makes acts be pretense ones.

Adults were very competent in identifying pretense versus real acts even in the absence of content cues. When judging an act as pretense, adults appealed to the characteristics of the act that they believed to be deviant from regular features of the real counterpart. They were most likely to appeal to the nonstandard movements of the character for their pretense interpretations. Adults' attention to the deviant features of the pretense behavior is consistent with the notion that recognition of an activity in the simulative mode often relies on the contrast between the simulation and the counterpart from which it derives [27].

Five-year-old children were relatively competent in identifying pretense versus real acts in the absence of content cues, although their performance was significantly less apt than that of adults. In particular, children in both Studies 1 and 2 falsely claimed that real acts were pretense approximately half the time. Such errors might have resulted from the absence of content cues in the video clips. By 5 years of age, children appear to associate a lack of necessary materials with pretense; when they cannot see whether the real content is there, they guess (50-50) and make their pretend-real judgment based on whatever their guess is.

In line with this possibility, even 2-year-olds can associate real content with an adult performing a real act and link imaginary or substitute content with a pretending adult [28, 29]. In the current studies, information about content was eliminated from the video clips. Thus, when the necessary content appears to be "missing," children might take its absence as a cue to pretense. The fact that around 30% of the time children claimed missing content was the relevant cue when making a pretense interpretation supports this explanation. This is especially interesting given that adults had previewed the test video clips and ascertained that one could not see or hear any direct perceptual information indicating the presence or absence of content in the clips. In this case, then, children's theories about what makes an act a pretense one appear to have trumped the reality of what they could see or hear.

Adults appealing to behavioral markers of pretense and children appealing to missing content suggest that they place differing weights on content versus behavioral cues in their conception of what makes an act a pretense one. For adults, deviant content might be an important marker of pretense, but how a person acts is also clearly an important determinant of whether an act is pretend or real, and when information about content is not available, adults rely on variations in a person's movements. Five-year-olds, however, appear to view deviant content as a more important marker of pretense than behavioral signs. No matter whether or not they can perceive the information about content, if the real content appears to be "missing" in some way, they are likely to judge the act as pretense, paying little attention to the behavioral cues of the person.

These findings might suggest something about how the intuitive theories of pretense held by young children differ from those held by adults. Intuitive theories are lay people's everyday understandings of information in certain domains (e.g., biology, and psychology). These theories have causal powers and serve to guide our interpretations and predictions of events within those domains [30–34]. As many researchers have suggested, intuitive theories imply that children interpret evidence based on their domain-appropriate beliefs and that evidence can help children shape or modify their existing beliefs (e.g., [31, 35]). An understanding of pretense is certainly part of adults' intuitive psychological theories; this understanding should be comprised of causal representations of several dimensions, such as why people pretend (and how it relates to other mental states and the world), how people pretend (including its mental origins and physical manifestations), what makes an act *appear* to be pretense, and what will follow from a pretense premise (psychologically and physically).

The current findings indicate that in children's intuitive theories, an absence of necessary materials could be the most important marker of pretense. Children even claim it is a cue when it is not actually accessible. In contrast, at least when content cues are not available, adults privilege behavioral signs as the *right* cues to pretense. This does not suggest that deviant content or behavioral signs are actually the defining features of pretense. What defines pretense is the underlying intention to pretend; without such intention, the behavior is not pretense (e.g., [1, 9, 36]). A real act can be intended or unintended, but in either case the underlying causes are different from what leads to pretense acts.

The present findings suggest two future paths for research. First, we examined a specific pretense situation: mothers pretending to have snacks in front of their toddlers. Although this pretense situation is prevalent in many cultures and very frequent in young children's early experience, future work is required to examine whether the present findings can be generalized to pretense situations other than snacking behavior. The second direction for research is what goes along with children moving from a content- to behavior-based interpretation of pretense. It is possible that the shift occurs sometime between 5 and 7, since by the age of 7 children's judgments are as apt as those of adults even in the absence of content [17].

In conclusion, the present study examines what kinds of evidence children and adults find most pertinent to judging an act as pretend or real. Our findings suggest that, like adults, by 5 years of age children hold intuitive theories of what makes an act a pretense one in the form of contrasts between pretense and its real counterpart. However, in contrast to adults, children appear to place greater weight on deviant content than on behavioral signs to the extent that they even claim to use deviant content when it is imperceptible.

References

[1] A. S. Lillard, "Pretend play skills and the child's theory of mind," *Child development*, vol. 64, no. 2, pp. 348–371, 1993.

[2] J. Belsky and R. K. Most, "From exploration to play: a cross-sectional study of infant free play behavior," *Developmental Psychology*, vol. 17, no. 5, pp. 630–639, 1981.

[3] I. Bretherton, "Representing the social world in symbolic play: reality and fantasy," in *Symbolic Play: The Development of Social Understanding*, I. Bretherton, Ed., pp. 3–41, Academic Press, Orlando, Fla, USA, 1984.

[4] G. G. Fein, "Pretend play in childhood: an integrative review," *Child Development*, vol. 52, pp. 1095–1118, 1981.

[5] L. Nicolich, "Beyond sensorimotor intelligence: assessment of symbolic maturity through analysis of pretend play," *Merrill-Palmer Quarterly*, vol. 23, no. 2, pp. 89–99, 1977.

[6] W. L. Haight and P. J. Miller, *Pretending at Home: Early Development in a Sociocultural Context*, SUNY Press, Albany, NY, USA, 1993.

[7] K. L. Walton, *Mimesis as Make-Believe*, Harvard University Press, Cambridge, Mass, USA, 1990.

[8] A. M. Leslie, "Pretense and representation: the origin of 'theory of mind,'" *Psychological Review*, vol. 94, pp. 412–426, 1987.

[9] A. S. Lillard, "Wanting to be it: children's understanding of intentions underlying pretense," *Child Development*, vol. 69, no. 4, pp. 981–993, 1998.

[10] H. Rakoczy, M. Tomasello, and T. Striano, "Young children know that trying is not pretending: a test of the "ehaving-as-if" construal of children's early concept of pretense," *Developmental Psychology*, vol. 40, no. 3, pp. 388–399, 2004.

[11] D. M. Sobel, "Children's knowledge of the relation between intentional action and pretending," *Cognitive Development*, vol. 22, no. 1, pp. 130–141, 2007.

[12] A. S. Lillard and D. C. Witherington, "Mothers' behavior modifications during pretense and their possible signal value for toddlers," *Developmental Psychology*, vol. 40, no. 1, pp. 95–113, 2004.

[13] P. H. Weiss, M. Jeannerod, Y. Paulignan, and H. J. Freund, "Is the organisation of goal-directed action modality specific? A common temporal structure," *Neuropsychologia*, vol. 38, no. 8, pp. 1136–1147, 2000.

[14] M. Bekoff, "Social communication in canids: evidence for the evolution of a stereotyped mammalian display," *Science*, vol. 197, no. 4308, pp. 1097–1099, 1977.

[15] A. S. Lillard, T. Nishida, D. Massaro, A. Vaish, L. Ma, and G. McRoberts, "Signs of pretense across age and scenario," *Infancy*, vol. 11, no. 1, pp. 1–30, 2007.

[16] J. S. DeLoache and B. Plaetzer, "Tea for two: joint mother-child symbolic play," in *Proceedings of the Biennial Meeting for the Society for Research in Child Development*, Toronto, Canada, 1985.

[17] R. A. Richert and A. S. Lillard, "Observers' proficiency at identifying pretense acts based on behavioral cues," *Cognitive Development*, vol. 19, no. 2, pp. 223–240, 2004.

[18] J. D. Bransford, J. R. Barclay, and J. J. Franks, "Sentence memory: a constructive versus interpretive approach," *Cognitive Psychology*, vol. 2, pp. 331–350, 1972.

[19] S.-E. Clausen, *Applied Correspondence Analysis: An Introduction*, Sage, Thousand Oaks, Calif, USA, 1998.

[20] B. S. Everitt, *The Analysis of Contingency Tables. Monographs on Statistics and Applied Probability*, vol. 4, Chapman & Hall/CRC, Washington, DC, USA, 1992.

[21] R. Baillargeon, "Object permanence in 3 1/2- and 4 1/2-month-old infants," *Developmental Psychology*, vol. 23, no. 5, pp. 655–664, 1987.

[22] E. S. Spelke, K. Breinlinger, J. Macomber, and K. Jacobson, "Origins of knowledge," *Psychological Review*, vol. 99, no. 4, pp. 605–632, 1992.

[23] J. H. Flavell, E. R. Flavell, F. Green, and J. E. Korfmacher, "Do young children think of television images as pictures or real objects," *Journal of Broadcasting & Electronics Media*, vol. 34, pp. 399–419, 1990.

[24] A. Dorr, "No shortcuts to judging reality," in *Children's Understanding of Television: Research on Attention and Comprehension*, J. Bryant and D. R. Anderson, Eds., pp. 199–220, Academic Press, New York, NY, USA, 1983.

[25] C. Hoffner, J. Cantor, and D. M. Badzinski, "Children's understanding of adverbs denoting degree of likelihood," *Journal of child language*, vol. 17, no. 1, pp. 217–231, 1990.

[26] S. R. Beck, E. J. Robinson, D. J. Carroll, and I. A. Apperly, "Children's thinking about counterfactuals and future hypotheticals as possibilities," *Child Development*, vol. 77, no. 2, pp. 413–426, 2006.

[27] C. Garvey, *Play*, Harvard University Press, Cambridge, Mass, USA, 1977.

[28] L. Ma and A. S. Lillard, "Where is the real cheese? Young children's ability to discriminate between real and pretend acts," *Child Development*, vol. 77, no. 6, pp. 1762–1777, 2006.

[29] L. Ma and A. S. Lillard, "Two-year-olds' understanding of real-pretend contrasts: the case of real versus substitute content," in *Proceedings of the Biennial Meeting of Society of Research in Child Development*, Boston, Mass, USA, 2007.

[30] S. Carey, *Conceptual Change in Childhood*, MIT Press, Cambridge, Mass, USA, 1985.

[31] A. Gopnik and A. N. Meltzoff, *Words, Thoughts, and Theories*, MIT Press, Cambridge, Mass, USA, 1997.

[32] K. Inagaki and G. Hatano, "Young children's conception of the biological world," *Current Directions in Psychological Science*, vol. 15, no. 4, pp. 177–181, 2006.

[33] F. C. Keil, "The origins of an autonomous biology," in *Modularity and Constraints in Language and Cognition: The Minnesota Symposia on Child Psychology*, M. R. Gunnar and M. Maratsos, Eds., vol. 25, pp. 103–137, Erlbaum, Hillsdale, NJ, USA, 1992.

[34] H. M. Wellman and S. A. Gelman, "Cognitive development: foundational theories of core domains," *Annual Review of Psychology*, vol. 43, no. 1, pp. 337–375, 1992.

[35] L. E. Schulz, E. B. Bonawitz, and T. L. Griffiths, "Can being scared cause tummy aches? Naive theories, ambiguous evidence, and preschoolers' causal inferences," *Developmental Psychology*, vol. 43, no. 5, pp. 1124–1139, 2007.

[36] A. K. Hickling, H. M. Wellman, and G. M. Gottfried, "Preschoolers' understanding of others' mental attitudes towards pretend happenings," *British Journal of Developmental Psychology*, vol. 15, no. 3, pp. 339–354, 1997.

Modelling the Trend and Determinants of Breastfeeding Initiation in Nigeria

Waheed Babatunde Yahya[1] and Samson Babatunde Adebayo[2]

[1] *Department of Statistics, University of Ilorin, PMB 1515, 640001 Ilorin, Nigeria*
[2] *Planning, Research and Statistics Directorate, National Agency for Food and Drugs Administration and Control, Wuse Zone 7, Abuja, Nigeria*

Correspondence should be addressed to Waheed Babatunde Yahya; wb yahya@daad-alumni.de

Academic Editor: Jeffrey W. Fagen

This paper examined the general trend of timing of breastfeeding initiation among nursing mothers in Nigeria. The time of initiating the first breast milk to an infant by his/her mother is measured as whether it is immediate (before the first hour of birth) or delayed (after the first hour of birth), and the impacts of some socioeconomic and maternal factors on this are determined. Results from this study showed that mother's age at birth, her enhanced educational status, mothers' domiciling in urban areas, singleton birth, and mother's frequent antenatal visits among others contributed positively to early initiation of breastfeeding by Nigerian nursing mothers ($P < 0.05$). In the contrary, delivery through caesarean operation, nursing mothers that delivers at homes instead of hospitals, and the current birth being the first from a mother are all found to militate against early initiation of breastfeeding ($P < 0.05$) among others. General results showed that early breastfeeding initiation experience among nursing mothers in Nigeria significantly improves over time between 1990 and 2008 ($P < 0.05$), although following a sinusoidal pattern. Four waves of national data from the Nigerian Demographic and Health Surveys for 1990, 1999, 2003, and 2008 were employed in the study.

1. Introduction

Early introduction of breast milk to newly-born babies immediately after delivery has been shown in many studies to be capable of giving the babies the required immunity to diseases through mother's antibodies, and this in turn, lowers the risks of early childhood deaths [1–6]. This is largely due to the possibility of ingesting maternal colostrum into the babies few hours after parturition. The colostrum is a liquid mixture that is rich in protein, sugar, vitamins, minerals, and antibodies which a child needs to facilitate his/her growth and survivorship. Some other health benefits derivable from feeding a child with early breast milk have been reported by Feachem and Koblinsky [7], Jason et al. [8], and Agunbiade and Ogunleye [9]. In their different studies, they reported, among other things, that early breastfeeding of infants reduces the risk of having diarrhoea which is a major cause of infant and childhood death in sub-Sahara African and other developing countries. In a related study, Clemens et al. [3] found that early initiation of breast milk actually reduces the risk of diarrhoea among rural Egyptian children.

The literature has it that social support received by mothers during childbirth is a catalyst for early initiation of breastfeeding in Nigeria [10]. Many studies have equally showed that successful timely breastfeeding largely depends on maternal related factors such as mother's age at the birth of the baby, mother's health, and her educational status [11–13], as well as some other socioeconomic factors. However, studies on timing of breastfeeding initiation that monitor the trend and consider the hierarchical nature of data collection are scarcely available, especially for Nigeria. The study here therefore is intended to explore the general trend of timing of initiation of the first breast milk to infants in Nigeria over time and identifying those sociodemographic and maternal factors that are determinants of timing of breastfeeding initiation among Nigerian mothers. The impacts of some of the identified risk factors of timing of breastfeeding initiation shall also be examined. 2 2 2 2 2

The data employed for this study are from the four waves of the Nigeria Demographic and Health Surveys (NDHS) for 1990, 1999, 2003, and 2008 which are national population based surveys conducted through a multistage sampling technique. The surveys included women of reproductive ages 15–49 years and men age 15–59 years. For detailed description of survey methodology, see National Population Commission (Nigeria) and ORC Macro [14–16]. Child recode data of the surveys were used for all analyses.

The principal objective of the Nigeria Demographic and Health Surveys is to provide current and reliable data on fertility and family planning behaviour, child mortality, children's nutritional status, the utilization of maternal, and child health services, as well as knowledge and attitudes towards HIV/AIDS.

Apart from fertility and mortality variables, information about the timing of initiation of breastfeeding by women of reproductive age is also available in the data. Traditional statistical techniques assume that individual observations (responses) are independent from one another. However, due to the hierarchical nature through which these data were collected, it is sometimes appropriate to assume that responses from individuals that are within the same clusters might be correlated and those in different clusters are uncorrelated. Therefore, breastfeeding attitudes of respondents (nursing mothers) that belong to the same cluster are assumed to be correlated but uncorrelated between different clusters. Hence, a generalized logistic regression (GLR) approach that would account for "*within cluster*" correlation is used to monitor the trend of early breastfeeding behaviour of nursing mothers and explore the possible relationships between timing of breastfeeding initiation and its determinants within the hierarchical nature of the data. Findings from this work will provide information that will assist policy makers in assessing impact of previous interventions on improving timing of breastfeeding initiation and attitude about child breastfeeding among child-bearing women of reproductive age in Nigeria. These will further assist health administrators, policy makers, and government in designing appropriate interventions that can assist in improving the breastfeeding attitude of nursing mothers in Nigeria.

2. Materials and Methods

The NDHS data for 1990, 1999, 2003, and 2008 contained sociodemographic and maternal related responses from 7,902, 3,552, 5,138, and 28,647 mothers of reproductive ages, respectively. Thus, a total of 45,239 mothers were involved in the four NDHS data sets combined. Out of this figure, information on timing of breastfeeding initiation was available for only 30,475 of the respondents. Also, complete information over all the factors considered in this study is only available for 25,233 respondents, and as a result, the remaining 20,006 respondents with incomplete information were excluded from the final analysis. The mean age of mothers in the study is 29.27 years with a standard deviation of 6.86. The minimum and maximum ages of mothers involved in this study are 13 years and 49 years, respectively.

Similar to Adebayo [4], a question on when child was put to breast after birth was used to determine the child's age at breastfeeding initiation. The age at which a child was given the first breast milk plays a vital role in determining his/her health status as well as that of his/her mother. Early initiation of breastfeeding could help mother's uterus to retract, which can reduce postpartum blood loss which is a major complication after birth that might result into maternal mortality [4]. Thus, the child's age at which he/she was given the first breast milk determines the timing of his/her breastfeeding initiation. In this paper, timing of breastfeeding initiation was measured based on the following binary categorical scale: 0 if "*Immediate*" (i.e., if the first breastfeeding was initiated to baby within the first one hour of birth) and 1 if "*delayed*" (i.e., if the time of the first breastfeeding initiation is one hour or more after birth).

Apart from timing of breastfeeding initiation which is the response variable here, information on the following independent variables was also available in the data, and they were therefore included in data analysis. These are mother's age at birth (mab), mother's and her partner's levels of educational attainment which are categorized into "no education," "primary," "secondary," and "higher" educational status with "no education" being the reference category. As employed in many studies [11–13], mother's age at birth of the child was categorized into six using class interval of five. This yielded the following classes of mother's age (in years) as used in this study: 15–19, 20–24, 25–29, 30–34, 35–39, and ≥40 with group 15–19 years being the reference category.

Others factors considered are child's sex, locality (urban or rural) where mother domiciled at the birth of the child, method of delivery (caesarean or normal), place of delivery (homes or hospitals), and birth type (singleton or multiple birth) with male, rural, normal, home, and multiple birth being the respective reference categories. Information on whether a mother received delivery assistance or not was equally available and incorporated in the analysis. Also, a variable that captures the number of antennal visits by nursing mothers was included in this study. This was later categorized into whether a nursing mother ever had antenatal visits or never had it (the reference category). We also included variable on birth order which indicates whether the current child from a nursing mother is the first or not (the reference category).

Based on the 36 states and the federal capital territory (FCT) Abuja that make up the Federal Republic of Nigeria, the entire country has been divided into six mutually exclusive geopolitical zones comprising the North-East, North-West, North-Central, South-East, South-West, and South-South zones. While all these geopolitical zones may be similar in term of belonging to the same federation unit of Nigeria, each of them is unique in term of their sociocultural characteristics. Given this background, it is therefore necessary to compare the breastfeeding initiation behaviour of child-bearing mothers from these six different geopolitical zones. This was fully captured and discussed in this study.

The distributions of mothers in this study based on their timing of breastfeeding experience, and the identified sociodemographic and biological factors are presented in Table 1.

To be able to monitor the trend of early breastfeeding behaviour of nursing mothers, three dummy variables were created for years of study beginning from 1990 to 2008 with 1990 being the reference category. This enables easy examination and comparisons of trends of breastfeeding initiation behaviour of nursing mothers in Nigeria from 1990 to 1999, 1990 to 2003, and 1990 to 2008. The timing of breastfeeding behaviours of all the 30,457 mothers between 1990 and 2008 are summarized in Table 2.

One of the metric covariates considered in this study is parity which indicates the total number of live births that already had by a mother including the current birth.

All the categorical predictor variables and metric covariate described previously were modelled nonlinearly on timing of breastfeeding initiation using binary logistic regression model [17–22]. The response variable $Y_i = (0, 1)$, $i = 1, \ldots, n$, is indexed to be 0 if the ith nursing mother breastfed her baby within the first one hour of birth (i.e., timing of breastfeeding is early or immediate) and 1 if she breastfed her baby after one hour or more of birth (i.e., timing of breastfeeding is delayed or late). That is,

$$Y_i = \begin{cases} 0 : \text{if timing of breastfeeding initiation is early} \\ \quad \text{(immediate)}, \\ 1 : \text{if timing of breastfeeding initiation is delayed} \\ \quad \text{(late)}. \end{cases} \tag{1}$$

Finally, in order to reduce recall bias that are often associated with analysis of cross-sectional data, we adjusted for the variable that indexes the number of children that are living with the respondents including the last birth as well as the one that represents the current births (number of births in the past year) in the analysis. Most of the analyses carried out in this paper were performed using STATA/SE 10.0 and SPSS 17.0 softwares. Data management was performed with SPSS and Microsoft Excel packages.

3. Data Analysis and Results

Analysis of all the four waves of the NDHS data and the results obtained are presented in this section.

From the distribution of the breastfeeding initiation behaviours of all the 30,475 mothers of reproductive ages that are involved in this study as presented in Table 1, it is observed that initiation of breastfeeding was delayed in about two-thirds (63%) of the infants. The implication of this is that only about a third of the respondents' babies received the needed colostrum at birth. As a consequence, there is a higher likelihood of early introduction of other supplements by mothers which can increase the risks of a child contracting infections that could lead to infant and childhood death.

In epidemiological literature, place of delivery, maternal educational attainment, place/locality of residence, and mother's age at birth of the child among other factors have been found to be associated with timing of breastfeeding initiation [23, 24]. From the descriptive statistics in Table 1, it is revealed that almost 7 out of every 10 births took place at homes, outside the hospitals. (Homes include mothers' homes and other traditional delivery homes, while hospitals include government and private hospitals, health centres, health posts, and clinics, as well as other public or private health services centres.) About 70% of the infants were born in the rural communities of Nigeria, and breastfeeding initiation was delayed in about two-thirds of this number. Also, breastfeeding initiation was delayed in about 70% of babies from illiterate parents, while about 70% of teenage mothers (age from 15 to 19 years) equally had delayed breastfeeding initiation experience.

Two-third of mothers with twin/multiple births have delayed timing of breastfeeding initiation, while about 70% of the inexperienced mothers that just had their first babies also initiated the first breast milk so lately. Almost 80% of mothers in the study received assistance during delivery. Two-third of the remaining 20% who did not receive delivery assistance delayed initiation of breastfeeding to their babies.

With respect to the six geopolitical zones in Nigeria, mothers from the North Eastern zone had the worst breastfeeding initiation behaviour with more than 70% of mothers from that region delayed initiation of breastfeeding after childbirth. The North Central had the best breastfeeding initiation experience with only 48% of mothers from that zone delayed breastfeeding initiation followed by the South-South zone having about 53% delayed cases.

About two-third of mothers in this study did not have antenatal visits prior to childbirth almost 70% of which delayed initiation of breastfeeding.

In terms trend of breastfeeding initiation behaviour of mothers over time, the summary statistics in Table 2 revealed an improvement in breastfeeding behaviour of mothers from the year 1990 to 1999 in which the percentage of mothers that delayed breastfeeding initiation dropped from around 69% in 1990 to 59% in 1999. However, this apparent improvement in breastfeeding initiation performance was not sustained for long before the percentage of mothers who delayed breastfeeding initiation went up to around 68% in 2003 and dropped again to around 61% in 2008. This shows an apparent improvement in breastfeeding initiation behaviours of mothers between 1990 and 1999 and between 2003 and 2008. Apparently similar breastfeeding initiation behaviours were exhibited by mothers in the years 1990 and 2003 among the early and late initiators of breastfeeding as shown by the bar chat of number of breastfeeding initiators in Figure 1. The general sinusoidal trend in breastfeeding initiation behaviours of mothers between 1990 and 2008 is graphically presented in Figure 2.

Except for child's sex and birth type (singleton or twin/multiple), the result from Pearson chi-square test of bivariate association between each of the previous identified factors and timing of breastfeeding initiation periods (early or immediate and late or delayed) is significant at 5% level ($P < 0.0001$). The P values of these tests are provided in Tables 1 and 2.

The results of the logit model that shows the relationship between all the previous categorical factors (and metrical

TABLE 1: Frequency (percentage in parenthesis) distribution of determinants of breastfeeding initiation across the three levels of breastfeeding initiation periods for 30,475 surveyed samples.

Determinants (factors)	Factors' levels	Timing of breastfeeding initiation Early (0) 11,278 (37%)	Delayed (1) 19,197 (63%)	Total 30,475 (100%)	P value
Child's sex	Male (ref)	5,660 (36.7%)	9,769 (63.3%)	15,429 (50.6%)	0.237*
	Female	5,618 (37.3%)	9,428 (62.7%)	15,046 (49.4%)	
Mother's educational status	No education (ref)	5138 (33.0%)	10,424 (67.0%)	15,562 (51.1%)	<0.001
	Primary	2,890 (40.3%)	4,273 (59.7%)	7,163 (23.5%)	
	Secondary	2,615 (40.3%)	3,873 (59.7%)	6,488 (21.3%)	
	Higher	635 (50.3%)	627 (49.7%)	1,262 (4.1%)	
Partner's educational status	No education (ref)	4,111 (32.5%)	8,539 (67.5%)	12,650 (42.7%)	<0.001
	Primary	2,528 (37.6%)	4,189 (62.4%)	6,717 (22.7%)	
	Secondary	2,888 (40.0%)	4,334 (60.0%)	7,222 (24.4%)	
	Higher	1,433 (47.7%)	1,571 (52.3%)	3,004 (10.2%)	
Locality	Urban (ref)	3,554 (39.4%)	5,472 (60.6%)	9,026 (29.6%)	<0.001
	Rural	7,724 (36.0%)	13,725 (64.0%)	21,449 (70.4%)	
Place of delivery	Hospitals (ref)	4,300 (42.0%)	5,948 (58.0%)	10,248 (34.3%)	<0.001
	Homes	6,745 (34.3%)	12,911 (65.7%)	19,656 (65.7%)	
Method of delivery	Normal (ref)	11,006 (37.1%)	18,654 (62.9%)	29,660 (97.9%)	<0.001
	Caesarean	201 (31.9%)	429 (68.1%)	630 (2.1%)	
Birth type	Twin/multiple (ref)	241 (35.5%)	437 (64.5%)	678 (2.2%)	0.425*
	Singleton	11,037 (37.0%)	18,760 (63.0%)	29,797 (97.8%)	
Mother's age at birth (mab)	15–19 years (ref)	621 (28.8%)	1,534 (71.2%)	2,155 (7.1%)	<0.001
	20–24 years	2,117 (34.4%)	4,035 (65.6%)	6,152 (20.2%)	
	25–29 years	3,239 (38.7%)	5,130 (61.3%)	8,369 (27.5%)	
	30–34 years	2,424 (39.0%)	3,787 (61.0%)	6,211 (20.4%)	
	35–39 years	1,678 (38.9%)	2,634 (61.1%)	4,312 (14.1%)	
	40–44 years	829 (36.5%)	1,440 (63.5%)	2,269 (7.4%)	
	≥40 years	370 (36.7%)	637 (63.3%)	1007 (3.3%)	
Birth order	2nd or higher order	9,484 (37.9%)	15,556 (62.1%)	25,040 (82.2%)	<0.001
	1st born	1,794 (33.0%)	3,641 (67.0%)	5,435 (17.8%)	
Assisted delivery	Assisted	9,341 (37.7%)	1,542 (62.3%)	24,762 (81.5%)	<0.001
	Not assisted	1,908 (34.0%)	3,710 (66.0%)	5,618 (18.5%)	
Geopolitical zones	North-Central	3,090 (51.8%)	2,880 (48.2%)	5,970 (19.5%)	<0.001
	North-East	1,866 (26.5%)	5,179 (73.5%)	7,045 (23.1%)	
	North-West	2,562 (32.2%)	5,404 (67.8%)	7,966 (26.1%)	
	South-East	1,371 (37.2%)	2,315 (62.8%)	3,686 (10.5%)	
	South-South	1,482 (47.4%)	1,644 (52.6%)	3,126 (10.3%)	
	South-West	907 (33.8%)	1,775 (66.2%)	2,682 (8.8%)	
Antenatal visits	No (ref)	3,424 (32.8%)	7,024 (67.2%)	10,448 (39.2%)	<0.001
	Yes	6,355 (39.2%)	9,854 (60.8%)	16,209 (60.8%)	

The P value is from Pearson chi-square test of independence. The symbol $^{(*)}$ indicates that the chi-square test of independence is not significant at 5% level. (ref) indicates the reference category of a factor as used in fitting the logit model.

covariates) and timing of breastfeeding initiation period as represented by (1) based on the four waves of the NDHS data for 1990, 1999, 2003, and 2008 are presented in Table 3. Except for birth type (Singleton or Twin/Multiple birth), only the results of factors that are statistically significant in the model at 5% level are presented due to space. Results in Table 3 contained the estimated *odds ratios (OR)*, *standard errors* of the estimated regression parameters, the P values to justify the significance or otherwise of each categorical factor, or metrical covariates in the model, as well as the 95% confidence intervals of the estimated odds ratios. Finally, the table also reported the percentage change in odds ratios (PCOR) for a unit change in the level of each of the risk factors. The PCOR measures the percentage increase (+) or decrease (−) in the risk of delaying breastfeeding initiation due to the influence of the level of the respective risk factor.

TABLE 2: Frequency distribution (percentage in parenthesis) of all the 30,475 nursing mothers by their timing of breastfeeding initiation behaviours from 1990 to 2008. The chi-square test of association between timing of breastfeeding initiation and years of study is statistically significant ($P < 0.001$).

Factor	Timing of breastfeeding initiation Early (0)	Delayed (1)	Total	P value
Year				
1990 (ref)	1,505 (31.4%)	3,283 (68.6%)	4,788 (15.71%)	<0.001
1999	1,319 (40.6%)	1,927 (59.4%)	3,246 (10.61%)	
2003	1,593 (32.4%)	3,329 (67.6%)	4,922 (16.15%)	
2008	6,861 (39.2%)	10,658 (60.8%)	17,519 (57.49%)	
Total	11,278 (37.0%)	19,197 (63.0%)	30,475 (100.0%)	

TABLE 3: Results of logistic regression model of timing of breastfeeding initiation on some sociodemographic and maternal factors. The odds ratio (OR), standard error, P value, 95% confidence intervals, and the percentage change in odds ratio for unit change in the level of each of the risk factors are presented.

Risk factor	Risk factor levels	Odds ratio (OR) exp(B)	s.e.(B)	P value	95% C.I. for exp(B) Lower	Upper	% change in OR
Year	Year 1990 (ref)						
	Year 1999	0.726	0.049	<0.001	0.659	0.799	−27.4
	Year 2008	0.718	0.032	<0.001	0.674	0.765	−28.2
Mother's education status	No Education (ref)						
	Higher	0.769	0.076	0.001	0.663	0.892	−23.1
Partner's education status	No Education (ref)						
	Higher	0.740	0.050	<0.001	0.672	0.816	−26.0
Locality	Urban (ref)						
	Rural	1.119	0.033	0.001	1.049	1.194	+11.9
Mother's age at birth	15–19 years (ref)						
	25–29 years	0.923	0.031	0.010	0.868	0.981	−7.7
	>40 years	1.144	0.045	0.003	1.047	1.249	+14.4
Birth order	2nd and higher (ref)						
	First born	1.153	0.043	0.001	1.060	1.255	+15.3
Place of delivery	Hospitals (ref)						
	Homes	1.117	0.036	0.002	1.040	1.199	+11.7
Method of delivery	Normal (ref)						
	Caesarean	1.581	0.100	<0.001	1.299	1.925	+58.1
Got delivery assistance	No (ref)						
	Yes	0.914	0.038	0.018	0.848	0.985	−8.6
Antenatal visits	No (ref)						
	Yes	0.916	0.035	0.013	0.855	0.981	−8.4
Geopolitical zones	North-Central (ref)						
	North-West	2.202	0.041	<0.001	2.031	2.386	+120.2
	North-East	3.094	0.041	<0.001	2.854	3.355	+209.4
	South-East	1.902	0.049	<0.001	1.727	2.094	+90.2
	South-South	1.387	0.051	<0.001	1.254	1.534	+38.7
	South-West	2.657	0.058	<0.001	2.370	2.979	+165.7
Birth type	Twin/Multiple (ref)						
	Singleton	0.834	0.100	0.069*	0.691	1.032	−16.6
Number of children living with mothers		0.951	0.009	<0.001	0.934	0.968	−4.9
Number of births in past year		1.073	0.027	0.010	1.017	1.131	+7.3
Constant		1.428	0.124	0.004			

The positive (+) or negative (−) signs represent positive or negative % changes in the OR which, respectively, reflected an increased or decreased risk of delaying breastfeeding initiation by nursing mothers due to the impact of the associated factor level. *indicates that the result is significant at 10% level.

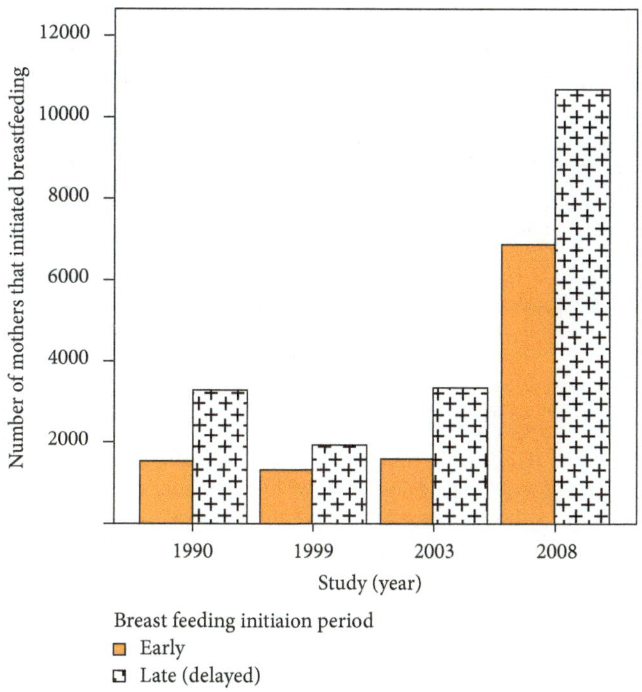

FIGURE 1: Bar chart of number of nursing mothers with early and delayed initiation of breastfeeding from 1990 and 2008. Breastfeeding behaviours of mothers among the early and late initiators of breastfeeding were apparently similar in 1990 and 2003.

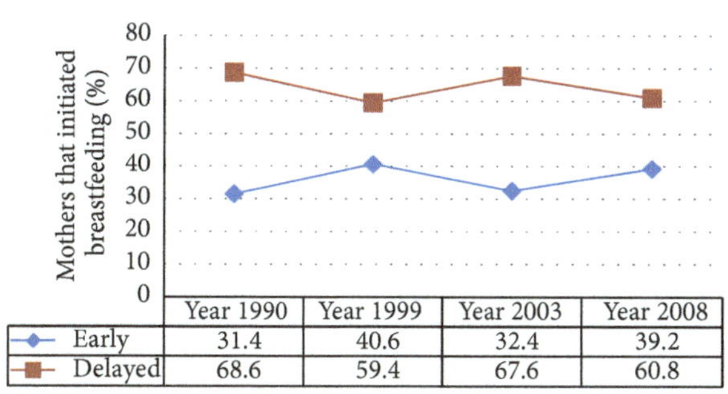

FIGURE 2: The line graph of percentage of mothers with early and late (delayed) initiation of breastfeeding from 1990 to 2008. The graph shows a sinusoidal trend in breastfeeding initiation behaviours of mothers over the period with apparently similar experience recorded in 1990 and 2003 among the early and late breastfeeding initiators.

The results in Table 3 show the influence of each factor or metrical covariate on timing of breastfeeding initiation by nursing mothers in Nigeria. All the estimated odds ratios were statistically significant at 5% level. Full interpretations and conclusions based on these results are presented in the next two sections.

4. Interpretation of Results and Discussions

Except for sex, parity, and birth type, logistic regression results in Table 3 generally revealed significant relationship between the two levels of timing of breastfeeding initiation (immediate or delayed) and all the identified sociodemographic factors ($P < 0.05$). The influence of each factor on the two levels of timing of breastfeeding initiation is determined by the percentage change in its odds ratios (OR) as presented in the last column of Table 3.

According to the results in Table 3, mothers' educational status and that of their partners are positively associated with timing of breastfeeding initiation in Nigeria. More specifically, mothers with higher level of education have about 23% reduced risk of delaying breastfeeding initiation than their illiterate counterparts (OR = 0.769, $P < 0.001$). In the same manner, mothers whose husband (partner) have higher level of education also have lower propensity for delaying breastfeeding initiation with a reduced odds of about 26%.

In terms of locality where mother domiciled up to the time the baby was delivered, and the results showed that nursing mothers that delivered in the rural communities have higher risk of about 12% of delaying breastfeeding initiation than their counterpart that domiciled in urban communities where basic sociomedical amenities are available (OR = 1.119, $P = 0.001$).

Considering the ages of mothers at the birth of their babies, results in Table 3 showed that middle-aged mothers of ages between 25 and 29 years have a significant lower risk of delaying breastfeeding initiation relative to their teenage counterparts (OR = 0.923, $P = 0.010$). On the other hand, old mothers of more than 40 years of age have an increased odds of about 14% for delaying breastfeeding initiation (OR = 1.144, $P = 0.003$). Furthermore, inexperienced mothers that just had their first baby delivery (first born) have higher relative risk of about 15% for delaying breastfeeding initiation than experienced mothers that were having their second or more number of children (OR = 1.153, $P = 0.001$).

Mothers that delivered their babies at homes have an increased relative risk of about 12% of delaying early initiation of breastfeeding than mothers that delivered in the hospitals (or clinics) (OR = 1.117, $P = 0.002$). Also, mothers that were delivered of their babies through caesarean section have about 58% increased risk of delaying early introduction of the first breast milk to their babies as compared to mothers who had vaginal (normal) delivery (OR = 1.581, $P < 0.001$). Mothers that received antenatal care have relative reduced risks (odds) of about 8% of delaying breastfeeding initiation than mothers without antenatal care (OR = 0.916, $P = 0.013$). Furthermore, delivery assistance received by mothers at birth is positively associated with their attitudes toward early initiation of breastfeeding (OR = 0.914, $P = 0.018$).

In term of geopolitical zones, the timing of breastfeeding initiation behaviour of mothers across the six geopolitical zones differs. This is clearly presented by the bar graphs of proportions of early and late initiators of breastfeeding across the six geopolitical zones as shown in Figure 3.

Out of all the 30,475 mothers that are involved in this study, statistics from the bar graph in Figure 3 indicated that the North-Central zone has the highest percentage of early initiators of breastfeeding followed by the South-South with North-East having the least. In other words, the North-Eastern Nigeria has the highest percentage of late initiators of

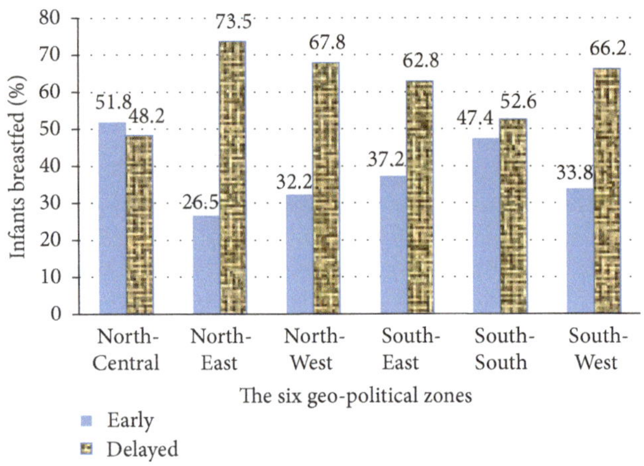

FIGURE 3: Bar chart of percentage of sampled mothers of reproductive ages with early and delayed initiation of breastfeeding across the six geopolitical zones based on the NDHS data for 1990, 1999, 2003, and 2008. The North-Central zone has the highest percentage of early breastfeeding initiators followed by the South-South with North-East being the least.

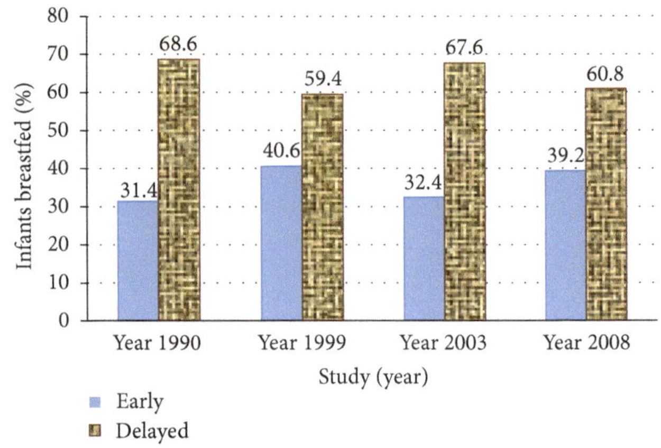

FIGURE 4: Bar chart of percentage of mothers of reproductive ages with early and delayed initiation of breastfeeding from 1990 and 2008. Breastfeeding behaviours of mothers among the early and late initiators of breastfeeding were apparently similar in 1990 and 2003.

breastfeeding among the nursing mothers in Nigeria followed by North-West, South-West, South-East, South-South, and North-Central in that order. More generally, the results from logit model in Table 3 showed that geopolitical zone of mothers is negatively associated with their breastfeeding initiation behaviours. In particular, mothers from the North-West geopolitical zone in Nigeria have increased odds (relative risks) of about 120% of delaying breastfeeding initiations relative to their counterpart in the North-Central zone (OR = 2.202, $P < 0.001$). Similarly, mothers from the North-East, South-East, South-South, and South-West zones have about 209%, 90%, 39%, and 165% increased relative risks of delaying breastfeeding initiation, respectively, as compared to mothers from the North-Central zone. Therefore, it could be inferred from the result of the logit model that the risk of delaying breastfeeding initiations by mothers of reproductive age in Nigeria is highest in the North-East (209%) followed by South-West (165%), North-West (120%), South-East (90%), and South-South (39%) in that order. These results agreed to a reasonable extent with the summary statistics of the NDHS data for 1990, 1999, 2003, and 2008 on the breastfeeding initiation behaviours of mothers of reproductive ages from the six geopolitical zones in Nigeria as represented by the bar graph in Figure 3.

As remarked earlier, the sinusoidal trend that characterized the breastfeeding initiation behaviours of mothers of reproductive age in Nigeria from 1990 to 2008 is shown clearly by the summary statistics in Table 2 which is again presented by the line graphs of early and late initiator of breastfeeding among mothers in Figure 2. However, the results from logit model indicated a positive association between the timing of breastfeeding initiation and years of study. In particular, the results showed that the relative risks (odds) of delaying initiation of the first breast milk to babies by their mothers significantly reduced by about 27% from 1990 to 1999 (OR = 0.726, $P < 0.001$) and by about 28% from 1990 to 2008 (OR = 0.718, $P < 0.001$). This result is supported by the multiple bar graphs of proportion of mothers that initiated breastfeeding within the first one hour of birth (early) and those that delayed initiation of breastfeeding (expressed in %) from 1990 to 2008 as shown in Figure 4. From these bar graphs, it can be observed that the percentage of mothers that delayed breastfeeding initiation dropped from 68.6% in 1990 to 59.4% in 1999 justifying why the estimated relative risk (odds ratio) for 1999 is 0.726 (about 27% reduced risk of delaying breastfeeding initiation). Similarly, the percentage of mothers that delayed breastfeeding initiation dropped from 68.6% in 1990 to 60.8% in 2008 equally justifying why the estimated relative risk (odds ratio) for 2008 is 0.718 (about 28% reduced risk of delaying breastfeeding initiation).

The odds ratio estimated from the logit model for the year 2003 was 1.013 which is not significant at 5% level ($P = 0.552$), and as such, it was removed from the analysis. The simple interpretation of this result is that there is no significant improvement in the breastfeeding initiation behaviours of mothers from 1990 (the base year) to 2003. This result is supported by the bar graphs display in Figure 3, and the statistics provided therein, in which the percentage of mothers that delayed breastfeeding initiation in 2003, computed as 67.6% is not significantly lower than the percentage of mothers that delayed breastfeeding initiation in 1990 (computed as 68.6%) as would have been expected ($P = 0.335$). This is an indication of no significant improvement in early initiation breastfeeding between 1990 and 2003. Hence, the nonsignificant result reported for year 2003 in the logit model.

The result from the estimated logit model in Table 3 also indicated that an increase in the number of births in the most recent time (birth in past year) would increase the relative risk of delaying breastfeeding initiation by about 7%. In the contrary, an increase in the number of children that are living with mothers of reproductive age would reduce the relative risk of delaying initiation of breastfeeding.

More generally, the estimated confident intervals for all the factors and metric covariates give more credence to the stability of the regression results provided by the logit model.

5. Conclusions

The amount of health benefits derived from breastfeeding is influenced by age of the child at initiation of breastfeeding, the duration and intensity of breastfeeding, and age at which the child starts to receive supplementary foods and other liquids as well as the types of supplementary liquids and foods received. Delay in breastfeeding initiation will obviously increase the chance of giving the babies other (prelacteal) liquid supplementations that can enhance infection which in turn could lower the chance of child's survival. Lack of early initiation of breastfeeding in Nigeria can be attributable to the country's worst record in reduction of under-five mortality rates as compared to some other African countries. Findings from this paper have provided information which permits opportunity of discerning the determinants of breastfeeding initiation in Nigeria.

Mother's educational status plays important role at determining the time a child is introduced to the first breast milk. Of the 30,475 mothers covered by this study, more than half (precisely 15,562) of them are illiterates who can neither read nor write. Unfortunately, about 67% (10,424) of these 15,562 illiterate mothers delayed initiation of the first breast milk to their babies beyond the first hour of birth. Although, it is established here that early initiation of the first breast milk by Nigerian nursing mothers improved significantly over time (between 1990 and 1999 and between 1990 and 2008). Obviously, this is not unconnected with apparent increase in literacy levels among women of reproductive age in Nigeria over time.

Not only that the localities where mothers domiciled up to the time of delivery play significant role at determining their breastfeeding initiation period after birth. About 70% of mothers in this study (precisely 21,449 women) live in the rural areas. Only about one-third of this number (precisely 7,724 women) initiated the first breast milk to their babies immediately after birth. By the results in Table 3, the relative risk of delaying breastfeeding initiation period beyond the first hour of birth increased by about 12% for women living in the rural areas compared to their counterparts living in the urban areas (OR = 1.119). All these results generally showed that localities where mothers domicile have significant impacts on timing of breastfeeding initiation.

Nursing mothers that live in urban areas at the time of delivery are more likely to initiate the first breast milk to their babies earlier than their rural counterparts, probably due to their accessibility to adequate information on the need for early initiation of breast milk and exclusive breastfeeding in general coupled with their relatively higher literacy levels. In view of this, intensive enlightenment programs are needed to sensitize prospective mothers living in the rural areas of the country on the importance and advantage of early initiation of the first breast milk to their babies immediately after birth. This would tremendously help at reducing the spate of neonatal deaths in Nigeria.

Pregnant women should be strongly encouraged to receive necessary antenatal treatments right from the time of conception. This will surely avail them the opportunity of receiving appropriate information on child and maternal care. All these shall immensely help at reducing several cases of complications at birth that often resulted to caesarean delivery which might in turn incapacitate mother at initiating the first breast milk to her baby immediately after the child birth.

Although appreciable improvement in the percentage of early initiators of breastfeeding among mothers of reproductive ages in Nigeria was recorded in the North-Central zone relative to others, the results generally showed that the current situation in which 3 out of every 5 nursing mothers in Nigeria delayed initiation of breastfeeding is still not impressive. This clearly fall short of the national objective of Healthy People 2010 for breastfeeding initiation [25] which expects 4 out of every 5 nursing mothers to initiate breastfeeding immediately after childbirth.

Finally, the pattern of breastfeeding behaviour of mothers of reproductive ages in Nigeria does not seem to follow a predictable trend. While some improvements in early breastfeeding initiation experience from mothers were recorded from 1990 to 1999, this apparent improvement was not sustained to 2003. However, possible improved trend in early breastfeeding initiation is expected in future given that promising improvement in timely breastfeeding initiation was again recorded in 2008. However, this optimistic result needs to be validated with future NDHS data sets.

References

[1] P. Ogra and D. Dayton, *Immunology of Breast Milk*, Raven Press, New York, NY, USA, 1979.

[2] A. S. Goldman, R. M. Goldblum, and L. A. Hanson, "Anti-inflammatory systems in human milk," *Advances in Experimental Medicine and Biology*, vol. 262, pp. 69–76, 1990.

[3] J. Clemens, R. A. Elyazeed, M. Rao et al., "Early initiation of breastfeeding and the risk of infant diarrhea in rural Egypt," *Pediatrics*, vol. 104, no. 1, article e3, 1999.

[4] S. B. Adebayo, "Bayesian geoadditive modelling of breastfeeding initiation in Nigeria," *Journal of Applied Econometrics*, vol. 19, no. 2, pp. 267–281, 2004.

[5] M. S. Kramer and R. Kakuma, "The optimal duration of exclusive breastfeeding: a systematic review," *Advances in Experimental Medicine and Biology*, vol. 554, pp. 63–77, 2004.

[6] K. M. Edmond, C. Zandoh, M. A. Quigley, S. Amenga-Etego, S. Owusu-Agyei, and B. R. Kirkwood, "Delayed breastfeeding initiation increases risk of neonatal mortality," *Pediatrics*, vol. 117, no. 3, pp. e380–e386, 2006.

[7] R. G. Feachem and M. A. Koblinsky, "Interventions for the control of diarrhoeal diseases among young children: promotion of breast-feeding," *Bulletin of the World Health Organization*, vol. 62, no. 2, pp. 271–291, 1984.

[8] J. M. Jason, P. Nieburg, and J. S. Marks, "Mortality and infectious disease associated with infant-feeding practices in developing countries," *Pediatrics*, vol. 74, no. 4, pp. 702–727, 1984.

[9] O. M. Agunbiade and O. V. Ogunleye, "Constraints to exclusive breastfeeding practice among breastfeeding mothers in

Southwest Nigeria: implications for scaling up," *International Breastfeeding Journal*, vol. 7, article 5, 2012.

[10] I. O. Morhason-Bello, B. O. Adedokun, and O. A. Ojengbede, "Social support during childbirth as a catalyst for early breast-feeding initiation for first-time Nigerian mothers," *International Breastfeeding Journal*, vol. 4, article 16, 2009.

[11] L. Dubois and M. Girard, "Social inequalities in infant feeding during the first year of life. The longitudinal study of child development in Québec (LSCDQ 1998–2002)," *Public Health Nutrition*, vol. 6, no. 8, pp. 773–783, 2003.

[12] B. Lande, L. Andersen, A. Bærug et al., "Infant feeding practices and associated factors in the first six months of life: The Norwegian Infant Feeding Survey," *Acta Paediatrics*, vol. 92, no. 2, pp. 152–161, 2003.

[13] J. A. Scott, C. W. Binns, W. H. Oddy, and K. I. Graham, "Predictors of breastfeeding duration: evidence from a cohort study," *Pediatrics*, vol. 117, no. 4, pp. e646–e655, 2006.

[14] National Population Commission [Nigeria], *Nigeria Demographic and Health Survey 1999*, National Population Commission and ORC/Macro, Calverton, Md, USA, 2000, http://www.measuredhs.com/.

[15] National Population Commission [Nigeria], *Nigeria Demographic and Health Survey 2003*, National Population Commission and ORC/Macro, Calverton, Md, USA, 2004, http://www.measuredhs.com/.

[16] National Population Commission [Nigeria], *Nigeria Demographic and Health Survey 2008*, National Population Commission and ORC/Macro, Calverton, Md, USA, 2009, http://www.measuredhs.com/.

[17] P. McCullagh, "Regression models for ordinal data (with discussion)," *Journal of the Royal Statistical Society B*, vol. 42, pp. 109–142, 1980.

[18] J. S. Long and J. Freese, *Regression Models for Categorical Dependent Variables Using STATA*, Stata Press, College Station, Tex, USA, 2nd edition, 2006.

[19] W. B. Yahya, *Genes Selection and Tumour Classifications in Cancer Research: A New Approach*, LAP LAMBERT Academic Publishing, Saarbrücken, Germany, 2012.

[20] W. B. Yahya, K. Ulm, L. Fahrmeir, and A. Hapfelmeier, "*k*-SS: a sequential feature selection and prediction method in microarray study," *International Journal of Artificial Intelligence*, vol. 6, no. S11, pp. 19–47, 2011.

[21] W. B. Yahya, M. O. Oladiipo, and E. T. Jolayemi, "A fast algorithm to construct neural networks classification models with high-dimensional genomic data," *Annals: Computer Science Series Journal*, vol. 10, no. 1, pp. 39–58, 2012.

[22] A. Hapfelmeier, W. B. Yahya, R. Robert, and K. Ulm, "Predictive modelling of gene expression data," in *Handbook of Statistics in Clinical Oncology*, J. Crowley and A. Hoering, Eds., pp. 463–475, Chapman and Hall/CRC, New York, NY, USA, 3rd edition, 2012.

[23] D. D. Awi and E. A. Alikor, "Barriers to timely initiation of breastfeeding among mothers of healthy full-term babies who deliver at the University of Port Harcourt Teaching Hospital," *Nigerian Journal of Clinical Practice*, vol. 9, no. 1, pp. 57–64, 2006.

[24] M. D. Awogbenja, "Factors influencing breastfeeding practices among mothers in Lafia Local government area of Nasarawa State, Nigeria," *PAT*, vol. 6, no. 2, pp. 126–138, 2010.

[25] Centers for Disease Control and Prevention (CDC), *Breastfeeding Report Card—United States, 2010*, 2010, http://www.cdc.gov.

Permissions

The contributors of this book come from diverse backgrounds, making this book a truly international effort. This book will bring forth new frontiers with its revolutionizing research information and detailed analysis of the nascent developments around the world.

We would like to thank all the contributing authors for lending their expertise to make the book truly unique. They have played a crucial role in the development of this book. Without their invaluable contributions this book wouldn't have been possible. They have made vital efforts to compile up to date information on the varied aspects of this subject to make this book a valuable addition to the collection of many professionals and students.

This book was conceptualized with the vision of imparting up-to-date information and advanced data in this field. To ensure the same, a matchless editorial board was set up. Every individual on the board went through rigorous rounds of assessment to prove their worth. After which they invested a large part of their time researching and compiling the most relevant data for our readers. Conferences and sessions were held from time to time between the editorial board and the contributing authors to present the data in the most comprehensible form. The editorial team has worked tirelessly to provide valuable and valid information to help people across the globe.

Every chapter published in this book has been scrutinized by our experts. Their significance has been extensively debated. The topics covered herein carry significant findings which will fuel the growth of the discipline. They may even be implemented as practical applications or may be referred to as a beginning point for another development. Chapters in this book were first published by Hindawi Publishing Corporation; hereby published with permission under the Creative Commons Attribution License or equivalent.

The editorial board has been involved in producing this book since its inception. They have spent rigorous hours researching and exploring the diverse topics which have resulted in the successful publishing of this book. They have passed on their knowledge of decades through this book. To expedite this challenging task, the publisher supported the team at every step. A small team of assistant editors was also appointed to further simplify the editing procedure and attain best results for the readers.

Our editorial team has been hand-picked from every corner of the world. Their multi-ethnicity adds dynamic inputs to the discussions which result in innovative outcomes. These outcomes are then further discussed with the researchers and contributors who give their valuable feedback and opinion regarding the same. The feedback is then collaborated with the researches and they are edited in a comprehensive manner to aid the understanding of the subject.

Apart from the editorial board, the designing team has also invested a significant amount of their time in understanding the subject and creating the most relevant covers. They scrutinized every image to scout for the most suitable representation of the subject and create an appropriate cover for the book.

The publishing team has been involved in this book since its early stages. They were actively engaged in every process, be it collecting the data, connecting with the contributors or procuring relevant information. The team has been an ardent support to the editorial, designing and production team. Their endless efforts to recruit the best for this project, has resulted in the accomplishment of this book. They are a veteran in the field of academics and their pool of knowledge is as vast as their experience in printing. Their expertise and guidance has proved useful at every step. Their uncompromising quality standards have made this book an exceptional effort. Their encouragement from time to time has been an inspiration for everyone.

The publisher and the editorial board hope that this book will prove to be a valuable piece of knowledge for researchers, students, practitioners and scholars across the globe.

List of Contributors

Daniel Paquette
Ecole de Psychoeducation, Universite de Montreal, Case postale 6128, Succursale Centre-Ville, Montreal, QC, Canada

Caroline Dumont
Departement de Psychologie, Universite de Montreal, Case postale 6128, Succursale Centre-Ville, Montreal, QC, Canada

Ann Dowker
Department of Experimental Psychology, University of Oxford, South Parks Road, Oxford OX1 3UD, UK

Karina Bennett and Louise Smith
St Hilda's College, Cowley Place, Oxford OX4 1DY, UK

Filippos Vlachos, Kiriazis Vaitsis and Argiris Karapetsas
Department of Special Education, University of Thessaly, Argonafton & Filellinon, 38221 Volos, Greece

Francois Gaillard
Institute of Psychology, University of Lausanne, Geopolis, 1015 Lausanne, Switzerland

Michele M. M. Mazzocco
Institute of Child Development, University of Minnesota, 51 East River Parkway, Minneapolis, MN 55455, USA
Johns Hopkins University School of Education Baltimore, MD 21218, USA

Laurie B. Hanich
Department of Educational Foundations, Millersville University of Pennsylvania, P.O. Box 1002, Millersville, PA 17551, USA

Maia M. Noeder
Department of Psychology, Case Western Reserve University, 10900 Euclid Avenue, Cleveland, OH 44106-7123, USA

Lauren A. Drvaric and Louis A. Schmidt
Department of Psychology, Neuroscience & Behavior, McMaster University, Hamilton, ON, Canada

Ryan J. Van Lieshout
Department of Psychiatry & Behavioral Neurosciences, McMaster University, Hamilton, ON, Canada

Kimberly G. Noble
Department of Pediatrics and GH Sergievsky Center, College of Physicians and Surgeons, Columbia University Medical Center, Columbia University New York, NY 10032, USA

Helena Duch, Maria Eugenia Darvique, Alexandra Grundleger, Carmen Rodriguez and Cassie Landers
Department of Population and Family Health, Mailman School of Public Health, Columbia University Medical Center, Columbia University New York, NY 10032, USA

Markus Jokela, Johanna Salo and Liisa Keltikangas-J¨arvinen
Unit of Personality, Work and Health Psychology, IBS, University of Helsinki, P.O. Box 9, 00014 University of Helsinki, Finland

Paivi Merjonen
Unit of Personality, Work and Health Psychology, IBS, University of Helsinki, P.O. Box 9, 00014 University of Helsinki, Finland
Department of Biological Psychology, VU University Amsterdam, 1081 BT Amsterdam, The Netherlands

Terho Lehtimaki
Laboratory of Atherosclerosis Genetics, Department of Clinical Chemistry, Centre for Laboratory Medicine, Tampere University Hospital, P.O. Box 66, 33101 Tampere, Finland
The School of Medicine, University of Tampere, 33014 Tampere, Finland

Jorma Viikari
Department of Medicine, University of Turku and Turku University Hospital, 20520 Turku, Finland

Olli T. Raitakari
Department of Clinical Physiology, Turku University Hospital and Research Centre of Applied and Preventive Cardiovascular Medicine, University of Turku, P.O. Box 52, 20521 Turku, Finland

Mirka Hintsanen
Unit of Personality, Work and Health Psychology, IBS, University of Helsinki, P.O. Box 9, 00014 University of Helsinki, Finland
Helsinki Collegium for Advanced Studies, 00014 University of Helsinki, Finland

Samantha Drain
Department of Psychology, University of Chester, Parkgate Road, Chester CH1 4BJ, UK

Paul E. Engelhardt
School of Psychology, University of East Anglia, Norwich Research Park, Elizabeth Fry Building 1.10, Norwich NR4 7TJ, UK

Lisa A. Wright and Rebecca B. McCathren
Kaplan University, Department of Educational Studies, Davenport, IA 52807, USA
University of Missouri, Department of Special Education, Columbia, MO 65211, USA

Laura Punaro and Robert Reeve
Melbourne School of Psychological Sciences, University of Melbourne, VIC 3010, Australia

Daniel Paquette
Ecole de Psychoeducation, Universite de Montreal, Case postale 6128, Succursale Centre-Ville, Montreal, QC, Canada

Marie-Noëlle Gagnon and Luc Bouchard
Departement de psychologie, Universite de Montreal, Case postale 6128, Succursale Centre-Ville, Montreal, QC, Canada

Marc Bigras
Departement de psychologie, Universite du Quebec a Montreal, Case postale 8888, Succursale Centre-Ville, Montreal, QC, Canada

Barry H. Schneider
School of psychology, University of Ottawa, Ottawa, Canada

Daniel J. O'Rourke, Ronald E. Smith and Frank L. Smoll
Department of Psychology, University of Washington, Seattle, WA 98195-1525, USA

Sean P. Cumming
School of Health, University of Bath, Bath BA2 7AY, UK

Steve Chinn
Faculty of Education, Health and Sciences, University of Derby, Derby DE22 1GB, UK

Paul R. Bruening and Patricia J. Brooks
Department of Psychology, College of Staten Island, City University of New York, 2800 Victory Boulevard, 4S-108, Staten Island, NY 10314, USA

Louis Alfieri
Learning Research and Development Center, University of Pittsburgh, 3939 O'Hara Street, Pittsburgh, PA 15260, USA

Vera Kempe
Division of Psychology, University of Abertay Dundee, Bell Street, Dundee, Scotland DD1 1HG, UK

Ineta Dabasinskiene
Division of Humanities, Vytautas Magnus University, Donelaicio 58, 44248 Kaunas, Lithuania

Amber A. Ankowski, Catherine M. Sandhofer and Aaron P. Blaisdell
Department of Psychology, University of California, Los Angeles, CA 90095, USA

Emily E. Thom
Department of Child and Adolescent Development, California State University, Northridge, CA 91330, USA

Yu Guan and Daniela Corbetta
Department of Psychology, The University of Tennessee, Knoxville, TN 37996-0900, USA

Katherine M. Robinson and Adam K. Dube
Department of Psychology Campion College at the University of Regina, 3737 Wascana Parkway, Regina, SK, Canada S4S 0A2

Yusuke Moriguchi
Department of School Education, Joetsu University of Education, Joetsu 943-8512, Japan
Japan Science and Technology Agency, Precursory Research for Embryonic Science and Technology, Tokyo 102-0076, Japan

Reiko Matsunaka
Department of General Systems Studies, Graduate School of Arts and Sciences, The University of Tokyo, Tokyo 153-8902, Japan

Shoji Itakura
Department of Psychology, Graduate School of Letters, Kyoto University, Kyoto, Japan

Kazuo Hiraki
The Interfaculty Initiative in Information Studies, The University of Tokyo, Tokyo 113-0033, Japan

Lili Ma
Department of Psychology, Ryerson University, 350 Victoria Street, Toronto, ON, Canada

Angeline S. Lillard
Department of Psychology, University of Virginia, P.O. Box 400400, Charlottesville, VA 22904-4400, USA

Waheed Babatunde Yahya
Department of Statistics, University of Ilorin, PMB 1515, 640001 Ilorin, Nigeria

Samson Babatunde Adebayo
Planning, Research and Statistics Directorate, National Agency for Food and Drugs Administration and Control, Wuse Zone 7, Abuja, Nigeria